New and Emerging Issues in Latinx Health

Airín D. Martínez · Scott D. Rhodes
Editors

New and Emerging Issues in Latinx Health

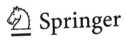

Editors
Airín D. Martínez
Department of Health Promotion and Policy,
School of Public Health and Health Sciences
University of Massachusetts-Amherst
Amherst, MA, USA

Scott D. Rhodes
Department of Social Sciences
and Health Policy
Wake Forest School of Medicine
Winston-Salem, NC, USA

ISBN 978-3-030-24045-5   ISBN 978-3-030-24043-1 (eBook)
https://doi.org/10.1007/978-3-030-24043-1

© Springer Nature Switzerland AG 2020

This work is subject to copyright. All rights are reserved by the Publisher, whether the whole or part of the material is concerned, specifically the rights of translation, reprinting, reuse of illustrations, recitation, broadcasting, reproduction on microfilms or in any other physical way, and transmission or information storage and retrieval, electronic adaptation, computer software, or by similar or dissimilar methodology now known or hereafter developed.

The use of general descriptive names, registered names, trademarks, service marks, etc. in this publication does not imply, even in the absence of a specific statement, that such names are exempt from the relevant protective laws and regulations and therefore free for general use.

The publisher, the authors and the editors are safe to assume that the advice and information in this book are believed to be true and accurate at the date of publication. Neither the publisher nor the authors or the editors give a warranty, expressed or implied, with respect to the material contained herein or for any errors or omissions that may have been made. The publisher remains neutral with regard to jurisdictional claims in published maps and institutional affiliations.

This Springer imprint is published by the registered company Springer Nature Switzerland AG
The registered company address is: Gewerbestrasse 11, 6330 Cham, Switzerland

We dedicate this edited volume to the dynamic US Latinx population with its rich diversity and profound assets; participants and partners in the studies and projects we are part of who continue to trust us, share with us, and teach us so much; our colleagues who contributed such important perspectives on Latinx health; other colleagues; and our families.

A special dedication to my husband, Balázs Kovács, and my mother, Christina Martínez, for keeping me grounded and for their continuous support.
—Airín D. Martínez

A special dedication to my husband, Glen Troiano, whose unconditional love and ongoing support sustain me, and to my mother and siblings who continue to influence my thinking in such profound ways.
—Scott D. Rhodes

Foreword

The information and opinions expressed in this Foreword are those of the author and do not necessarily represent the official position of the Centers for Disease Control and Prevention.

W. K. Kellogg's Health Scholars Program gave me the opportunity to conduct community-based participatory research (CBPR). For several years, I implemented principles of CBPR in Detroit, Michigan, and enjoyed establishing equitable partnerships to collectively identify public health issues, jointly plan research projects, and ensure that every aspect of the work benefited the community. Drs. Airín D. Martínez and Scott D. Rhodes were also Kellogg Scholars trained in CBPR and have implemented many CBPR projects with some of the most disenfranchised populations. Dr. Martínez has emerged as a preeminent thought leader in interpreting the layered relationships between immigration and health of Latinx immigrants. At Wake Forest School of Medicine, Dr. Rhodes has established a successful body of research on Latinx health that spans many topics but with a focus on immigrant health, sexual and gender minorities, sexual health, and access to care. They have dedicated their careers to resolving some of the most complex problems in public health and know how to leverage power and use their voices to elevate those of the most disenfranchised communities in the USA.

This book highlights epidemiologic data and real-world examples that researchers, public health and medical students, college and university faculty, public health practitioners, clinicians, and policymakers can learn from and apply to their own work with Latinx communities and other populations in the USA. For someone new to public health, research, or the field of Latinx health, this book can serve as a starting place—an invaluable resource to understand the current and most critical health issues affecting a heterogeneous Latinx population. For those with an advanced understanding, this book can be a guide to developing state-of-the-science interventions, programs, and research agendas and inform policies to improve health and well-being.

Nearly two decades have passed since the publication of the seminal compilation, *Health Issues in the Latino Community*, edited by Marilyn Aguirre-Molina, Carlos W. Molina, and Ruth Enid Zambrana. During this time, the Latinx population in the USA has directly and indirectly benefited from tremendous achievements in population health, public health, and medicine. The systematic effort to improve population health in the USA has centered on the expansion and improvement of clinical services, increasing access to health insurance, reducing under-insurance, and making significant investments in prevention at the population level. Our public health and healthcare systems have embraced many technological advances. For example, geospatial information systems have merged with traditional public health surveillance systems, population surveys, vital records, and other strategies to yield real-time multilevel data by zip code. These advances have yielded critical data on the traditional concepts in epidemiology: (1) person, (2) place, and (3) time. Based on these data, we know racial and ethnic populations in the USA continue to experience profound health disparities across the leading causes of morbidity and mortality; unfortunately, in many cases, those disparities are widening.

Typical comparisons between Latinx populations and non-Hispanic white and black populations paint the forest and hide the trees. The Latinx population is highly heterogeneous. Researchers and practitioners have suggested moving away from general comparisons and instead improving major surveillance systems by adding three additional variables: (1) country of origin, (2) native language spoken, and (3) nativity. The goal of this more nuanced approach is to paint the trees by conducting subpopulation analysis of the Latinx population and learning about differences in their behaviors, chronic health conditions, and use of preventive services. This book will help the reader understand the limitations of analyses that generalize the Latinx population as a monolithic group (e.g., "Hispanics") and the importance of conducting more in-depth analyses. Contributors in this book outline how to work with Latinx subpopulations to ensure more insightful discovery and create interventions to prevent and control diseases, including the modification of built environments. Specifically, the editors have framed this book around many new and emerging issues that affect the health and well-being of a heterogeneous and growing US population of 50 million persons.

What are the drivers of these new and emerging issues in the USA? For the next 20 years, the US-born Latinx population is destined to transform every aspect of our society and influence American culture. Larger than the foreign-born Latinx immigrant population, the US-born Latinx population constitutes a significant percentage of distinct generations (e.g., Millennial, post-Millennial/Generation Z, and Generation Alpha) and represents a large percentage of babies born in the past five years. These young persons have distinctive characteristics that influence their culture and health; for example, they live in homes where Spanish is spoken, have parents with ancestry to Latin America, are accustomed to households with various immigration statuses, and most importantly, are American "kids." Thus, we are in a great position to begin to understand their reality and to collectively improve upstream determinants of health, develop culturally congruent prevention materials, and invest in programs that stress health during early childhood and that follow them to young adulthood and across the entire life course.

Another emerging issue is migration of Latinx populations into southern and midwestern states instead of their traditional settlement in southwestern and northeastern states and cities. These new destinations offer more work opportunities

Foreword

but much less infrastructure, social capital, and settings to receive linguistically and culturally congruent health care. For many Latinx persons, health and well-being are profoundly influenced by the stress and hardship of having to understand a new culture and language, racial and ethnic intolerance, stratified socioeconomic layers, weather patterns, and navigating a complex healthcare system. Will these new destinations for Latinx populations lead to different patterns in the causes of death, disease prevalence, and behavioral and environmental risk factors? The contributors of each chapter explore the implications of migration into new destinations and its relationship to public health and healthcare system.

The chapters in this book illustrate the heterogeneity of the Latinx population and provide strategies to mitigate the challenges of migrating to new destinations. Professionals in population, public, and community health will find the information useful to enhance their repertoire of skills to work effectively across subpopulations. Although CBPR is not the main focus in this book, the complexity of Latinx social determinants of health can be effectively and efficiently investigated through participatory approaches. Moreover, we need to develop interventions within this community that reflect cultural, demographic, and geographic differences, which are small to the untrained eye but of great importance in shaping the future health status of the USA as a whole. My own hope for readers of this book is that it spawns renewed interest in Latinx health among researchers, public health and medical students, college and university faculty, public health practitioners, clinicians, and policymakers; increases understanding of the data regarding the multi-level factors influencing Latinx health and well-being; and generates innovative ideas to develop culturally congruent tools, programs, interventions, and policies to promote protective factors that are common among Latinx communities: strong family ties, hard work, and the love of being Americano!

Carlos S. Zometa, Ph.D., MSPH
Health Scientist, Center for State, Tribal, Local,
and Territorial Support, Centers for Disease
Control and Prevention, Atlanta, GA, USA
hlm7@cdc.gov

Preface

When we received the green light from Springer to produce this edited volume on Latinx health, it was seven months before the 2016 US General Election. We never imagined how the election of Donald J. Trump and his administration's subsequent policies and practices would make our volume both much more pertinent and much more controversial. With this edited volume, we re-introduce to the US public, including academic and government researchers, practitioners in the field, students, and Latinx community members, the demographic composition of the Latinx population in the USA, what the health needs and priorities of this population are, and which multilevel factors influence these needs and priorities. We also explore what is needed to promote health equity among the Latinx population given the current contentious sociopolitical context. Of course, this sociopolitical context extends beyond immigration-related issues and undermines evidence-based public health and science and policymaking related to reproductive health; protections for low-income, racial/ethnic, sexual and gender minorities; immigration enforcement; and climate change research, among others.

We had two goals when we initially developed the proposal for this edited volume. First, we sought to provide a comprehensive resource that summarized the current state of Latinx health in the USA for researchers, practitioners, students, and community members. It has been over 15 years since the most recent comprehensive edited volumes were published that were exclusively dedicated to Latinx health in the US context. These volumes include Chong's (2002) *The Latino Patient: A Cultural Guide for Health Care Providers*, Ianotta's (2002) *Emerging Issues in Hispanic Health: Summary of a Workshop*, and of course, Aguirre-Molina, Molina, and Zambrana's (2002) *Health Issues in the Latino Community*. There have been several edited volumes that have followed, either with a more general approach to minority health, including that of Latinx persons (LaVeist, 2005), or with a sharper focus on specific health outcomes like mental health (e.g., González & González-Ramos, 2005; Organista, 2007). There have also been demographic-specific edited volumes focusing on Latinx men's (e.g., Aguirre-Molina, Borrell, & Vega, 2011), children's (e.g., Pérez-Escamilla & Melgar-Quiñonez, 2011), or older adults' (e.g., Angel & Angel, 2014) health. There was also an edited volume about social justice issues that the Latinx community faces, which included a section on the barriers to health and health care (Gutiérrez, 2015). We hope this particular volume provides readers with a diverse set of theories, research approaches, and practices that will encourage researchers, practitioners, students, and community members to address Latinx health, in the USA and across the Americas.

Second, we sought to inspire and shape the future of Latinx health research by encouraging others to take an interest in less examined subpopulations such as older adults, persons with disabilities, sexual and gender minority persons, and children and youth. In "Part I: The Health Status of Latinx Persons in the United States", we provide a review of the most up-to-date data on the health status of Latinx persons in multiple health arenas including cancer, chronic disease (Baquera & Parra-Medina, Chap. 2), disabilities (Balcazar, Magaña, & Suarez-Balcazar, Chap. 6), sexually transmitted infections (Rhodes et al., Chap. 10), occupational injuries and fatalities (Quandt & Arcury, Chap. 9), and substance use (Marsiglia & Kiehne, Chap. 5). These specific health outcomes were selected because the Latinx population in the USA suffers disproportionately from these particular conditions and/or they remain largely invisible in these areas of research for various reasons, which we discuss further in the Introduction. Furthermore, the chapters also focus on multilevel determinants of health, including biological, individual-level, and social determinants. As has been well established, the factors that influence health and well-being are complex and influence one another in unique ways. There is no one pathway to health and well-being, but there certainly are underlying factors that influence health and well-being, subtly or profoundly.

More importantly, we hope to inspire researchers, practitioners, students, and community members to work toward improving Latinx health with novel and multidisciplinary theoretical and methodological tools that address the heterogeneities in Latinx persons' health status. We included "Part II: Communities, Systems, and Structures," which identifies often mentioned but inadequately explored and rarely addressed social determinants of Latinx health. We included the chapters from experts in the field on health insurance reform and the Affordable Care Act (Hall & Mann-Jackson, Chap. 11), racial and ethnic discrimination (LeBrón & Viruell-Fuentes, Chap. 14), immigration enforcement policies (Kline & Castañeda, Chap. 12), the built, social, and natural environments (Lara-Valencia & García-Pérez, Chap. 13), expansions of acculturation (Martínez, Chap. 15), and politics, representation, and leadership (Rodriguez-Diaz, Chap. 16).

It is important to note that some colleagues, experts in their fields, were nervous about contributing to this volume. We heard from colleagues who did not want to be aligned with a scholarly product that had potential to be targeted. Immigration and immigration reform continue to be "hot button" issues in the USA. Federal immigration enforcement policies, including border enforcement measures by Customs and Border Protection (CBP), have led to an increase in racial profiling, border killings, detainment, the separation of families, overcrowding in border facilities, and denial of due process rights. As this book goes to press, we continue to hear cries for a wall across the US southern border and representatives from the

Immigration and Customs Enforcement (ICE) agency talk of a "new normal" in which health centers, hospitals, clinics, schools, and churches are places that are no longer safe spaces for immigrants or those who are racially profiled to be immigrants. These trends promote fear at all levels including among researchers, practitioners, and students.

This edited volume could not be completed without the support of many people. First, we thank our Publishing Editor at Springer, Janet Kim, who has been exceedingly supportive and patient with the production of this volume. We encountered several technical and personal challenges to produce this volume, but she always centered us and helped us push forward to its completion. Second, we thank Lori Alexander for providing copyedits to the chapters in this volume. She served as the third set of eyes we needed. We also thank the volume's contributors who produced chapters about topics they are not only uniquely knowledgeable about, but also passionate about to support the advancement of health equity in diverse Latinx communities. In an era where journal articles and extramural funding reign supreme in academic advancement, we appreciate their efforts to support the production of an accessible resource about Latinx health. Lastly, we thank the emerging Latinx population in the USA for inspiring us all, e.g., researchers, practitioners, students, faculty, and community members, to ensure that we are doing the best to promote health and well-being among this population through sound science, state-of-the-art practices, and supportive policies. We must continue to take risks and forge new ground for our Latinx families, friends, neighbors, colleagues, communities of identity, and population at large.

Amherst, MA, USA Airín D. Martínez, Ph.D.
Winston-Salem, NC, USA Scott D. Rhodes, Ph.D., MPH

Contents

1 **Introduction: Disentangling Language and the Social Determinants of Latinx Health in the United States** 1
Airín D. Martínez and Scott D. Rhodes

Part I The Health Status of Latinx Persons in the United States

2 **Chronic Disease and the Latinx Population: Threats, Challenges, and Opportunities** 19
Barbara Baquero and Deborah M. Parra-Medina

3 **Mental Health Issues Within Latinx Populations: Evaluating the State of the Field** 45
Esther J. Calzada, Lauren E. Gulbas, Carolina Hausmann-Stabile, Su Yeong Kim and Jodi Berger Cardoso

4 **Latinx Child Health: Challenges and Opportunities to Build a Healthy Future** 63
Julie M. Linton and J. Raul Gutierrez

5 **Substance Use Among Latinx Adolescents in the USA: Scope, Theory, Interventions, and Next Steps** 97
Flavio F. Marsiglia and Elizabeth Kiehne

6 **Disability Among the Latinx Population: Epidemiology and Empowerment Interventions** 127
Fabricio E. Balcazar, Sandra Magaña and Yolanda Suarez-Balcazar

7 **Aging and Health in the Latinx Population in the USA: Changing Demographics, Social Vulnerabilities, and the Aim of Quality of Life** 145
Iveris L. Martinez and Adriana Baron

8   Health Threats that Can Affect Hispanic/Latino Migrants
    and Immigrants 169
    Thomas M. Painter

9   The Status of Latinx Occupational Health 197
    Sara A. Quandt and Thomas A. Arcury

10 The Health and Well-Being of Latinx Sexual and Gender
    Minorities in the USA: A Call to Action 217
    Scott D. Rhodes, Lilli Mann-Jackson, Jorge Alonzo, Jonathan C. Bell,
    Amanda E. Tanner, Omar Martínez, Florence M. Simán,
    Timothy S. Oh, Benjamin D. Smart, Jesus Felizzola
    and Ronald A. Brooks

Part II Communities, Systems, and Structures

11 Health Insurance Reform and the Latinx Population 239
    Mark A. Hall and Lilli Mann-Jackson

12 Immigration Enforcement Policies and Latinx Health:
    State of Knowledge 253
    Nolan Kline and Heide Castañeda

13 Three Ecologies of the Urban Environment and the Health
    of Latinx Communities 271
    Francisco Lara-Valencia and Hilda García-Pérez

14 Racial/Ethnic Discrimination, Intersectionality, and Latina/o
    Health 295
    Alana M. W. LeBrón and Edna A. Viruell-Fuentes

15 Divergent Dilemma: The Reconceptualization and Critical
    Use of Acculturation in Latinx Health Research 321
    Airín D. Martínez

16 Health Is Political: Advocacy and Mobilization
    for Latinx Health 349
    Carlos E. Rodríguez-Díaz

Index 363

Editors and Contributors

About the Editors

Airín D. Martinez, Ph.D. is Assistant Professor in the Department of Health Promotion and Policy at the School of Public Health and Health Sciences at the University of Massachusetts-Amherst. Prior to this appointment, she was Assistant Professor in the School of Transborder Studies at Arizona State University. She is a medical sociologist by training, with a Ph.D. from the Sociology Program at the University of California, San Francisco. She completed her postdoctoral training in community-based participatory research through the W.K. Kellogg Health Scholars Program at the Johns Hopkins Bloomberg School of Public Health.

Her independent research has included a situational analysis of comiendo bien (eating well) among Latinx immigrant families in San Francisco, where she identified the transnational processes that sustain and transform practices of healthy eating. She has also collaborated with multidisciplinary teams to conduct participatory research examining the relationship between health and place, cardiovascular disease, and occupational health risks among Latinx immigrants. Her current research uses an ecosocial approach to examine how the local implementation of immigration enforcement policies shapes chronic disease risk in Latinx mixed-status families.

Scott D. Rhodes, Ph.D., MPH is Professor in and Chair of the Department of Social Science and Health Policy, Wake Forest School of Medicine, Winston-Salem, NC. He also directs the Program in Community Engagement within the Wake Forest Clinical and Translational Science Institute.

He explores immigration policy enforcement, healthcare access, and health outcomes among Latinx populations in the USA. He has developed, implemented, and evaluated >10 evidence-based interventions designed to promote sexual health among Latinx and African American/Black populations.

He has published numerous articles and chapters on the health of vulnerable populations, including immigrants, Latinx persons, and sexual and gender minorities. He edited a book titled, Innovations in HIV Prevention Research and Practice through Community Engagement (Springer, 2014).

Contributors

Jorge Alonzo Department of Social Sciences and Health Policy, Wake Forest School of Medicine, Winston-Salem, NC, USA

Thomas A. Arcury Department of Family and Community Medicine, Wake Forest School of Medicine, Medical Center Boulevard, Winston-Salem, NC, USA

Fabricio E. Balcazar Department of Disability and Human Development, University of Illinois-Chicago, Chicago, IL, USA

Barbara Baquero The University of Washington, Seattle, WA, USA; The University of Iowa, College of Public Health, Iowa City, IA, USA

Adriana Baron Benjamin Leon Center for Geriatric Education and Research, Florida International University, Miami, FL, USA

Jonathan C. Bell Department of Social Sciences and Health Policy, Wake Forest School of Medicine, Winston-Salem, NC, USA

Jodi Berger Cardoso Graduate College of Social Work, University of Houston, Houston, TX, USA

Ronald A. Brooks Department of Family Medicine, UCLA David Geffen School of Medicine, Los Angeles, CA, USA

Esther J. Calzada Steve Hicks School of Social Work, University of Texas-Austin, Austin, TX, USA

Heide Castañeda Department of Anthropology, University of South Florida, Tampa, FL, USA

Jesus Felizzola Department of Psychology, George Washington University, Washington, DC, USA

Hilda García-Pérez Department of Population Studies, El Colegio de la Frontera Norte, Nogales, Sonora, Mexico

Lauren E. Gulbas Steve Hicks School of Social Work, University of Texas-Austin, Austin, TX, USA

J. Raul Gutierrez Department of Pediatrics, Zuckerberg San Francisco General Children's Health Center, University of California, San Francisco, CA, USA

Editors and Contributors

Mark A. Hall Wake Forest University School of Law, Winston-Salem, NC, USA; Department of Social Sciences and Health Policy, Wake Forest School of Medicine, Winston-Salem, NC, USA

Carolina Hausmann-Stabile Graduate School of Social Work and Social Research, Bryn Mawr College, Bryn Mawr, PA, USA

Elizabeth Kiehne School of Social Work, Phoenix, AZ, USA

Su Yeong Kim Department of Human Development and Family Sciences, University of Texas-Austin, Austin, TX, USA

Nolan Kline Department of Anthropology, Rollins College, Winter Park, FL, USA

Francisco Lara-Valencia School of Transborder Studies, Arizona State University, Tempe, AZ, USA

Alana M. W. LeBrón Department of Population Health and Disease Prevention & Department of Chicano/Latino Studies, University of California, Irvine, CA, USA

Julie M. Linton University of South Carolina School of Medicine, Greenville, USA;
Department of Pediatrics, Prisma Health Children's Hospital-Upstate, Greenville, SC, USA

Sandra Magaña Steve Hicks School of Social Work, University of Texas-Austin, Austin, USA

Lilli Mann-Jackson Department of Social Sciences and Health Policy, Wake Forest School of Medicine, Winston-Salem, NC, USA

Flavio F. Marsiglia School of Social Work, Phoenix, AZ, USA

Airín D. Martínez School of Public Health & Health Sciences, University of Massachusetts-Amherst, Amherst, MA, USA

Iveris L. Martinez Center for Successful Aging, California State University, Long Beach, CA, USA

Omar Martínez School of Social Work, Temple University, Philadelphia, PA, USA

Timothy S. Oh McGaw Medical Center of Northwestern University, Chicago, IL, USA

Thomas M. Painter Division of HIV/AIDS Prevention, U.S. Centers for Disease Control and Prevention, Atlanta, GA, USA

Deborah M. Parra-Medina Department of Mexican American and Latina/o Studies, University of Texas-San Antonio, San Antonio, TX, USA

Sara A. Quandt Department of Epidemiology and Prevention, Wake Forest School of Medicine, Winston-Salem, NC, USA

Scott D. Rhodes Department of Social Sciences and Health Policy, Wake Forest School of Medicine, Winston-Salem, NC, USA

Carlos E. Rodríguez-Díaz Department of Prevention and Community Health, George Washington University, Washington, DC, USA

Florence M. Simán El Pueblo, Inc., Raleigh, NC, USA

Benjamin D. Smart Wake Forest School of Medicine, Winston-Salem, NC, USA

Yolanda Suarez-Balcazar Department of Occupational Therapy, University of Illinois-Chicago, Chicago, IL, USA

Amanda E. Tanner Department of Public Health Education, University of North Carolina Greensboro, Greensboro, NC, USA

Edna A. Viruell-Fuentes Department of Latina/Latino Studies, University of Illinois, Urbana-Champaign, IL, USA

List of Figures

Fig. 4.1	Percent of the total population of the Latinx population by US State. *Source* Adapted from Annie E. Casey Foundation (2017)	64
Fig. 11.1	Insurance coverage before and after implementation of the ACA. *Source* Authors' computations based on US census data	242
Fig. 13.1	Urban environment–health nexus. *Source* Adapted from Galea et al. (2005) and from Klitzman et al. (2006)	276
Fig. 13.2	Concentration of Latinx populations in the Phoenix Metropolitan Area in 2010. *Source* Lara-Valencia, & Garcia-Perez, (2018)	280

List of Tables

Table 1.1	Hispanic or Latinx living in the United States by country of origin	6
Table 3.1	Landmark epidemiological studies including Latinx participants (adult and pediatric samples)	47
Table 4.1	Definitions and legal statuses	65
Table 7.1	Comparative demography of Latino subgroups	148
Table 13.1	Sociodemographic characteristics of Latinx women interviewed	282

Chapter 1
Introduction: Disentangling Language and the Social Determinants of Latinx Health in the United States

Airín D. Martínez and Scott D. Rhodes

Abstract This book comes at a critical time in U.S. history. Currently, more than 18% of the U.S. population is Latinx, and by the year 2050, it is estimated that nearly 30% of the population will be Latinx. In our introduction, we first provide definitions and clarifications of the nomenclature used throughout this volume, particularly the use of the pan-ethnic label and identifier, "Latinx". Next, we describe some of the recent major demographic shifts within the Latinx population in the United States, focusing on the year 2000 to the present, and the implications these shifts have for Latinx health. Third, we outline major cross-cutting themes within this edited volume. We also demonstrate that this volume serves as a critical resource designed to enrich dialogue around the multilevel determinants of Latinx health. We conclude with a call to action for both increased culturally congruent and sound Latinx-focused research and the mentorship of Latinx early-career investigators.

Keywords Demographics · Latinx health · Social determinants of health · United States · Cultural congruence

The Latinx population has become the largest minority population in the United States. Currently, more than 18% of the U.S. population is Latinx, and by the year 2050, it is estimated that nearly 30% of the U.S. population will be Latinx. Moreover, the United States has the largest population of Latinx persons outside of Latin America. Clear definitions of "Latina", "Latino", "Hispanic", "Latinx", "immigrant", and "migrant" are important for identifying and understanding the health needs and priorities of the Latinx population in the United States and its subpopulations and communities. The term Hispanic has origins in Spanish colonization and refers to those persons who were born in Spain or were the progeny of Spanish parents. How-

---

A. D. Martínez (✉)
School of Public Health and Health Sciences, University of Massachusetts-Amherst, Amherst, MA, USA
e-mail: admartinez@umass.edu

S. D. Rhodes
Department of Social Sciences and Health Policy, Wake Forest School of Medicine, Winston-Salem, NC, USA
e-mail: srhodes@wakehealth.edu

© Springer Nature Switzerland AG 2020
A. D. Martínez and S. D. Rhodes (eds.), *New and Emerging Issues in Latinx Health*, https://doi.org/10.1007/978-3-030-24043-1_1

ever, in the 1970s, Hispanic was the label adopted by the Nixon Administration to distinguish those persons in the United States who had descendants from Spanish-speaking Latin American countries (Oboler, 1995) or Spain (Gracia, 2000).

Chicana/o/x[1] and Puerto Rican organizers in the 1970s advocated for a categorical designation that distinguished them from the mainstream non-Latinx White population in order to account for disparities occurring in their communities. They did not, however, advocate for the label "Hispanic". In 1977, the U.S. Office of Management and Budget (OMB) issued Statistical Directive No. 15, which instituted the four legal administrative racial group classifications and the only ethnic group classification, Hispanic, used today by all state and federal agencies. In fact, the OMB took the suggestion from the king of Spain at the time, Juan Carlos I, to use Hispanic to designate all those persons whose culture or origin is Spanish, regardless of race (Toro, 1998). Although the term Latino was more popular during the 1970s, Juan Carlos I advised the OMB against its use because he claimed Latino sounded too similar to the word "Ladino", the Sephardic Jewish-Castilian language, which at one time was spoken throughout the Mediterranean (Alcoff, 2005, citing Toro, 1998). As Alcoff (2005) writes, "Maybe this issue was huge in the mind of the king of Spain, but it seems hardly uppermost in the minds of most Latinos today" (p. 403).

The term Hispanic was used for the first time in the 1980 U.S. Census (Cohn, 2010). Therefore, Hispanic is utilized as an administrative ethnic category imposed by the U.S. government primarily for federal agencies to describe subgroups within the U.S. population and account for differences and disparities within the population. With the help of television networks like Univision, corporate marketing (Dávila, 2012), the U.S. Census, and political campaigns (McConnell & Delgado-Romero, 2004; Beltrán, 2005), Hispanic transformed into an umbrella term to describe this group of English- and Spanish-speaking persons with Latin American origin or descent and to frame an imagined unitary consciousness (Oboler, 1995).

Latina, Latino, and its gender-neutral English variant "Latin" are rooted in colonial French epistemology, which constructed Latina/o to differentiate Anglo-Saxon Americans, from non-Anglo-Saxon Americans. Any New World country that spoke a Latin-based language (e.g., French, Spanish, or Portuguese) could use the label of Latina/o, but not necessarily Hispanic because they did not share a history of Spanish colonization. For example, according to these guidelines a Haitian, a Brazilian, and a Puerto Rican can all be considered Latino, but neither Haitians nor Brazilians can be considered Hispanic because the primary colonizing languages of those nations are

---

[1] Chicana/o/x refers to an identity position, a cultural/ethnic group, and political movement that originated in the United States to represent Mexican Americans. Some argue that Chicana/o/x culture and identity were in formation since the signing of the Treaty of Guadalupe Hidalgo (Anzaldúa, 1987; Aldama & Quiñonez, 2002) when the border between the United States and Mexico was constructed, militarized, medicalized, and racialized. The Chicana/o/x culture became institutionalized in the mid-twentieth century in the southwestern United States as Chicanas/os/x organized for civil rights and economic and social justice and were formulating ethnic studies and scholarship about their political movements, media and expressive culture, language, and identity formation as a marginalized racial/ethnic group. Many still use this term today to identify themselves. However, because it is exclusive to those who are U.S.-born Mexican persons and Mexican-born naturalized U.S. citizens, we do not use it as an umbrella term for all subgroups of Latinx persons.

not Spanish (Gracia, 2000; de Alba, 2003). For the past 35 years, the use of Latina/o has become more popular in both everyday vernacular and for legal administrative purposes. The 2000 U.S. Census aggregated Hispanic with Latino to constitute the Hispanic/Latino ethnic category widely used today (Cohn, 2010).

Hispanic/Latino is the only ethnic category on the U.S. Census. As a result of relegating Hispanic/Latino persons to an ethnicity, health researchers have often ignored that the Hispanic/Latino population in the United States is also a highly racialized group at risk for discrimination. The consequences of designating Hispanics/Latinos as an ethnic group have minimized related research, including health-related research, to cultural explanations; much less attention has been placed on the determinants of health and institutional forms of racism that result in adverse health outcomes within this population (For an overview, see Chap. 14 in this volume).

Come Latinx

We, the editors, find ourselves in an important historical junction, as the adoption of a new pan-ethnic label is occurring among Latinx persons inside and outside the Americas. We do not want to enter a linguistic or political debate about the use of Latinx to change the use of gender in every article or noun in the Spanish language or change how persons choose to identify themselves. In this edited volume, most contributors use the pan-ethnic identifier, Latinx, as an intersectional inclusive identifier to represent a multilingual, multiracial, and multinational group with descendants from the U.S. territory of Puerto Rico, Spanish-speaking Latin American countries, and/or indigenous populations in the Americas (Scharrón-del Río & Aja, 2015). The "a/o" at the end of Latina/o recognizes the feminine and masculine genders used in the Spanish language. However, Latinx emerged from Latinx lesbian, gay, bisexual, transgender, and queer (LGBTQ) communities in the United States and Latin America during the mid-2000s. Some members of these communities sought to acknowledge the fluidity of gender and sexuality and to disrupt male dominance employed in the Spanish language and practice in society (Vidal-Ortiz & Martínez, 2018; Scharrón-del Río, & Aja, 2015).

Although a history and discussion about the active use of Latina/o/x (see Vidal-Ortiz & Martínez, 2018, for a more detailed discussion) in Latinx health and public health research are beyond the scope of this volume, we are health researchers with histories in and active engagement with community-engaged research and, more precisely, community-based participatory research (CBPR). Briefly, CBPR is a research approach that is based on producing an equitable research collaboration that includes representatives from community organizations with their broad experiences working in and on behalf of communities and community members affected by the particular health issue or social problem under study in all aspects of the research process—from research question development to study design and implementation to interpretation and dissemination of results—in partnership with researchers and investigators (Rhodes et al., 2018). Thus, we are heavily invested in acknowledging the diversity within marginalized communities, specifically Latinx communities, in order to address structural sources of health inequities. Using Latinx is not an attempt to erase the terms, Hispanic, Latina/o, or other variations (e.g., Chicanx or Latin@), but rather using Latinx is designed to signal the need to approach the Latinx population as heterogeneous, and to directly recognize that throughout the life course, gender and sexual identity, expression, and behavior may be fluid. Furthermore, some persons, Latinx or not, identify as non-binary; thus, the term Latinx tends to be more inclusive. The use of Latinx also signals our desire to identify, prevent, and reverse health inequities in the Latinx population by acknowledging multiple systems of oppression that produce intra-group differences that may make traditional public health and healthcare approaches for this group problematic.

As readers will learn in the various chapters in this volume, when we examine the health outcomes of Latinx persons living in different regions in the United States and from distinct national origins, age groups, or genders, we find that there are vast differences between subgroups; disparities that may initially be invisible emerge. For example, in large epidemiological surveys like the Behavioral Risk Factor Surveillance Survey (BRFSS), identifying as Hispanic/Latino may be related to positive health status indicators like longer life expectancy, but this can also overshadow the negative health outcomes that result from ignoring the fluidity of sexuality, such as the late diagnosis of sexually transmitted infections and HIV among Latinx gay, bisexual, and other men who have sex with men.

We use Latinx with an understanding that the pan-ethnic label and political identifier may not gain popularity or endure in U.S. or Latin American racial and ethnic nomenclature. We know of community organizations that have adopted and promoted the use of Latinx and after a few years returned to the use of Latina and Latino based on feedback from younger Latinx persons who may find identity with the gendered terms. Nevertheless, we do recognize the many forms of marginalization and discrimination that sexual and gender non-conforming Latinx person's experience, including in health research.

We have chosen to move forward with language that is inevitably changing and evolving. A few contributors to this volume continued to use Latina/o, when referring to a specific gender or the Latinx population as a whole, partly out of habit and partly out of the limitations imposed by their institutional affiliations. Contributors of this edited volume also continued to use Hispanic and/or Latina/o when referencing specific datasets or publications with these identifiers, such as the Hispanic Health and Nutrition Examination Survey (HHANES) or the Hispanic Community Health Survey/Study of Latinos (HCHS/SOL). This is important because we do not want to erase this history and the importance these studies have in influencing Latinx health research and practice and Latinx health overall during the past 40 years. We also want to be true to the sample and how it was described and operationalized by those conducting the research.

Finally, an immigrant refers to an individual who migrates to another country to live. In this volume, this "other" country is often the United States. A migrant refers to a person who has temporarily moved to another country to work, reunite with family, seek refuge, or is in transit to another country for temporary residence or permanent destination. It is important to recognize that not all Latinx immigrants and migrants want to settle into the United States permanently.

The Latinx Population in the United States: Basic Demographic Characteristics

The Latinx population is the largest racial/ethnic minority group in the United States accounting for 18.1% of the total U.S. population (US Census Bureau, 2017). Since 1960, persons indicating on the U.S. Census that they were of Spanish, Latin American, Mexican, or Puerto Rican origin has increased from 6.3 million to more than 58 million persons. The majority of Latinx persons are U.S.-born citizens (~39.1 million; 66.5%), while Latinx immigrants account for 33.5% of the Latinx population (~19.7 million). Latinx immigrants make up the majority of the foreign-born population in the United States at about 40% (American Community Survey, 2017). However, contrary to some of the erroneous assertions by some in the media and some within the Trump administration, the proportion of the Latin Americans migrating to the United States has been declining since 2008 (Flores, 2017). Between 2000 and 2015, the increase in the Latinx population can be attributed primarily to births, not immigration, as in previous decades (Flores, 2017). Of the U.S. Latinx population, the majority identify as Mexican (62.3%), with the second highest representation among Puerto Ricans and Central Americans (both at 9.5%), followed by South Americans (6.3%) and Cubans (3.9%) (See Table 1.1).

Overall the Latinx population in the United States is a young population. The median age of the Latinx population in the United States is 28 years (US Census Bureau, 2017). However, there are differences between the U.S.-born and foreign-born populations, with U.S.-born Latinx persons being much younger, having a median age of 19, while the median age of Latinx immigrants is 42. The U.S.-born Latinx population is also much younger than the U.S.-born Asian (median age: 36), U.S.-born non-Hispanic Black (median age: 34), and U.S.-born non-Hispanic White (median age: 43) populations (US Census Bureau, 2015). Knowing that the majority of U.S.-born Latinx persons are young, we must create conditions in which they have opportunities to live in communities that promote positive health behaviors, good health, and quality of life in their early childhood and throughout their development because they will make up a sizeable proportion of future labor force in the United States.

The smallest proportion of the U.S. Latinx population is that of older adults, 65 years or older, at just under 3% (US Census Bureau, 2017), but as Martinez and Baron assert (Chap. 7), the proportion of the Latinx aging population will rapidly increase. In two decades or less, if Latinx immigrants decide to retire in the United States, it is unclear whether the U.S. healthcare delivery system and long-term care institutions will be prepared to meet the needs of this population. We must consider these demographic shifts in the Latinx population in order to prepare for a growth

Table 1.1 Hispanic or Latinx living in the United States by country of origin

	Estimate	Percentage (%)
Total Hispanic or Latinx	58,846,134	
Mexican	36,668,018	62.3
Puerto Rican	5,588,664	9.5
Cuban	2,315,863	3.9
Dominican (Dominican Republic)	2,081,419	3.5
Central American	5,562,327	9.5
Costa Rican	153,317	0.26
Guatemalan	1,456,965	2.5
Honduran	945,916	1.6
Nicaraguan	444,585	0.76
Panamanian	208,423	0.35
Salvadoran	2,310,784	3.9
Other Central American	42,337	0.07
South American	3,721,161	6.3
Argentinian	278,825	0.47
Bolivian	106,583	0.02
Chilean	157,375	0.26
Colombian	1,222,960	2.1
Ecuadorian	735,165	1.2
Paraguayan	27,625	0.05
Peruvian	679,340	1.2
Uruguayan	69,332	0.12
Venezuelan	418,366	0.71
Other South American	25,590	0.04
Other Hispanic or Latinx[*]	2,908,682	4.9

Source 2017 ACS 1-Year Estimates, Data Table B03001
[*]Includes Spaniard, Spanish, Spanish American, and all other Hispanic or Latinx persons

in the aging population and to provide enriching and safe environments for Latinx children to live with their families. Demographic shifts should inspire us to not only be able to treat Latinx patients when they fall ill, but to create equitable conditions that will promote their health and well-being throughout the life course.

While Latinx persons also have the longest life expectancies in the United States in comparison to the all racial groups, longer life expectancies do not necessarily translate into better quality of life and or less morbidity in older age. As, Martinez and Baron note, "… disability rates are slightly higher for Latinx older adults (39%) than non-Hispanic older adults (35.4%)." The proportion of the older population reporting one or more disabilities is considerably higher among Puerto Ricans, Dominicans, and Mexican Americans (42.8, 40.3, and 40.2%, respectively)."

Socioeconomic status (SES), including occupation, education, and income, and its byproducts (e.g., social and cultural capital, civic engagement, home ownership, neighborhood of residence, and health insurance status), are important social determinants of health because they relate to material and social resources and opportunities and capacities to be healthy. SES and its byproducts are also necessary to secure an overall population that can promote and maintain an economically productive and modern society (Foucault, 1984). While individuals may have other forms of resources (including inherited wealth), occupation, education, and income are simple and common variables used to measure and compare the health status of racial and ethnic groups in the United States.

The occupational and income statuses of the Latinx population have not experienced drastic changes in the past 12 years. The proportion of Latinx women who worked in managerial occupations (often the highest paying occupations) only rose 4% between 2005 and 2017, from 22.6 to 27%. The proportion of Latinx men who worked in managerial occupations rose even less, from 18 to 21.4% during the same time period. According to 2017 American Community Survey estimates, Latinx women primarily worked in service occupations (30.9%) and Latinx men primarily worked in natural resources, construction, and maintenance occupations (25.8%). In 2017, it was estimated that the majority of Latinx immigrants worked in service occupations (29%) (US Census Bureau, 2017). Given that the majority of the U.S. Latinx population works in service occupations, it is not surprising that 19.3% of Latinx persons live at or below the U.S. poverty level, in comparison to 9.6% of the White population (US Census Bureau, 2017). However, Latinx persons living at or below the poverty level are slightly lower than those living at or below the poverty level within the Black population (23%).

Despite one-fifth of the Latinx population living at or below the federal poverty level, there have been strides in educational attainment among the Latinx population. For example, the percentage of Latinx women with a Bachelor's degree or higher has almost doubled (47.9%) between 2005 and 2017. While there are more Latinx women with a Bachelor's degree or higher, Latinx men had a 56.2% increase in Bachelor's degrees or higher between 2005 and 2017. Higher educational attainment is related to lower death rates from common chronic and acute conditions, increased access to care, receiving better quality of care, overall better health outcomes, and longer life expectancy (Telfair & Shelton, 2012). Higher educational attainment shapes future occupational opportunities and is related to increased earnings, cultural and social capital, residence in better quality homes and safer neighborhoods, and access to healthier foods, just to name a few of the positive health outcomes associated with educational attainment (Telfair & Shelton, 2012).

Twenty-one percent of the Latinx population in the United States remains uninsured, and the Latinx population has the highest uninsured rate of any racial/ethnic group under the age of 65 in the United States. This high percentage results in part from the types of occupations in which they often work; these occupations tend not to provide employer-sponsored health insurance (Garrett & Gangopadhyaya, 2016). Furthermore, as Hall and Mann-Jackson outline (Chap. 11) Latinx individuals, among full-time employees, have the lowest earnings of any racial/ethnic group (Stepler & Brown, 2016). In other words, when faced with the option to buy private health insurance from their employer or the Affordable Care Act (ACA) Healthcare Marketplace, it can be too expensive to purchase for themselves or their families. Furthermore, a large proportion of the uninsured Latinx population are Latinx immigrants who often do not qualify for Medicaid or private insurance through the ACA Healthcare Marketplace.

While the U.S. Latinx population faces significant barriers in accessing health care because of the lack of health insurance, health insurance does not tell the complete story. Other barriers to accessing health care in the United States include the lack of culturally sensitive health care, language-concordant providers, time, and reliable transportation.

Many of the contributors to this volume, whether writing about a specific health outcome, a Latinx population subgroup, or critical determinants of health, reference the important demographic shift in terms of where Latinx populations are settling and living: traditional gateways versus new destinations. New destinations was a concept introduced by sociologists Victor Zuñiga and Rubén Hernández-León, in their edited volume, *New Destinations: Mexican Immigration in the United States* (2005), which refers to a demographic phenomenon that commenced in the 1990s in which immigrants, primarily from Mexico and Central America, were migrating and settling in new, nontraditional destinations in the United States. These destinations were primarily located in the South and in the Midwest (Marrow, 2011; Massey, 2008). These destinations presented new job opportunities and lower costs of living than traditional destinations such as New York, Los Angeles, Chicago, Houston, and Miami (Card & Lewis, 2007). Social scientists and demographers have broadly examined how the presence of Latinx populations in these areas have enriched and revitalized local economies and cultures or produced a backlash of anti-immigrant sentiment that resulted in more restrictive immigration enforcement policies in these states (Marrow, 2011; Massey, 2008). However, more recently, multidisciplinary scholars in health are examining the health of Latinx populations in new destinations and how the determinants of health in new destinations are distinct from those of traditional immigrant destinations.

Considering whether Latinx populations live in new or traditional destinations is important because each geographic location has distinct community and social structures and institutional arrangements to address the needs and priorities of the Latinx population. For example, new destinations tend to have fewer bilingual service providers and community-based and advocacy organizations for Latinx persons. Thus, those living in new destinations may have limited available resources and lack access to health and social services that promote health and prevent adverse health outcomes. However, social ties in these new destinations may in fact be stronger.

Interestingly, Latinx life expectancy and mortality rates appear to be better than those of non-Hispanic Whites, particularly living in new destinations, because new destinations are often areas with decades of economic decline (Brazil, 2017). Given these socioeconomic conditions and the lack of health services in these areas, Whites have experienced higher mortality rates and lower life expectancies. So, Latinx persons may look much healthier next to this reference group. Unfortunately, new epidemiological studies (e.g., HCHS/SOL) that are collecting critical data on key Latinx subgroups are not capturing the health and conditions of Latinx populations living in new destinations, like those in the South and Midwest.

In each chapter of this volume, contributors have identified immigration and/or documentation status of Latinx persons as an important variable to consider in research because being unauthorized in the United States excludes one from public and private health and social services, and in the majority of states, state-issued documents like driver's licenses. U.S.-born and authorized immigrant family members in mixed immigration status households suffer profoundly as well. The words "immigration" and "documentation status" were often used in this volume interchangeably by the authors to refer to a foreign-born person's legal authorization to live and/or work in the United States.

Moreover, a discussion of unauthorized immigration among the U.S. Latinx population is important because as many contributors note, the current U.S. president, Donald J. Trump, has escalated the xenophobia of Latin Americans by implementing policies that separate Latinx migrant children from their parents and has sent thousands of troops to the U.S.-Mexico border to deter a caravan of Honduran migrants from seeking asylum in the United States, among other practices his first two years in office. The number of unauthorized immigrants in the country is estimated to be 10.6 million persons, which is low compared to 2009 at 12 million (Padford & Budiman, 2018). Mexican immigrants represent about half of all unauthorized migrants in the United States (Padford & Budiman, 2018). However, some argue that there may be anywhere between 16 and 26 million unauthorized immigrants in the country; it is difficult to know given that undocumented immigrants tend to be an invisible population (Fazel-Zarandi, Feinstein, & Kaplan, 2018). Although these new estimates are still under debate (see Capps, Gelatt, Van Hook, & Fix, 2018), time will tell what the larger consequences of anti-immigrant policies and overall anti-immigration sentiment will be on Latinx health, particularly that of the U.S.-born Latinx population.

It is also estimated that 16 million people in the United States live in a household with an unauthorized immigrant. Of these 16 million, about 6 million are the children of at least one unauthorized immigrant parent (Mathema, 2017). Therefore, there are many Latinx households of mixed immigration status (also termed "mixed-status families"). U.S. citizen and legal permanent resident family members in mixed-status households are often not enrolled in public health insurance programs like Medicaid or Medicare nor are they enrolled in publicly funded food assistance programs like Supplemental Nutrition Assistance Program (SNAP). Participation in these programs is known to mitigate the negative health effects of poverty. Moreover, the implementation of immigration enforcement policies and the exclusion of mixed-status families from social institutions may also further marginalize Latinx persons who are living with an unauthorized family member, or are unauthorized themselves, by removing them from support systems and social networks that help most people mitigate stress and be resilient in the face of adversity (Rhodes et al.,

2015; Martínez, Ruelas, & Granger, 2018). Kline and Castañeda's chapter in this volume (Chap. 12) provides an overview of the research that examines immigration status as a social determinant of health, the implications immigration enforcement policies have on Latinx persons and communities, and they identify future directions for this research.

Political participation, representation, and leadership are related to health through the benefits from civic engagement and community building and voting for politicians who promote the distribution of resources to policies that promote health and social equity (Rodriguez, Geronimus, Bound, & Dorling, 2015). As one can discern from the demographic data, Latinx persons are heterogeneous by ethnic affiliation (identify with Hispanic versus Latina/o/x), national origin and descent, documentation status, language use, racialized position (pre- and post-migration), immigrant generational status, and in their politics. Much of the heterogeneity in Latinx political participation stems from their immigrant generational status, reasons for migration, economic and political context in their country of origin, history of and current civic participation, their personal political affiliations, and their age at arrival to United States (Tran, 2017). Latinx political participation consists of voting, civic engagement, volunteering for campaign efforts, participating in political protest or public rallies, communicating with politicians, and fundraising for political causes or candidates (Beltrán, 2005; DeSipio, 2006; Tran, 2017).

When we examine Latinx persons' voting behavior, we see that despite the fact that there are 40 million Latinx persons in the United States, only about 50% are eligible to vote. Some are ineligible to vote because they are noncitizens, while many are under the voting age of 18. Because race and ethnicity are inadequately collected by the Bureau of Justice Statistics, it is difficult to know how many Latinx persons are kept from voting due to felony disenfranchisement, in which persons in prison or who are on parole or probation are restricted from voting in 18 states (Uggen, Larson, & Shannon, 2016). Eight hundred thousand Latinx millennials were eligible to vote for the November 2018 midterm elections, but since youth are less likely to vote (DeSipio, 2006), it is difficult to discern whether they will in fact change the demographic landscape of the electorate and become the Latinx bloc that Democrats or Republicans desire.

Political representation of the U.S. Latinx population is complicated to generalize not only because of the heterogeneities within this population, but also because there are few politicians and appointed leaders who identify as Latinx. Latinx politicians represent 8.6% of elected members in the U.S. Congress (National Association of Latino Elected and Appointed Officials, 2018). When we think about Latinx representation in leadership positions at federal agencies, their numbers are low, too. Although there have been gains in the number of elected officials in more recent elections, less than 0.02% of all elected officials at the state and federal level self-identify as Hispanic or Latina/o/x. For this reason, Carlos E. Rodriguez-Díaz's chapter (Chap. 16) is so important to end our edited volume. From a human rights perspective and health-in-all-policies approach, Rodriguez-Díaz examines how the disenfranchisement of Puerto Ricans on the island has stimulated more CBPR and intervention efforts that address health disparities that result from exclusionary or inadequate laws and policies. Generally, without participation and representation of Latinx persons in interventions and policy-making decisions in their local areas, there is little hope that Latinx persons and their allies will be able to improve their social position in the United States, much less their health status.

We write this section on Latinx changing demographics to demonstrate the heterogeneities in Latinx communities, but also what they share. Each contributor has made a concerted effort to describe heterogeneities in relation to Latinx persons' health status, risk factors, and social determinants of health, not just by Latinx nationality, but also by age, gender, socioeconomic status, U.S. region, and even whether they live in a new versus traditional destination for Latinx migrants. As such, we want readers of this volume to realize that the epidemiological trinity of "age, sex/gender and race" is not sufficiently comprehensive to elucidate the complexities of Latinx health disparities and Latinx resilience.

Overarching and Cross-Cutting Themes

Throughout this volume, contributors share their research perspectives, experiences, and insights. Several overarching and cross-cutting themes emerged across the chapters. First, there is a need to apply theory and conceptual frameworks from multiple disciplines to address the complex health issues of the Latinx population in the United States. Concepts of acculturation and assimilation and considerations related to "traditional" or assumed Latinx values, such as machismo, fatalism, and familism, deserve more comprehensive exploration. This research must be conducted through careful partnerships with Latinx persons themselves to move beyond stereotyping. While research is meant to generalize, overgeneralizations lead to inadequate and thus insufficient understandings and inappropriate next steps, further contributing to disparities and inequities. Moreover, research is needed that moves beyond western European ways of conceptualizing the world and incorporating perspectives from Latin America and the Caribbean, including theories of dependency, liberation, popular education, critical and militant sociology, and community social psychology.

A second important theme that emerged from this volume is the need to identify and harness datasets that can provide critical insights into the health and well-being of the Latinx population, as well as various subgroups including critical variables such as country of origin, immigration status, sexual orientation, and gender identity. Furthermore, well-designed studies are needed to add to our increasing understanding of Latinx health. These studies must be theoretically sound, building off our current foundation and moving the science in new directions. We cannot continue to extrapolate on the state of Latinx health as we have in the past. Studies that explore US regional differences are desperately needed. Currently, the larger studies such as the HCHS/SOL have four field centers (Miami, FL, San Diego, CA, Chicago, IL, and the Bronx, NY). None of these centers reflect the current demographic trends of immigrant Latinx settlement in the United States. While these centers reflect important established Latinx communities, more research is needed in the Midwest and

South, regions that have states with some of the fastest growing Latinx populations in the country.

Another key theme emerging from this volume is the profound need to move beyond formative research and move toward intervention research. The development, implementation, and evaluation of interventions designed to promote health and well-being are needed at multiple levels, including intrapersonal, interpersonal, social and environmental, community, structural, and policy levels. While there is rich discussion within health literature regarding the various levels of determinants of health, efforts to intervene tend to remain focused on intrapersonal and interpersonal levels. The social determinants of health tend to be less focused on in intervention research, perhaps because intervening on these determinants is more difficult to evaluate; the outcomes tend to be more distal. However, innovations are needed in terms of strategies to positively intervene on the social determinants of health and the evaluation of these strategies.

Finally, we must include Latinx persons as partners in research and practice. Despite "being from the community," very few Latinx researchers reflect the communities that are most affected by health inequities. Through no fault of their own, all researchers become different from the communities they come from; thus, the inclusion of Latinx partners in research is necessary to ensure authentic understandings of the needs and priorities of Latinx communities. Community-engaged research, which includes various levels of community involvement and participation and CBPR that implies shared leadership and or even community-led research, is needed within Latinx health to ensure that the needs and priorities of community members and community assets are identified, understood, and harnessed.

Final Thoughts

We produce this volume knowing that we are providing an updated snapshot of the current health status of the Latinx population; we hope this will provide the stimulus and vision needed to spark further health research and interventions that are conducted through a comprehensive framework of broad determinants of health. We also want readers, including researchers, practitioners, and students, to incorporate other conceptual frameworks to examine the health status of Latinx populations and compare Latinx in the United States to those in Latin America.

We are aware that this volume could expand further on all topics including maternal health, sexual and reproductive health, and veterans' health. These are topics of great importance. Despite our multiple attempts to find contributors with expertise in some of these topics in the Latinx population, we had little success producing a substantial list of potential contributors. Only a handful of thought leaders (researchers and practitioners) in each topic area are carrying the heavy lifting in their fields, even for the topics represented in this volume. The limited number of health and social science researchers of Latinx health and well-being is clearly a barrier to Latinx health equity. Without the necessary research, it is next to impossible to create change. We call upon established scholars in Latinx health or in positions of leadership to train and support the next generation of racial/ethnic researchers and practitioners to examine and address Latinx health. We also call upon established scholars to support the training and retention of Latinx health scholars and support their application to higher-level occupational positions in academia, local and state public health departments, and federal agencies dedicated to science, medicine, and public health.

Thus, in addition to the profound need for research within Latinx health, we call on Latinx health scholars to ensure that the next generation of Latinx health researchers and public health practitioners have innovative theoretical and methodological tools to examine and reverse the many racial, economic, and social injustices that the Latinx population faces. This requires encouraging young scholars to pursue novel questions that are distinct from and expand on the current foundation and understanding of Latinx health. It also requires the leadership in Latinx health to support young and mid-level scholars when they pursue positions of leadership in national professional associations and at federal agencies.

References

Alcoff, L. M. (2005). Latino vs. Hispanic: The politics of ethnic names. *Philosophy & Social Criticism, 31*(4), 395–407.

Aldama, A. J., & Quiñonez, N. H. (2002). *Decolonial voices: Chicana and Chicano cultural studies in the 21st century*. Bloomington: Indiana University Press.

Anzaldúa, G. (1987). *Borderlands: la frontera* (Vol. 3). San Francisco: Aunt Lute.

Beltrán, C. (2005). *The trouble with unity: Latino politics and the creation of identity*. New York: Oxford University Press on Demand.

Brazil, N. (2017). Spatial variation in the Hispanic paradox: mortality rates in new and established Hispanic US destinations. *Population, Space & Place, 23*(1), e1968.

Bureau of Labor Statistics, U.S. Department of Labor, *The Economics Daily*, Hispanics and Latinos in industries and occupations. Retrieved from https://www.bls.gov/opub/ted/2015/hispanics-and-latinos-in-industries-and-occupations.htm.

Capps, R., Gelatt, J., Van Hook, J., & Fix, M. (2018). Commentary on "The number of undocumented immigrants in the United States: Estimates based on demographic modeling with data from 1990–2016". *PLoS ONE, 13*(9), e0204199.

Card, D., & Lewis, E. G. (2007). The diffusion of Mexican immigrants during the 1990s: Explanations and impacts. *Mexican immigration to the United States* (pp. 193–228). Chicago: University of Chicago Press.

Centers for Disease Control & Prevention. Office of Management and Budget (OMB) Directive No. 15 Race and Ethnic Standards for Federal Statistics and Administrative Reporting, May 12, 1977. Access on January 9, 2018 from https://wonder.cdc.gov/wonder/help/populations/bridged-race/directive15.html.

Cohn, D. (2010). *Census history: Counting Hispanics*, March 10, 2010. Washington, D.C.: Pew Research Center.

Dávila, A. (2012). *Latinos, Inc: The marketing and making of peoples*. Berkeley: University of California Press.

de Alba, A. G. (2003). The Chicana/Latina dyad, or identity and perception. *Latino Studies, 1*(1), 106–114.

DeSipio, L. (2006). Transnational politics and civic engagement: Do home country political ties limit Latino immigrant pursuit of U.S. civic engagement and citizenship? In T. Lee, S. K. Ramakrishnan, & R. Ramírez (Eds.), *Transforming politics, transforming America: The political and civic incorporation of immigrants in the United States* (pp. 106–126). Charlottesville: University of Virginia.

Fazel-Zarandi, M. M., Feinstein, J. S., & Kaplan, E. H. (2018). The number of undocumented immigrants in the United States: Estimates based on demographic modeling with data from 1990 to 2016. *PLoS ONE, 13*(9), e0201193.

Flores, A. (2017). Facts on U.S. Latinos, 2015: Statistical portrait of Hispanics in the United States, September 18, 2017. Washington, D.C.: Pew Research Center.

Foucault, M. (1984). The politics of health in the eighteenth century. In P. Rabinow (Ed.), *The Foucault Reader* (pp. 273–289). New York: Pantheon Press.

Garrett, B., & Gangopadhyaya, A. (2016). *Who gained health insurance coverage under the ACA, and where do they live?*. Washington, DC: Urban Institute.

Gracia, J. (2000). *Hispanic/Latino identity: A philosophical perspective*. Malden, MA: Blackwell.

Marrow, H. (2011). *New destination dreaming: Immigration, race, and legal status in the rural American South*. Palo Alto, CA: Stanford University Press.

Massey, D. S. (Ed.). (2008). *New faces in new places: The changing geography of American immigration*. New York: Russell Sage Foundation.

Mathema, S. (2017). *Keeping families: Together why all Americans should care about what happens to unauthorized immigrants*. Center for American Progress, March 16, 2017. Washington, D.C. Center for American Progress.

McConnell, E. D., & Delgado-Romero, E. A. (2004). Latino panethnicity: reality or methodological construction? *Sociological Focus, 37*(4), 297–312.

National Association of Latino Elected and Appointed Officials. (2018). Latino Elected Officials in America, October 28, 2018. Washington, D.C.

Oboler, S. (1995). *Ethnic labels, Latino lives: Identity and the politics of (re) presentation in the United States*. Minneapolis: University of Minnesota Press.

Padford, J., & Budiman, A. (2018). *Facts on U.S. Immigrants, 2016: Statistical Portrait of the foreign-born population in the United States*. Washington, D.C.: Pew Research Center.

Rhodes, S. D., Alonzo, J., Mann-Jackson, L., Tanner, A. E., Vissman, A. T., Martinez, O., et al. (2018). Selling the product: Strategies to increase recruitment and retention of Spanish-speaking Latinos in biomedical research. *Journal of Clinical and Translational Science, 2*(3), 147–155.

Rhodes, S. D., Mann, L., Simán, F. M., Song, E., Alonzo, J., Downs, M., et al. (2015). The impact of local immigration enforcement policies on the health of immigrant Hispanics/Latinos in the United States. *American Journal of Public Health, 105*(2), 329–337.

Rodriguez, J. M., Geronimus, A. T., Bound, J., & Dorling, D. (2015). Black lives matter: Differential mortality and the racial composition of the US electorate, 1970–2004. *Social Science and Medicine, 136–137*, 193–199.

Scharrón-del Río, M. R., & Aja, A. A. (2015). The case FOR 'Latinx': Why intersectionality is not a choice. *Latino Rebels, 5*.

Stepler, R., & Brown, A. (2016). *Statistical portrait of Hispanics in the United States*. Washington, D.C.: Pew Research Center.

Telfair, J., & Shelton, T. L. (2012). Educational attainment as a social determinant of health. *North Carolina Medical Journal, 73*(5), 358–365.

Toro, L. A. (1998). Race, identity, and "box checking": The Hispanic classification in OMB directive no. 15. In R. Delgado & J. Stefancic (Eds.), *The Latino condition: A critical reader* (pp. 52–59). New York: New York University Press.

Tran, V. C. (2017). Beyond the ballot box: Age-at-arrival, civic institutions and political participation among Latinos. *Journal of Ethnic and Migration Studies, 43*(5), 766–790.

Uggen, C., Larson, R., & Shannon, S. (2016). Lost Voters: State-level estimates of felony disenfranchisement, 2016. The Sentencing Project, Washington, D.C., October 6, 2016. Retrieved from https://www.sentencingproject.org/publications/6-million-lost-voters-state-level-estimates-felony-disenfranchisement-2016/.

United States Census Bureau. (2017). Hispanic or Latino Origin by Specific Origin: 2017 American Community Survey 1-Year Estimates. Retrieved from https://factfinder.census.gov/faces/tableservices/jsf/pages/productview.xhtml?pid=ACS_17_1YR_B03001&prodType=table.

United States Census Bureau. (2015). Hispanic or Latino Origin by Specific Origin: 2015 American Community Survey 5-Year Estimates. Retrieved from https://factfinder.census.gov/faces/tableservices/jsf/pages/productview.xhtml?pid=ACS_17_1YR_B03001&prodType=table.

Vidal-Ortiz, S., & Martínez, J. (2018). Latinx thoughts: Latinidad with an X. *Latino Studies, 16*(3), 384–395.

Zuñiga, V., & Hernández-León, R. (2005). *New destinations: Mexican immigration in the United States*. New York: Russell Sage Foundation.

Part I
The Health Status of Latinx Persons in the United States

Chapter 2
Chronic Disease and the Latinx Population: Threats, Challenges, and Opportunities

Barbara Baquero and Deborah M. Parra-Medina

Abstract Compared with other ethnic/racial and socioeconomic groups, the US Latinx population is disproportionately affected by chronic diseases. In this chapter, we describe the epidemiology of chronic diseases and related health behaviors among this population. We then explore social, economic, cultural, and environmental factors and behaviors associated with the risks for cancer and chronic diseases for Latinx persons and the protective factors that can be harnessed to reverse the high prevalence of many diseases, such as cancer, asthma, and type 2 diabetes. We also propose and describe select health behavior theories that can inform the development of interventions and provide examples of effective interventions that have helped prevent and control cancer and chronic diseases in the Latinx population. Lastly, we discuss future priorities for research in the prevention of cancer and chronic diseases and interventions to address health disparities among Latinx persons.

Keywords Latinx chronic disease · Health behavior theories · Modifiable risk factors · Prevention · Social determinants

Chronic diseases, including cancer, heart disease, stroke, type 2 diabetes, and obesity, are strikingly common in the United States. Half of all US adults, or almost 117 million people, have at least one chronic health problem (Centers for Disease Control and Prevention (CDC), 2016a). Seven of the top ten causes of death are chronic diseases (CDC, 2016a). However, chronic diseases are mostly preventable. Most of the social, economic, cultural, and environmental factors and behaviors associated with the development of chronic disease are modifiable risks; therefore, these diseases and their consequences to communities are preventable.

Compared with other ethnic/racial and socioeconomic groups, the US Latinx population is disproportionately affected by chronic diseases (American Cancer Society,

B. Baquero (✉)
The University of Washington, Washington, DC, USA
e-mail: bbaquero@uw.edu

The University of Iowa, Iowa City, IA, USA

D. M. Parra-Medina
University of Texas-San Antonio, San Antonio, TX, USA

2015). For example, cancer and heart disease are the leading causes of death among Latinx persons, and the rates of obesity, uncontrolled blood pressure, and diabetes are higher than those for non-Hispanic white persons (CDC, 2015b). The risk of cancer and chronic diseases differs among Latinx subgroups. Latinx persons of Mexican or Puerto Rican origin are more likely to die from diabetes than other Latinx persons, and infections related to cancers are higher for foreign-born Latinx individuals (CDC, 2015b). The urgent and widening disparities that Latinx persons face require a continued commitment from researchers, community advocates, and practitioners to reduce the risks factors threatening this population. The development and testing of new culturally, structurally, and socially salient interventions are needed to address the persistent, pervasive risks for Latinx persons. In addition, sustaining interventions with demonstrated ability to advance health are needed, as well as the adaptation, implementation, and evaluation of successful interventions designed for other communities to meet the needs and resources of the Latinx population.

In this chapter, we describe the epidemiology of chronic diseases and related health behaviors among the US Latinx population. We then explore social, economic, cultural, and environmental factors and behaviors associated with the risks for cancer and chronic diseases for Latinx individuals and the protective factors that can be harnessed to reverse the high prevalence of many diseases, such as cancer, asthma, and type 2 diabetes. We also propose and describe select health behavior theories that can inform the development of interventions and provide examples of effective interventions that have helped prevent and control cancer and chronic diseases in the Latinx population. Lastly, we discuss future priorities for research in the prevention of cancer and chronic diseases and interventions to address health disparities among Latinx persons.

Epidemiology of Chronic Diseases: Heterogeneity of the Latinx Population

We reviewed national databases for the years 2005–2017 to capture the state of cancer and chronic diseases and conditions for the US Latinx population and summarized the evidence by disease and Latinx subgroups, when available. Most of the reported data on Latinx persons are aggregated, which masks the differences among subgroups. For example, although Mexican and Puerto Rican populations, among populations of other nationalities, are generally grouped under "Hispanic" or "Latino," cancer-related mortality rates for Mexican persons are 12% lower than those for Puerto Rican persons who live on the mainland (American Cancer Society, 2015). Disaggregating or deconstructing health data from these larger categories of "Hispanic" or "Latino" is important because the Latinx population is a heterogeneous group that may share linguistic and historical roots, but differ in many important factors related to effective public health interventions. We must understand and examine the diversity of Latinx individuals to address the root causes of the health disparities they confront. Rates of cancer and chronic diseases and conditions among Latinx persons differ according to many dimensions, such as country of origin, place of birth, citizenship, language, race, culture, number of years in the United States, immigration or generation status, and demographics. We describe and examine, when available, subgroup differences in cancer and chronic diseases and conditions by socioeconomic, country of origin, and immigration status.

Cancer

According to 2015 data from the American Cancer Society, cancer is diagnosed in almost 30% of Latinx persons in the United States in their lifetime (American Cancer Society, 2015). Although the incidence rate for cancer in the Latinx population is lower than that in the white and non-Hispanic black (black) populations, the most common cancers are more likely to be diagnosed at advanced stages in the Latinx population compared with these same other populations. Since 2009, cancer has replaced heart disease as the leading cause of death among Latinx persons in the United States and accounted for approximately 22% of all Latinx deaths in the country in 2012 (American Cancer Society, 2015). Relative to other racial/ethnic populations, the mortality rates associated with specific types of cancer (breast, uterine, cervical, and gastrointestinal) are more likely to be higher in the Latinx population (American Cancer Society, 2015). In summary, different types of cancer disparities exist among Latinx subgroups, as described here.

Breast cancer. In 2015, breast cancer was the most common cancer in US-born Latina women, with 19,800 cases diagnosed (American Cancer Society, 2015). Within Latinx subgroups, incidence rates vary by nationality, country of origin, and environment (i.e., housing, neighborhood, employment conditions) (Stern et al., 2016). The incidence rate is lower for women who live in Puerto Rico than for Puerto Rican women who live in the mainland United States (Stern et al., 2016). Country of birth and migration history are also associated with breast cancer risks in Latinx women. The risk of breast cancer is lower for foreign-born Latina women than for US-born Latina women, regardless of socioeconomic status (Stern et al., 2016). Among Latina women who reside in Florida, the rate of breast cancer is higher for women of Puerto Rican or Cuban origin than for women of Mexican and other Latinx origins (Stern et al., 2016). Longer residency in the United States is associated with an increased risk for the development of breast cancer (Stern et al., 2016).

Prostate and colorectal cancer. The most common cancer among Latino men is prostate cancer, with an incidence rate of 13,000 in 2015; however, the incidence is lower among Latino men than among black and white men (American Cancer Society, 2015). Among Latino subgroups, the prevalence of prostate cancer is lower for Mexican American men (US-born Mexican descendent) and is slightly higher for Cuban-origin and Puerto Rican men compared with white men (Penedo et al., 2016; Stern et al., 2016).

After prostate and breast cancers, colorectal cancer is the most common cancer diagnosis for Latinx men and women (American Cancer Society, 2015). The American Cancer Society estimates that colorectal cancer was diagnosed in 6400 Latinx men and 5300 Latinx women in 2015 (American Cancer Society, 2015). In the Latinx population, colorectal cancer is the third leading cause of cancer-related death, due in part to the fact that cancer is likely to be diagnosed at a more advanced stage (American Cancer Society, 2015; Stern et al., 2016). The incidence and mortality rate for colorectal cancer are approximately 10–20% lower for the Latinx population than for the white population (Stern et al., 2016). However, the incidence rate differs significantly in the Latinx population according to socioeconomic status. For Latinx persons with a lower socioeconomic status, the incidence rate is lower (41 per 100,000 men and 28 per 100,000 women) than that for Latinx persons with a higher socioeconomic status (68 per 100,000 men and 43 per 100,000 women) (Stern et al., 2016). This pattern is notable because data on the incidence of colorectal cancer and socioeconomic status among the white and black populations demonstrate the opposite relationship; that is, a high socioeconomic status is associated with a lower incidence of colorectal cancer (Stern et al., 2016). The incidence rate of colorectal cancer in Latinx subgroups also varies according to the country of origin. For example, in California, the incidence of colorectal cancer is higher for men of Cuban origin than for men of Mexican origin (Stern et al., 2016). In Florida, the incidence rate of colorectal cancer is twice as high among Cuban-origin and Puerto Rican adults compared with Mexican adults (Stern et al., 2016).

Lung cancer. The rate of lung and bronchus cancer has been decreasing in recent years among all racial and ethnic groups in the United States. Compared with other racial and ethnic groups in this country, the prevalence of lung cancer is lowest for the Latinx population (American Cancer Society, 2016a). Nevertheless, with a prevalence of 9%, lung cancer is the third most common cancer diagnosis among Latino men (Siegel et al., 2015). Between 2008 and 2012, the rate of lung cancer (per 100,000) for Latinx persons was 43.3 for men and 26.0 for women (American Cancer Society, 2016a). The American Cancer Society estimates that in 2015, lung cancer was newly diagnosed in 5000 Latino men and in 4600 Latina women (American Cancer Society, 2015). Among women, mortality related to lung and bronchus cancer is second only to that related to breast cancer and accounts for 13% of deaths from cancer among Latinas (American Cancer Society, 2015). As with the incidence rates of lung and bronchus cancer, the mortality rate continues to decline for Latinx men but remains static for Latinx women (CDC, 2016c). Despite the lower incidence of lung cancer in the Latinx population compared with the white population (Siegel et al., 2015), the rates of lung cancer range widely among various Latinx subgroups. These varied patterns are related to different smoking patterns in diverse cultures and countries of origin. For example, the rate of smoking is historically high in Cuba, and lung cancer is much more likely to develop in men of Cuban origin (49.9 per 100,000) than in men of Mexican origin (27.1 per 100,000) (Siegel et al., 2015).

Liver cancer, chronic liver disease, and cirrhosis. The rate of liver cancer is disproportionately high in the Latinx population (American Cancer Society, 2016b). The number of deaths from chronic liver disease has declined within the general

US population since the late 2000s, but not within the Latinx population (Carrion, Ghanta, Carrasquillo, & Martin, 2011). Mortality related to chronic liver disease for Latinx persons is 13.7 per 100,000, which is about 50% higher than that for white persons (9.2 per 100,000) (Carrion et al., 2011). Among the general population in 2014, chronic liver disease and cirrhosis were the twelfth leading causes of death, whereas for the Latinx population it was the sixth (Heron, 2016). For Latinx persons, the 5-year survival rate after a liver cancer diagnosis is only 20% (American Cancer Society, 2016b). According to the Centers for Disease Control and Prevention (CDC), the 2013 rate of liver cancer among Latinx men was 19 per 100,000, which was the second highest in the United States (the highest rate was 19.1 for Asian/Pacific Islander men) (CDC, 2016b). In that same year, among all women, the incidence of liver cancer was higher for Latinx women (7.5 per 100,000) than for women in all other racial/ethnic populations (CDC, 2016b).

Liver disease increases the likelihood of the development of liver cancer (American Cancer Society, 2015). For example, hepatitis B and C viruses cause the majority of liver cancers, although both infections can be prevented through public health improvements (American Cancer Society, 2015). Among Latinx subgroups, the disparities are evident. The risk of liver cancer among Latinx persons born in the United States is twice as high compared with the risk for Latinx immigrants (Siegel et al., 2015). Among Puerto Rican persons, the rate of liver cancer is twice as high for persons who live in Florida than for those who live on the island (Siegel et al., 2015). In Texas, the incidence and mortality rate are higher for Latinx persons of Mexican descent than for the state's general population (Siegel et al., 2015).

Latinx persons die of cancer more than any other diseases, in part because cancer is more often diagnosed at an advance stage in this population. Furthermore, Latinx persons live in communities that may expose them to many of the known social, economic, and environmental factors associated with a higher risk of cancer, such as obesity, hepatitis C, alcohol use, and diabetes (Siegel et al., 2015). The disparities in cancer diagnoses also mask the heterogeneity of the community.

Cardiovascular Disease and Stroke

Cardiovascular disease (CVD) refers to several types of heart disease, including coronary artery disease, heart attack, and high blood pressure (CDC, 2015a). Coronary artery disease, defined as decreased blood flow to the heart, is the most common heart disease in the United States. CVD is very common in Latinx persons living in this country (Office of Minority Health, 2016c); 48.3% of Latinx men and 32.4% of Latinx women have CVD (Mozaffarian et al., 2016). CVD is the second leading cause of death in the Latinx population (CDC, 2016d), and the death rate is higher for Latinx women than Latinx men (Mozaffarian et al., 2016). Although heart disease is a major health concern for Latinx persons, the rates of CVD and CVD-related deaths are lower than the rates for white persons (Office of Minority Health, 2016c). The age-adjusted prevalence ratio for the Latinx and white populations is 0.9, meaning that CVD is slightly less likely to be diagnosed in Latinx persons (Office of Minority Health, 2016c).

According to the American Stroke Association, 2.8% of Latinx men and 2% of Latinx women have had a stroke within the past year (Mozaffarian et al., 2016). Rates of stroke are projected to increase nationwide, and the highest rates are expected to be among Latinx men (Mozaffarian et al., 2016), in part due to the higher prevalence of stroke-related conditions such as diabetes and metabolic syndrome. For instance, the average age at the time of the first stroke is 67 years among Latinx persons and 80 years among white persons (American Stroke Association, 2012).

High blood pressure is a major risk factor for both CVD and stroke. Among Latinx adults, 29.6% of men and 29.9% of women have high blood pressure (Mozaffarian et al., 2016). Although screening for high blood pressure, cholesterol levels, and other risk factors are necessary for diagnosis, a smaller percentage of Latinx adults receives screening compared with white adults. For example, among adults older than 20 years of age, 59.3% of Latinx individuals and 71.8% of white individuals were screened for cholesterol levels in 2011 and 2012 (Office of Minority Health, 2016c).

Evidence of CVD disparities among Latinx subgroups is limited. Within the US Latinx population, the Mexican American subgroup is the largest. As a result, there are more sources of health data to characterize this subgroup. For example, data from the 2010 National Health and Nutrition Examination Survey showed that the prevalence of CVD among Mexican American persons was 7% for men and 5% women (Balfour, Ruiz, Talavera, Allison, & Rodriguez, 2016). However, data are available to determine disparities on risk factors for CVD among Latinx subgroups. The Study of Latinos (SOL) is a federally funded study to address the limited data on health indicators among Latinx subgroups. Self-reported data from the SOL indicate that the prevalence of CVD for men and women of Puerto Rico, Dominican, and Cuban origin is 5%. Seven major biobehavioral risk factors for CVD are considered important: high cholesterol level, hypertension, diabetes, obesity, cigarette smoking, diet, and activity levels. For example, cholesterol levels are high in 48% of men of Dominican and Puerto Rican origin and in 55% of men of Central American origin. Among women, 31% of Latinx women from South America and 41% from Puerto Rico have high cholesterol levels. On average, 25% of Latinx men and 24% of Latinx women have hypertension. The prevalence of hypertension for Cuban-origin men is higher (29%) than that for men in all other Latinx subgroups. Among Latinx women, the rate of hypertension is highest for Puerto Rican women (29%) (Daviglus et al., 2012). We will discuss physical activity, smoking, and diet later in the chapter.

Asthma and Pulmonary Disease

Two million (5.8%) individuals in the Latinx population reported that they had asthma in 2014 (Office of Minority Health, 2016a). The prevalence of asthma is higher for Latinx women, as well as for women in the general population, than for men

(Akinbami, 2010). In addition, the rate of asthma is higher for low-income women and children (Centers for Disease Control and Prevention, 2011). Although the prevalence of asthma among Latinx adults (5.8%) is lower than among white adults (7.6%), Latinx adults are slightly more likely to die from asthma (Office of Minority Health, 2016a). The rate of death related to asthma is 1.3 per 100,000 for the Latinx population as a whole and 1.1 for the white population (Office of Minority Health, 2016a). The number of hospital visits, an indicator that asthma is not managed adequately, is also higher for Latinx persons. Compared with white persons, Latinx persons are 60% more likely to visit the hospital for asthma (Office of Minority Health, 2016a).

For persons of Puerto Rican descent, the prevalence of asthma (16.1 per 10,000) is almost twice that for the overall Latinx population (Office of Minority Health, 2016a), and the prevalence of asthma attacks is also highest (Akinbami, 2010). Furthermore, Puerto Rican children are three times more likely to have asthma than white children (Office of Minority Health, 2016a). Among all Latinx subgroups, the prevalence of asthma is lowest for the Mexican-origin population (5.4%). The risk of asthma is greater for Mexican-origin persons born in the United States than foreign-born Mexican persons (Rosser, Forno, Cooper, & Celedón, 2014).

The broad range of disparities in asthma/pulmonary disease among Latinx subgroups in the United States is related to differences in exposure to tobacco smoke and other pollutants, genetic susceptibility, access to health care, and other factors (Brehm & Celedón, 2008). Data from the SOL show that, among Latinx subgroups, the rate of asthma is highest for the Puerto Rican subgroup (36.5%). The rates of asthma are higher for Latinx persons born in the United States and persons who had immigrated as children compared with persons who had immigrated as adults or were foreign-born. Other pulmonary diseases, such as chronic obstructive pulmonary disorder, a disease characterized by wheezing and difficulty breathing (National Heart, Lung, & Blood Institute, 2017), follow several patterns. Among Latinx subgroups, the disease is more prevalent among persons of Puerto Rican (14.1%) and Cuban (9.8%) origin (Barr et al., 2016).

Diabetes

Diabetes is a chronic condition that occurs when the level of sugar in the form of glucose in the blood is too high (National Institute of Diabetes and Digestive and Kidney Diseases, 2016). Diabetes is an underdiagnosed disease, and as a whole, Latinx individuals have a higher risk for type 2 diabetes mellitus than white individuals (American Diabetes Association, 2014). According to the American Diabetes Association, the prevalence of diagnosed and undiagnosed type 2 diabetes is 16.9% in the Latinx population and 10.2% in the white population (American Diabetes Association, 2014). The prevalence and incidence of diabetes increase dramatically with age; for Latinx adults 70 years and older, the prevalence is 50% for women and 44.3% for men (American Diabetes Association, 2014). Furthermore, the longer time foreign-born Latinx individuals live in the United States, the more likely it is that type 2 diabetes will develop (American Diabetes Association, 2014). Within the Latinx population, diabetes was the third leading cause of death for women and the fourth leading cause of death for men in 2015 (Go et al., 2013). Compared with white adults, Latinx adults are 50% more likely to die from diabetes (CDC, 2016c). Diabetes disparities among Latinx subgroups exist. For example, the prevalence of diabetes is lowest for Latinx persons from South America (10.2%) and is similar for persons of Mexican (18.3%), Dominican (18.1%), and Puerto Rican (18.1%) origin (Schneiderman et al., 2014).

Diabetes is associated with multiple health conditions, including chronic kidney disease, which can lead to kidney failure, end-stage renal disease requiring dialysis, and kidney transplantation (CDC, 2016c). These diabetes-related conditions develop at a higher rate among Latinx adults than among white adults. Latinx adults are twice as likely to have amputation of the lower extremity as a result of diabetes and more than three times as likely to have end-stage renal disease compared with white adults (Office of Minority Health, 2016b).

Summary

Cancer and chronic diseases disproportionally affect Latinx persons in the United States. Of the ten top causes of death in the Latinx population, six are chronic diseases. Not only are Latinx persons more likely to have chronic diseases, they also die from them at higher rates and younger ages compared with persons in other racial/ethnic groups. The disparities are even more pronounced when the data are reviewed across Latinx subgroups. Many of these intergroup and intragroup disparities are rooted in a multitude of factors that range from individual lifestyle health behaviors and social, cultural, economic, and environmental factors. In the next section, we discuss the most relevant factors associated with chronic diseases in the Latinx population.

Factors Associated with Chronic Diseases Within the Latinx Population

Unhealthy diet and physical inactivity, combined with smoking, account for one-third of all deaths in the United States (Bauer, Briss, Goodman, & Bowman, 2014). In addition, social, cultural, political, and environmental factors interact with individual health behaviors to affect the rates of chronic diseases in the Latinx population. In particular, we focused on dietary intake and physical activity because they are direct risk factors for obesity. Obesity is a risk factor for 13 types of cancers, including the five most common cancers among Latinx persons, as well as diabetes, CVD, and asthma (CDC, 2017a, 2017b; National Heart, Lung, & Blood Institute, 1998), leading causes of death and disease in the Latinx population. Therefore, physical activity and dietary intake are directly and indirectly related to the prevention or onset of chronic diseases. In the following section, we discuss the impact of these behaviors on chronic diseases among Latinx individuals in the United States.

Lifestyle Health Behaviors Related to Chronic Disease

Physical activity. Regular physical activity is associated with prevention of chronic diseases and weight control (CDC, 2017c). Lack of physical activity and sedentary behavior, on the other hand, have been consistently documented as being associated with a higher risk for CVD, other chronic diseases, and obesity (CDC, 2017c). The CDC suggest that adults engage in at least 150 min of moderate physical activity or 75 min of vigorous physical activity every week, and practice muscle-strengthening activities two or more days per week to achieve health benefits. Individual physical activity level is reported in a variety of ways: meeting CDC's physical activity guidelines; average weekly minutes of moderate-to-vigorous physical activity; total minutes of physical activity per week; or by physical activity type (leisure, transportation, and work). On average, 23% of white adults and 18% of black adults meet the physical activity guidelines, compared with 16% of Latinx adults (CDC, 2017c). Specifically, 42.5% of Latinx men and 42.3% of Latinx women reported engaging in regular physical activity, defined as moderate-intensity activity for 30 min per day on at least five days per week or 20 min of vigorous-intensity activity on at least three days per week, whereas the rates are 52.5% for white men and 49.6% for white women (CDC, 2017e).

Lower rates of physical activity are related to social and cultural characteristics. (We will discuss these factors in a later section in the chapter.) Despite the fact that most adults in the United States do not meet the physical activity recommendation, the rates of physical activity are lower for Latinx adults than for adults in other racial/ethnic groups. For example, more Latinx men overall meet the physical activity recommendation than Latinx women (CDC, 2017c; Larsen, Pekmezi, Marquez, Benitez, & Marcus, 2013; Lee & Im, 2010), and younger Latinx adults are more likely to report meeting the physical activity recommendation than older Latinx adults (Arredondo et al., 2015).

On average, Latinx adults reported 23.8 min of moderate-to-vigorous physical activity (Palta et al., 2016). Among Latinx subgroups, 32.1% of Puerto Rican adults, 29.1% of Dominican-origin adults, and 15.3% of Cuban-origin adults report meeting the physical activity guideline (Palta et al., 2016). Puerto Rican and Dominican-origin adults report the most transportation-related physical activity, whereas adults of Mexican and Central American origin report the most work-related physical activity (90.7 and 93.2%, respectively) (Palta et al., 2016). Additionally, work-related physical activity and hours worked per week are positively associated with a higher risk of overweight and obesity among Latinx adults (Palta et al., 2016). The rate of self-reported moderate-to-vigorous physical activity is higher for Latinx adults of normal weight than for obese Latinx adults (Palta et al., 2016).

Diet and dietary patterns. Dietary intake has been consistently associated with risk for CVD, diabetes, and obesity (CDC, 2017c). However, few studies have focused on examining the link between diet quality and intake with chronic diseases in the US Latinx population.

Data from the SOL represent the latest and most comprehensive information on health behaviors and outcomes in the Latinx population in the United States (Siega-Riz et al., 2014). From these data, we learned that dietary intake differs significantly across Latinx subgroups. For example, adults of Central American or South American origin had higher fruit intake and Puerto Rican adults had the lowest fruit intake. Overall, the total vegetable intake ranged from 2.5 to 4.0 servings per day, with Cuban-origin adults having the highest vegetable intake and Dominican-origin and Puerto Rican adults having the lowest intake. Grains and refined grains comprised a large proportion of the Latinx diet in this representative sample. Red meat accounted for a greater proportion of meat intake in Latinx adults' diets and was higher for Cuban-origin adults (three servings per day) than for adults of Mexican, Central American, or South American origin (two servings per day). The consumption of fat was also highest in the Cuban subgroup (6.7 servings per day) and lowest in the Dominican subgroup (3.9 servings per day). Sugary beverage consumption ranged from 1.1 to 1.8 servings (eight ounces in a serving) per day. These data are crucial to understanding the risk of CVD, diabetes, and obesity in the Latinx population. First, the data demonstrate that the dietary patterns in some Latinx subgroups must be considered when developing health promotion and prevention efforts. In addition, these dietary data help to explain the high risk of chronic diseases among Latinx persons, as it is well documented that diets higher in fat, meats, and sugar are linked to cancer, diabetes, and CVD (Corsino et al., 2017; Medina-Inojosa, Jean, Cortes-Bergoderi, & Lopez-Jimenez, 2014; Pinheiro et al., 2017).

Unhealthy eating practices, such as eating away from home and eating fast food, have become more common among adults in the United States in recent decades. As of 2015, 50% of US adults reported eating three or more meals away from home per week and more than 35% reported eating two or more fast-food meals per week (Kant, Whitley, & Graubard, 2015). Diets dependent on away-from-home foods and fast foods are higher in fat, energy density, and portion size and lower in fiber content than meals prepared at home. Compared with white and black individuals, Latinx individuals eat fewer meals away from home or from fast-food restaurants (Dunn, Sharkey, & Horel, 2012; Fryer & Ervin, 2013), which could be protective. However, this finding varies within the Latinx population; some estimates indicate that, for middle-aged Latinx adults (40–59 years old) one-fifth of the calorie intake comes from fast-food meals (Fryer & Ervin, 2013).

Obesity. Obesity, which is defined as an unhealthy amount and distribution of body fat (National Cancer Institute, 2017), is measured by body mass index (BMI) and categorizes individuals as normal weight, overweight, or obese (CDC, 2017f). Obesity is directly related to diet quality and intake and physical activity, and is an important risk factor for cancer and many of the chronic diseases (e.g., diabetes, asthma, CVD) that affect the US Latinx population.

Obesity is one of the greatest threats to the health of the US Latinx population. Approximately, 77% of the population (almost 12 million Latinx individuals) are considered overweight or obese compared with 67.2% of the white population. The disparities are even greater among Latinx children: 38.9% of Latinx children are overweight or obese compared with 28.5% of white children (Trust for America's Health & Robert Wood Johnson Foundation, 2014).

Among Latinx persons, the rates of overweight and obesity vary according to many factors, including country of birth, acculturation status, and gender (Isasi et al., 2015). Data from the SOL showed that the rate of obesity was highest for Puerto Rican adults (both women and men) and was lowest for adults of South American origin. Latinx individuals who were born in the United States or who have lived in the country for more than 20 years are more likely to be obese than foreign-born Latinx individuals who have lived in the country for less than 20 years. Latinx adults who are more socially acculturated were less likely to be overweight, and adults who reported eating equal amounts of Latinx and American foods were more likely to be obese than Latinx adults who eat mostly Latinx foods (Isasi et al., 2015).

These data on the current levels of physical activity and dietary intake in the Latinx population are concerning. We chose to highlight these behaviors because they are directly and strongly associated with the risk for obesity and therefore increase the risk for chronic diseases. But in addition, physical activity and dietary intake are key health behaviors associated with the prevention and control of chronic diseases. Smoking and alcohol consumption are also important health behaviors for the prevention and control of chronic diseases.

Smoking and alcohol use. Smoking and alcohol use are important causes of chronic disease, and both are associated with specific cancers and CVD. Among the general Latinx population, rates of smoking and drinking are not substantially higher than the rates for the white population. However, when these behaviors are compared across Latinx subgroups, specific patterns are found. Overall, almost 21% of Latinx individuals smoke; the rates are highest in the Puerto Rican subgroup (28.5%), and lower in the Central and South American subgroups (20.2%), the Cuban subgroup (19.8%), and the Mexican subgroup (19.1%). Latinx men are more likely to smoke than Latinx women (16–9%, respectively) (CDC, 2017d).

A specific type of drinking behavior, binge drinking, is a serious problem in the Latinx population (Ornelas et al., 2016). In 2010, binge drinking, defined as five or more drinks per occasion for men and four or more for women, was reported by 18%, of Latinx adults, a rate higher than that for black adults (13%), but the same as that for white adults (CDC, 2012). Among the 5313 Latinx individuals in the SOL, 23% reported binge drinking in the past month and higher rates were found for younger men and were also associated with English speaking, single status, higher income, and an educational attainment of at least high school. More than 30% of Latinx adults of Mexican or Dominican heritage have reported binge drinking (Ornelas et al., 2016), and the rate of binge drinking in the past month is higher for foreign-born Latinx men (44% to 58%) than for all US men (23%) (Daniel-Ulloa et al., 2014).

Individual and Societal Factors Related to Chronic Disease

Socioeconomic and demographic factors. Socioeconomic status and demographic variables are strongly associated with chronic diseases and obesity in the Latinx population (Goldman, Kimbro, Turra, & Pebley, 2006; Sanchez-Vaznaugh, Kawachi, Subramanian, Sanchez, & Acevedo-Garcia, 2008, 2009). The relationships between education, gender, and income are well-established correlates of health status (Morales, Lara, Kington, Valdez, & Escarce, 2002; Wang & Beydoun, 2007). Evidence suggests that the socioeconomic gradient varies by immigrant versus US-born status for Latinx persons (Sanchez-Vaznaugh et al., 2009). Among women, lower socioeconomic status is strongly associated with higher BMI. Using data from National Health Interview Survey (NHIS) 1995–2007, researchers found that US-born Latinx persons were more likely to be obese than foreign-born Latinx persons. The findings also provide evidence for the moderation effect of place of birth (e.g., United States vs. foreign-born) by gender on obesity. Sanchez-Vaznaugh et al. (2008) found similar results with data from the California Health Interview Survey, with foreign-born Latinx men being more likely to be obese than Latinx women (Sanchez-Vaznaugh et al., 2008). Data from the National Latino and Asian American Survey (2002–2003) also indicate that Latinx men of all generations were more likely to be obese than Latinx women. Age is a demographic indicator associated with obesity and chronic diseases in the Latinx population. In a study of the social disparities in BMI across several adult age categories (20–39 years, 40–59 years, and older than 59 years) by gender, race/ethnicity, and socioeconomic status, researchers found that, among Latinx persons of Mexican origin, the proportion who were overweight and/or obese increased with age category (Wang & Beydoun, 2007). The Mexican American population in the SOL, older individuals were more likely to be obese than younger ones. In addition, NHANES data show that the rate of obesity was significantly higher among Mexican American women older than 50 years compared to whites and blacks (Sundquist & Winkleby, 1999).

Evidence suggests that marital status and obesity are moderated by gender and age among Mexican American adults. Younger married and widowed men are more likely to be obese than younger never-married men. The rate of obesity is higher for middle-aged and older married men than for men in all other marital status categories. For women, being married and middle-aged reduced the risk of obesity compared with single, widowed, and divorced women (Bowie, Juon, Rodriguez, & Cho, 2007).

Education, income, and household size have emerged as significant correlates of obesity in the Latinx population. For example, lower educational status and low income are associated with obesity (Sanchez-Vaznaugh et al., 2009). However, increased years of education are associated with obesity among third-generation Latinx persons and the education gradient effect on overweight and obesity is found among both white and Mexican-origin adults (Goldman et al., 2006). In the analysis of the data from the California Health Interview Survey, researchers found that, among Latinx women, rates of obesity increased dramatically for women with less than a high school education. Overall, there was a negative association between income and education and BMI; for example, the less the education and income, the higher the mean BMI in Latinx men in the sample (Sanchez-Vaznaugh et al., 2008). Despite the evidence, differences in BMI are not fully explained by individual socioeconomic status. Other factors such as lifestyle, social factors, and physical neighborhood environments may explain disparities in obesity rates in the Latinx population and, in particular, Mexican-immigrant and Mexican American subgroups (Wang & Beydoun, 2007).

Social and cultural factors. Many social and cultural factors are associated with the prevention and management of chronic diseases in the Latinx population. Cultural factors are thoughts, values, and shared group experiences that inform beliefs and behaviors. Cultural beliefs have an assigned value and evolve and endure over time. The Latinx culture in the United States serves as a template for social organization (Geertz, 1973). Social factors are related to culture and represent major characteristics of the US Latinx population. These factors are vital in addressing health disparities among Latinx individuals for several reasons. First, these factors cut across contexts and issues for Latinx persons. Second, many of these factors are salient to the unique cultural experience of Latinx individuals in the United States. Third, ignoring these factors or not acknowledging their effect on the health decisions of Latinx individuals can undermine our health promotion and disease prevention efforts (Arrellano, Elder, Sosa, Baquero, & Alcantara, 2016).

Acculturation is one of the strongest and most consistent factors associated with health outcomes for Latinx persons (Ayala et al., 2004; Cuy Castellanos, 2015). Acculturation is a proxy for a very complex process that Latinx persons experience when they migrate to the United States (Elder, Ayala, Parra-Medina, & Talavera, 2009). Other relevant factors that have emerged are perceived discrimination, experiences of racism and othering, immigration status, receiving and sending communities, collectivism, and familism (Acevedo-Garcia, Sanchez-Vaznaugh, Viruell-Fuentes, & Almeida, 2012). Next, we discuss acculturation in more detail and its association as a risk factor for obesity and many chronic diseases that affect the Latinx population.

Acculturation is defined as changes in behaviors and cultural patterns derived from continuous exposure to a dominant culture (Ayala et al., 2004; Marin & Gamba, 1996). Acculturation is a long-term and flexible process in which the individual moves among the multiple ethnic cultures continuously, and the combination of cultural and psychosocial changes penetrates every aspect of life. Latinx individuals in the United States acculturate to social norms, values, language, food, and traditions (Thomson & Hoffman-Goetz, 2009). There is ample evidence for the association of acculturation and chronic diseases (Marin & Gamba, 1996). However, less evidence exists on the mechanisms by which US cultural beliefs and practices shape health behaviors and outcomes of Latinx persons (for more discussion on acculturation See Chap. 15).

Mexican American acculturation, when measured as the preference for the English language, is associated with reduced BMI among Mexican American women. Second- and third-generation Latinx individuals were more likely to have higher BMI (Khan, Sobal, & Martorell, 1997). Data from NHANES 1988–1994 for more than 3000 Mexican American persons showed that acculturation was associated with abdominal obesity. The prevalence of obesity was higher for US-born Spanish-speaking women than for Mexican-born and US-born English-speaking women (Sundquist & Winkleby, 1999). In a study of persons of Mexican origin in Harris County, Texas, the number of years in the United States and the Bidimensional Acculturation Scale (BAS) for Hispanics (Marin & Gamba, 1996) were used as measures of acculturation to examine obesity rates. The risk of obesity was lower for Mexican-born respondents than for US-born respondents. Highly acculturated men (i.e., men with a higher BAS acculturation score [2.5 or higher]) were more likely to be obese. Mexican-immigrant women, more years in the United States was associated with higher BMI. Among women living in the US for 15 or years or longer weighed more than women who had immigrated less than 5 years previously (Ayala et al., 2004; Barcenas et al., 2007). Consistently, and regardless of the measure used for acculturation, it appears that acculturation and the behavioral changes related to immigrating to the United States are associated with obesity among Latinx individuals. Acculturation is one of the many risk factors that should be considered when addressing chronic disease in the Latinx population.

Political and economic factors. Political and economic factors are indirectly associated with chronic disease outcomes in the US Latinx population. Historical and political relationships between the United States and Latin American countries and immigration trajectories, status, and experiences influence the way Latinx persons access health services and interact with organizations and other community members. For example, Puerto Rican persons are US citizens by birth, and therefore, have most of the rights and benefits of a US citizen; however, the contrary is true for undocumented Latinx persons and their families. How Latinx individuals immigrate to the United States and where they settle can determine their political and economic capital. For example, Latinx persons who immigrate from Cuba and settle in the southeastern United States have access to strong long-standing economic influence, and social and instrumental support of the Cuban community and may not experience discrimination the same way as Mexican individuals who settle in Arizona and, despite the large Mexican community there, experience discrimination because that community has less political or economic power in that state. Latinx persons also have differential access to services and resources depending on the region of the United States in which they settle. For example, in traditional gateway states with long Latinx histories and large populations, such as New Mexico, California, and Texas, Latinx persons may access larger social networks and have access to more services and resources. The opposite may be true in new destinations and emergent states, such as Iowa, Nebraska, North Carolina, or Georgia, where Latinx populations have grown significantly since the late 1990s; these Latinx individuals were seeking better economic opportunities but found themselves with limited access to services and resources and small social networks. When chronic disease in the US Latinx population is studied and addressed, political and economic factors should be considered. Given that these factors are linked to social structures and policies that support and perpetuate health inequalities that affect Latinx individuals, these factors should be considered as part of multilevel and system-based interventions for preventing chronic diseases in Latinx populations.

Review of Relevant Conceptual/Theoretical Approaches

To address the complexity of the issues and factors related to controlling and preventing chronic diseases in the Latinx population, we must use multifactorial and multilevel approaches. We recommend the following core tenets in the development of interventions: (1) There are multiple levels of influence on health behaviors, (2) each of these levels interacts with one another to influence behaviors, and (3) health behaviors must be specified to identify the most relevant and modifiable correlates of influence. The following models and frameworks provide the conceptual and theoretical guidance to consider these tenets in the development of interventions.

Socioecological Model

One of the most commonly used models in health promotion interventions is the socioecological model, which postulates that individual-level behavior is influenced by multiple systems (Bronfenbrenner, 1981; Stoklos, Allen, & Bellingham, 1996). These systems include the macrosystem (society and laws), mesosystem (work and neighborhoods), and microsystem (family and individuals). These systems interact across the model, and the interactions influence individual-level behaviors. Thus, this model has been widely used in public health research. Although it is not specific to the Latinx population, it provides an overall view of systems and factors to consider when developing interventions to address the prevention of cancer and chronic diseases in Latinx individuals. Indeed, the socioecological model allows for the incorporation of other health behavior theories that may apply at any of the levels of influence.

Promoting Latinx Health Through Communities

In 2009, Elder and colleagues proposed a health communication model for interventions to improve health in the US Latinx population by adapting the socioecological model to incorporate the sociocultural characteristics of Latinx individuals in the United States in the framework to promote health. In this framework, the authors suggest that many of the socioeconomic and cultural factors that are related to the health of Latinx persons in this country are not easily changed or cannot be changed. Therefore, health promotion and disease prevention interventions should have a clear, effective message to individuals, their organizations, social networks, and communities. These messages go across and interact with the different levels of influence on individuals. Also, the framework incorporates the acculturation process and describes crucial factors associated with health promotion and disease prevention in the Latinx population. Furthermore, the authors suggest we consider country and culture of origin, socioeconomic and legal status, history of migration in community (mature, emerging, incipient) and acculturation, discrimination, perceived racism and othering, familism and collectivism, and gender and age issues on the channels or medium of communications, settings, sources, and messages we use for communicating with Latinx persons. Although these factors are complex, they are important to consider and we should determine their relative influence in designing interventions. In some instances, these factors may not be explicitly addressed in interventions, but they are important to recognize because they may play a role in addressing the prevention and control of cancer and chronic diseases in Latinx persons.

Cross-National Framework for Immigrant Health Research

In this framework, postulated by Acevedo-Garcia et al. (2012), a comprehensive approach to explaining immigrant health through a cross-national lens is proposed. The framework is derived from several theories on migration and immigrant health. At its core lies the belief that immigrants' health is embedded in both their sending country and their receiving community, and their experiences in both can have substantial effects on their health outcomes. This framework includes social determinants and health distributions in both the sending and the receiving countries, push-and-pull factors, health selection into migration, and life course experiences to understand health outcomes of Latinx individuals in the United States. Many of the risk or protective factors related to Latinx health can be linked to experiences or exposures from their sending countries and how Latinx persons express and process those experiences in the host society, which is often the United States. This framework extends our paradigms and offers new processes associated with Latinx health outcomes in the United States. Therefore, it is important to explain the burden of disease carried by Latinx individuals and develop strategies to address these chronic diseases (Acevedo-Garcia et al., 2012; Barnes, 2005).

Expanded Chronic Care Model

Another model that provides a multipronged approach to address the prevention and control of cancer and chronic diseases is the expanded chronic care model (ECCM). This model extends the original CCM, which was designed to address management of chronic disease at the clinic and individual levels. The CCM proposes that integrated strategies among the healthcare team and engaged and interactive patients can improve chronic disease outcomes. There is a robust body of evidence that this approach is successful at the clinic level and for individuals managing chronic diseases (Stellefson, Dipnarine, & Stopka, 2013). However, the CCM falls short in considering population health, which is the burden of chronic disease that communities and families carry. The expanded CCM incorporates concepts of population health promotion, conceptualized as improving social, economic, and environmental conditions of people's lives that support healthy lifestyles, and can increase the effectiveness of CCM by creating a continuum of prevention and care from community to clinic. This model may be helpful for the prevention and control of chronic diseases in the US Latinx population for several reasons. First, Latinx persons living with chronic diseases require intense medical and clinic care; second, the burden of disease affects not only the individual but also his or her family and communities; third, Latinx persons typically live in low-resourced communities, which increases their risk for disease. Applying this continuum of care from community prevention, improving resources for health and well-being, and integrating to clinic and ill-health management may prove most effective to prevent and control cancer and chronic diseases among Latinx individuals in the United States (Barr et al., 2003).

Community Health Worker Model

Community health workers (CHWs) are an established approach to addressing health disparities and promoting health and disease prevention in underserved communities (Rhodes, Foley, Zomea, & Bloom, 2008). CHWs are known as *promotoras,* lay health advisors, community health advisors, natural helpers, and other names, and they serve as a link between the community they belong to and the organizations and services provided to their community. In other words, CHWs are cultural and social brokers for their community (Ayala, Vaz, Earp, Elder, & Cherrington, 2010; Rhodes et al., 2008). They have been shown to be a feasible and effective strategy to address Latinx health disparities in the United States (Balcázar & de Heer, 2015; Norris et al., 2006). At its core, the CHW model works because there are community members who are naturally connected to other members of the community and who are trusted when these members seek advice, support, and aid. As cultural and language brokers, CHWs can negotiate barriers that limit Latinx persons' access to health care and serve as bridges between healthcare services and communities (Ayala et al., 2010). Over the years, the role of CHWs has expanded from health education activities to policy and community advocacy and from the delivery of healthcare services to case management and insurance broker. Reviews of the literature describing CHW roles and activities identify many of the roles that CHWs have been involved in, including promotion of healthy diet and physical activity, cancer screening, smoking cessation, cardiovascular health, management and prevention of diabetes (Rhodes, Foley, Zomea, & Bloom, 2008; Rowe et al., 2018).

Successful Research and Interventions

Successful health promotion and chronic disease prevention interventions for Latinx persons share several characteristics. First, these interventions are tailored to the geographic location where Latinx persons settle, attending to contextual, social, historical, and political influences of the region. Second, these interventions consider places where Latinx individuals live, work, and play; for example, churches, homes, community clinics, and soccer fields may play a role in the health of Latinx persons as important environments for health promotion. Third, these interventions apply extensive health communication strategies to reach and communicate health messages to the Latinx population. These communication strategies range from using the *promotora* (CHW) model to face-to-face interactions to emerging media (i.e., social media). Evidence from these interventions suggests that combining communication-related intervention approaches with the use of *promotoras* is an effective and viable strategy (Arrellano et al., 2016). The *promotora* model appears to be more successful than the other communication strategies, although the Latinx-targeted print materials were by far the most cost-effective (Ayala et al., 2010; Elder et al., 2009; Rhodes et al., 2008). Interventions developed for mature markets, or communities with a longer history of Latinx immigration, are not necessarily transferable to Latinx populations in other markets with more recent migration (Elder et al., 2009).

Reviews of the literature demonstrate acceptable levels of obesity-related improvements in the most recent studies. The interventions that were the most successful were implemented in healthcare settings, community centers, homes, and churches by a variety of groups, such as healthcare professionals, *promotoras*, and dietitians (Perez et al., 2013). Interventions that use the socioecological model to address interventions for the prevention and control of chronic diseases and obesity in the Latinx population are costly and complex to implement. However, tailoring interventions to Latinx individuals by involving bilingual/bicultural professionals, social support networks, key locations for participant recruitment, and intervention implementation, and actively engaging in a participatory research process are ways to increase the effectiveness of the intervention.

A Su Salud program successfully used mass media and emerging channels for cancer prevention and promotion of behavioral risk reduction (Ramirez & McAlister, 1988). Similar approaches were used to promote smoking cessation among Latinx persons (McAlister et al., 1992). Another example of a successful intervention to address cardiovascular risk is *Un Corazon Saludable: A Healthy Heart* (Harralson et al., 2007). The intervention addressed important risk factors such as BMI, abdominal fat, and blood pressure, in addition to depressive symptoms and perceived social support. The intervention was delivered in Latinx-owned places and Latinx neighborhoods.

Y Living was a culturally relevant family-based healthy lifestyle program designed collaboratively by the YMCA of greater San Antonio and researchers using a participatory planning and implementation process. The group-based education and physical activity sessions were delivered by trained bilingual/bicultural YMCA staff to families residing in high-risk San Antonio urban neighborhoods that were financially disadvantaged. Families received text messages aligned with the intervention program to reinforce key health education concepts, provide program reminders, and promote community events. Significant improvements in weight-related measures were found for adult participants (Parra-Medina, Liang, Yin, Esparza, & Lopez, 2015).

Vida Sana Hoy y Mañana was conducted in the southeastern United States, an emerging region for Latinx populations, and was successful at promoting and increasing fruit and vegetable intake to prevent cancer. Researchers worked with Latinx-owned small food stores (*tiendas*) to implement all activities, which were all conducted in Spanish and in the stores to reach Latinx customers (Ayala, Baquero, Laraia, Ji, & Linnan, 2013). In traditional destinations for Latinx persons such as Texas, we find successful interventions to promote behavioral risk factors, such as diet and physical activity. *Mi Casa, Mi Salud*, and *Pasos Adelante* were successful at improving health behaviors (diet and physical activity) and body composition markers. These interventions involved the use of evidence-based recommendations from the CDC Task Force on Community Preventive Services and trained *promotoras* to deliver the intervention (de Heer et al., 2015; Staten et al., 2012). An example of a promising intervention to address the high rates of diabetes among Latinx persons is a yearlong intervention in Texas as part of the Starr County Border Health Initiative. This effort included *promotoras*, a nurse case manager, and a research dietitian as part of the intervention team. *Promotoras* were the primary contact and conduit of the intervention activities and worked with the health professionals to deliver the educational sessions (Lucio et al., 2012).

Identifying Research and Intervention Needs and Priorities

Addressing disparities in chronic diseases in the Latinx population will take innovative approaches and long-term investment and engagement of many public health stakeholders, community leaders and organizations, and government agencies, as well as Latinx individuals and their families. At stake are the health and well-being of generations of individuals and communities. This challenge poses many opportunities and obstacles. Public health research and practice can contribute to solving some of these obstacles and provide effective and sustainable solutions and strategies. The continuance of research to address these challenges is crucial. We propose that research focuses first on theory development and model testing that adequately incorporates an evidence-based, theory-based hypothesis and well-defined constructs that capture the experiences of Latinx persons. These constructs and models should be primarily based on historical, cultural, and socioeconomic experiences of Latinx persons and abandon attempts to adapt or interpret Latinx health behaviors based on theories and models developed from a white dominant perspective. We described several models in this chapter that incorporate these experiences and factors and draw from a broader and deeper array of behavior and social sciences, such as policy, immigration, sociology, and anthropology.

Second, to truly and permanently address the root causes of health disparities, public health researchers must collaborate with researchers in other disciplines and areas of expertise to focus on advancing health equity, contributing to social justice efforts, and engaging in community-based participatory research. If we do not combine our effective health behavior interventions with larger social and structural efforts to mitigate and eliminate the root causes of these disparities, our public health efforts will fall short and provide only short-term benefit. Smoking cessation, active lifestyles, and healthy diets cut across the various chronic diseases, and improving these factors in the Latinx population can help prevent the incidence of new cases of chronic diseases and alleviate the burden of disease among people for whom the burden is disproportionate.

Third, intervention research should consider innovative channels of communication and strategies that can reach the heterogeneity of the Latinx community in the United States. As we demonstrated in this chapter, not all Latinx individuals experience chronic diseases in the same way. Multiple factors have an impact on their health outcomes and interaction with the US public health and healthcare system. For example, Latinx health experiences are influenced by the receiving and sending communities. Latinx individuals who have been well established in their communities for several generations will face very different challenges, have access to very different resources, and therefore experience different accesses to health care than recent immigrants.

Fourth and lastly, we submit that researchers and practitioners invested in addressing health disparities in cancer and chronic diseases in the Latinx population study the issues through a transnational lens. Individual behaviors reflect previous and present experiences, and these experiences will consist of immigrant experiences in their sending and receiving regions. Increased access to social media and the Internet also holds underexplored potential to reach Latinx populations across regional boundaries and enhances access to family, traditions, and services. The unique experiences of Latinx individuals and their relationship with health outcomes do not come from only their country of origin or years in the United States, but from the accumulation of all these experiences.

Health promotion is the process of enabling people to increase control over, and to improve, their health. It moves beyond a focus on individual behavior toward a wide range of social and environmental interventions. Health promotion represents a comprehensive social and political process, embracing not only actions directed at strengthening the skills and empowering the capabilities of individuals but also actions directed toward changing social, environmental, and economic conditions, so as to alleviate their impact on public and individual health. Participation is essential to sustain health promotion action. To make "the healthy choice the easy choice," as the axiom goes, it is necessary to provide readily available, accessible, and appealing health programs. However, an appropriate health program or message for Latinx populations in the United States cannot be the same from one community to the next, or even similar to those aimed at the general population. In this regard, health promotion efforts to improve chronic disease cannot be exactly replicated across communities, and the barriers to healthy practices facing people living in their communities must be addressed.

Reaching Latinx communities remains a challenge. Many programs use a one-size-fits-all approach across communities that, in practice, fits none. Community-based participatory approaches offer an opportunity to respond to the community's needs and have been shown to successfully design and implement culturally appropriate programs and interventions that meet the needs and concerns of specific communities.

Public health researchers and community members can combine their knowledge and assets to work together as colleagues on the development of relevant programs and policies. Community involvement leverages community members' diverse skills, knowledge, and expertise that can lead to enhanced and more trusting communication and relationships between public health and community partners; more culturally appropriate interventions; greater community interest and support; and ideally, more sustainable strategies for improved health and well-being.

References

Acevedo-Garcia, D., Sanchez-Vaznaugh, E. V., Viruell-Fuentes, E. A., & Almeida, J. (2012). Integrating social epidemiology into immigrant health research: A cross-national framework. *Social Science and Medicine, 75*(12), 2060. https://doi.org/10.1016/j.socscimed.2012.04.040.

Akinbami, L. (2010). *Asthma prevalence, health care use and mortality: United States, 2003–05.* Atlanta, GA: CDC. http://www.cdc.gov/nchs/data/hestat/asthma03-05/asthma03-05.htm.

American Cancer Society. (2015). *Cancer facts & figures for Hispanics/Latinos 2015–2017.* Atlanta, GA: American Cancer Society.

American Cancer Society. (2016a). *Cancer facts & figures 2016.* Atlanta, GA: American Cancer Society.

American Cancer Society. (2016b). *Liver cancer.* Atlanta, GA: American Cancer Society.

American Diabetes Association. (2014). *Diabetes among Hispanics: All are not equal.* Alexandria, Virginia: American Diabetes Association.

American Stroke Association. (2012). *Stroke among Hispanics.* Dallas, TX: American Stroke Association. http://www.strokeassociation.org/STROKEORG/AboutStroke/UnderstandingRisk/Stroke-Among-Hispanics_UCM_310393_Article.jsp-.WAAAyXqH-Sw.

Arredondo, E. M., Sotres-Alvarez, D., Stoutenberg, M., Davis, S. M., Crespo, N. C., Carnethon, M. R., ... Evenson, K. R. (2015). Physical activity levels in U.S. Latino/Hispanic adults: Results from the Hispanic community health study/study of Latinos. *American Journal of Preventive Medicine, 50*(4), 500–508. https://doi.org/10.1016/j.amepre.2015.08.029.

Arrellano, L., Elder, J., Sosa, E., Baquero, B., & Alcantara, C. (2016). Health promotion among Latino adults: Conceptual frameworks, relevant pathways and future directions. *Journal of Latina/o Psychology, 4*(2), 83–87. https://doi.org/10.1037/lat0000051.

Ayala, G. X., Baquero, B., Laraia, B. A., Ji, M., & Linnan, L. (2013). Efficacy of a store-based environmental change intervention compared with a delayed treatment control condition on store customers' intake of fruits and vegetables. *Public Health Nutrition,* 1. https://doi.org/10.1017/s1368980013000955.

Ayala, G. X., Elder, J. P., Campbell, N. R., Slymen, D. J., Roy, N., Engelberg, M., et al. (2004). Correlates of body mass index and waist-to-hip ratio among Mexican women in the United States: Implications for intervention development. *Women's Health Issues, 14*(5), 155. https://doi.org/10.1016/j.whi.2004.07.003.

Ayala, G. X., Vaz, L., Earp, J. A., Elder, J. P., & Cherrington, A. (2010). Outcome effectiveness of the lay health advisor model among Latinos in the United States: An examination by role. *Health Education Research, 25*(5), 815. https://doi.org/10.1093/her/cyq035.

Balcázar, H. G., & de Heer, H. D. (2015). Community health workers as partners in the management of non-communicable diseases. *The Lancet Global Health, 3*(9), e508–e509. https://doi.org/10.1016/S2214-109X(15)00142-4.

Balfour, P. C., Ruiz, J. M., Talavera, G. A., Allison, M. A., & Rodriguez, C. J. (2016). Cardiovascular disease in Hispanics/Latinos in the United States. *Journal of Latina/o Psychology, 4*(2), 98–113. https://doi.org/10.1037/lat0000056.

Barcenas, C. H., Wilkinson, A. V., Strom, S. S., Cao, Y., Saunders, K. C., Mahabir, S., et al. (2007). Birthplace, years of residence in the United States, and obesity among Mexican-American adults. *Obesity, 15*(4), 1043–1052. https://doi.org/10.1038/oby.2007.537.

Barnes, N. (2005). *Transnational networks and community-based organizations: The dynamics of AIDS activism in Tijuana and Mexico City*. (3167838 Ph.D.), University of California, San Diego, Ann Arbor. ProQuest Dissertations & Theses A&I; ProQuest Dissertations & Theses Full Text database.

Barr, R. G., Avilés-Santa, L., Davis, S. M., Aldrich, T. K., Gonzalez, F., Henderson, A. G., ... Loredo, J. S. (2016). Pulmonary disease and age at immigration among Hispanics. Results from the Hispanic community health study/study of Latinos. *American Journal of Respiratory and Critical Care Medicine, 193*(4), 386–395.

Barr, V. J., Robinson, S., Marin-Link, B., Underhill, L., Dotts, A., Ravensdale, D., & Salivaras, S. (2003). The expanded Chronic Care Model: An integration of concepts and strategies from population health promotion and the Chronic Care Model. *Healthcare Quarterly, 7*(1).

Bauer, U. E., Briss, P. A., Goodman, R. A., & Bowman, B. A. (2014). Prevention of chronic disease in the 21st century: Elimination of the leading preventable causes of premature death and disability in the USA. *The Lancet, 384*(9937), 45–52.

Bowie, J. V., Juon, H.-S., Rodriguez, E. M., & Cho, J. (2007). Peer reviewed: Factors associated with overweight and obesity among Mexican Americans and Central Americans: Results from the 2001 California Health Interview Survey. *Preventing Chronic Disease, 4*(1).

Brehm, J. M., & Celedón, J. C. (2008). Chronic obstructive pulmonary disease in Hispanics. *American Journal of Respiratory and Critical Care Medicine, 177*.

Bronfenbrenner, U. (1981). Children and families: 1984? *Society, 18*(2), 38–41.

Carrion, A. F., Ghanta, R., Carrasquillo, O., & Martin, P. (2011). Chronic liver disease in the Hispanic population of the United States. *Clinical Gastroenterology and Hepatology, 9*(10), 834–853.

Centers for Disease Control and Prevention. (2011). *CDC health disparities and inequalities report—United States, 2011*. Atlanta, GA: Centers for Disease Control and Prevention.

Centers for Disease Control and Prevention. (2012). Vital signs: Binge drinking prevalence, frequency, and intensity among adults-United States, 2010. *Morbidity and Mortality Weekly Report, 61*(1), 14.

Centers for Disease Control and Prevention. (2015a). About heart disease. https://www.cdc.gov/heartdisease/about.htm.

Centers for Disease Control and Prevention. (2015b). *CDC vital signs—Hispanic health*. http://www.cdc.gov/vitalsigns/hispanic-health/.

Centers for Disease Control and Prevention. (2016a). *Chronic diseases: The leading causes of death and disability in the United States*. http://www.cdc.gov/chronicdisease/overview/.

Centers for Disease Control and Prevention. (2016b). *Liver cancer*. Atlanta, GA: Centers for Disease Control and Prevention.

Centers for Disease Control and Prevention. (2016c). *Lung cancer rates by race and ethnicity*. Atlanta, GA: Centers for Disease Control and Prevention. http://www.cdc.gov/cancer/lung/statistics/race.htm.

Centers for Disease Control and Prevention. (2016d). *Men and heart disease fact sheet*. Atlanta, GA: Centers for Disease Control and Prevention.

Centers for Disease Control and Prevention. (2017a). *Adult obesity facts*. Atlanta, GA: Centers for Disease Control and Prevention. https://www.cdc.gov/obesity/data/adult.html.

Centers for Disease Control and Prevention. (2017b). *Cancers Associated with Overweigth and Obesity Make up 40 percent of Cancers Diagnosed in the United States*. Retrieved from https://www.cdc.gov/media/releases/2017/p1003-vs-cancer-obesity.html.

Centers for Disease Control and Prevention. (2017c). Facts about physical activity|Physical Activity|CDC. *Physical Activity*. https://www.cdc.gov/physicalactivity/data/facts.htm.

Centers for Disease Control and Prevention. (2017d). Hispanics/Latinos and tobacco use. Retrieved from https://www.cdc.gov/tobacco/disparities/hispanics-latinos/index.htm.

Centers for Disease Control and Prevention. (2017e). How much physical activity do adults need?|Physical Activity|CDC. *Physical Activity.* https://www.cdc.gov/physicalactivity/basics/adults/index.htm.

Centers for Disease Control and Prevention. (2017f). *Overweight and obesity.* https://www.cdc.gov/obesity.

Corsino, L., Sotres-Alvarez, D., Butera, N. M., Siega-Riz, A. M., Palacios, C., Pérez, C. M., et al. (2017). Association of the DASH dietary pattern with insulin resistance and diabetes in US Hispanic/Latino adults: Results from the Hispanic Community Health Study/Study of Latinos (HCHS/SOL). *BMJ Open Diabetes Research and Care, 5*(1), e000402.

Cuy Castellanos, D. (2015). Dietary acculturation in Latinos/Hispanics in the United States. *American Journal of Lifestyle Medicine, 9*(1), 31–36. https://doi.org/10.1177/1559827614552960.

Daniel-Ulloa, J., Reboussin, B. A., Gilbert, P. A., Mann, L., Alonzo, J., Downs, M., et al. (2014). Predictors of heavy episodic drinking and weekly drunkenness among immigrant Latinos in North Carolina. *American Journal of Men's Health, 8*(4), 339–348.

Daviglus, M. L., Talavera, G. A., Avilés-Santa, M., et al. (2012). Prevalence of major cardiovascular risk factors and cardiovascular diseases among Hispanic/Latino individuals of diverse backgrounds in the United States. *Journal of the American Medical Association, 308*(17), 1775–1784. https://doi.org/10.1001/jama.2012.14517.

de Heer, H. D., Balcazar, H. G., Wise, S., Redelfs, A. H., Rosenthal, E. L., & Duarte, M. O. (2015). Improved cardiovascular risk among Hispanic border participants of the Mi Corazón Mi Comunidad Promotores De Salud Model: The HEART II cohort intervention study 2009–2013. *Frontiers in Public Health, 3.*

Dunn, R. A., Sharkey, J. R., & Horel, S. (2012). The effect of fast-food availability on fast-food consumption and obesity among rural residents: An analysis by race/ethnicity. *Economics & Human Biology, 10*(1), 1–13. https://doi.org/10.1016/j.ehb.2011.09.005.

Elder, J. P., Ayala, G. X., Parra-Medina, D., & Talavera, G. A. (2009). Health communication in the Latino community: Issues and approaches. *Annual Review of Public Health, 30,* 227. https://doi.org/10.1146/annurev.publhealth.031308.100300.

Fryer, C. D., & Ervin, R. B. (2013). *Caloric intake from fast food among adults: United States 2007–2010.* https://www.cdc.gov/nchs/products/databriefs/db114.htm.

Geertz, C. (1973). *The interpretation of cultures* (Vol. 5019): Basic Books.

Go, A. S., Mozaffarian, D., Roger, V. L., Benjamin, E. J., Berry, J. D., Borden, W. B., … Turner, M. B. (2013). Hispanics/Latinos & Cardiovascular Diseases: American Heart Association.

Goldman, N., Kimbro, R. T., Turra, C. M., & Pebley, A. R. (2006). Socioeconomic gradients in health for white and Mexican-origin populations. *American Journal of Public Health, 96*(12), 2186–2193. https://doi.org/10.2105/ajph.2005.062752.

Harralson, T. L., Emig, J. C., Polansky, M., Walker, R. E., Cruz, J. O., & Garcia-Leeds, C. (2007). Un Corazon Saludable: Factors influencing outcomes of an exercise program designed to impact cardiac and metabolic risks among urban Latinas. *Journal of Community Health, 32*(6), 401. https://doi.org/10.1007/s10900-007-9059-3.

Heron, M. (2016). Deaths: Leading Causes for 2014. *National Vital Statistics Reports, 65,* 1–95. https://www.cdc.gov/nchs/data/nvsr/nvsr65/nvsr65_05.pdf.

Isasi, C. R., Ayala, G. X., Sotres-Alvarez, D., Madanat, H., Penedo, F., Loria, C. M., … Siega-Riz, A. M. (2015). Is acculturation related to obesity in Hispanic/Latino adults? Results from the Hispanic community health study/study of Latinos. *Journal of Obesity.*

Kant, A. K., Whitley, M. I., & Graubard, B. I. (2015). Away from home meals: associations with biomarkers of chronic disease and dietary intake in American adults, NHANES 2005–2010. *International Journal of Obesity, 39*(5), 820–827. https://doi.org/10.1038/ijo.2014.183.

Khan, L., Sobal, J., & Martorell, R. (1997). Acculturation, socioeconomic status, and obesity in Mexican Americans, Cuban Americans, and Puerto Ricans. *International Journal of Obesity & Related Metabolic Disorders, 21*(2).

Larsen, B. A., Pekmezi, D., Marquez, B., Benitez, T. J., & Marcus, B. H. (2013). Physical activity in Latinas: Social and environmental influences. *Women's Health (London, England), 9*(2). https://doi.org/10.2217/whe.2213.2219. https://doi.org/10.2217/whe.13.9.

Lee, S. H., & Im, E.-O. (2010). Ethnic differences in exercise and leisure time physical activity among midlife women. *Journal of Advanced Nursing, 66*(4), 814–827. https://doi.org/10.1111/j.1365-2648.2009.05242.x.

Lucio, R., Zuniga, G., Seol, Y., Garza, N., Mier, N., & Trevino, L. (2012). Incoporating what *promotoras* learn: Becoming role models to effect positive change. *Journal of Community Health, 37*(5), 1026–1031. https://doi.org/10.1007/s10900-011-9526-8.

Marin, G., & Gamba, R. J. (1996). A new measurement of acculturation for Hispanics: The Bidimensional Acculturation Scale for Hispanics (BAS). *Hispanic Journal of Behavioral Sciences, 18*(3), 297. https://doi.org/10.1177/07399863960183002.

McAlister, A. L., Ramirez, A. G., Amezcua, C., Pulley, L., Stern, M. P., & Mercado, S. (1992). Smoking cessation in Texas-Mexico border communities: A quasi-experimental panel study. *American Journal of Health Promotion, 6*(4), 274–279.

Medina-Inojosa, J., Jean, N., Cortes-Bergoderi, M., & Lopez-Jimenez, F. (2014). The Hispanic paradox in cardiovascular disease and total mortality. *Progress in Cardiovascular Diseases, 57*(3), 286–292.

Morales, L. S., Lara, M., Kington, R. S., Valdez, R. O., & Escarce, J. J. (2002). Socioeconomic, cultural, and behavioral factors affecting Hispanic health outcomes. *Journal of Health Care for the Poor and Underserved, 13*(4), 477.

Mozaffarian, D., Benjamin E. J., Go, A. S., Arnett, D. K. Blaha, M. J., Cushman M., ... Turner, M. B. (2016). Heart disease and stroke statistics–2016 update: a report from the American Heart Association. *Circulation, 133*(4), e38–e360.

National Cancer Institute. (2017). Obesity and cancer. https://www.cancer.gov/about-cancer/causes-prevention/risk/obesity/obesity-fact-sheet.

National Heart, Lung, & Blood Institute. (1998). *Clinical guidelines on the identification, evaluation, and treatment of overweight and obesity in adults–the evidence report*. (98-4083). Washington, DC: U.S Department of Health and Human Services. https://www.nhlbi.nih.gov/files/docs/guidelines/obesity_guidelines_archive.pdf.

National Heart, Lung, & Blood Institute. (2017). What is COPD? https://www.nhlbi.nih.gov/health/health-topics/topics/copd/.

National Institute of Diabetes and Digestive and Kidney Diseases. (2016). What is diabetes? https://www.niddk.nih.gov/health-information/diabetes/overview/what-is-diabetes.

Norris, S. L., Chowdhury, F. M., Van Le, K., Horsley, T., Brownstein, J. N., Zhang, X., et al. (2006). Effectiveness of community health workers in the care of persons with diabetes. *Diabetic Medicine, 23*(5), 544–556.

Office of Minority Health. (2016a). *Asthma and Hispanic Americans*. http://minorityhealth.hhs.gov/omh/browse.aspx?lvl=4&lvlid=60.

Office of Minority Health. (2016b). *Diabetes and Hispanic Americans*. http://minorityhealth.hhs.gov/omh/browse.aspx?lvl=4&lvlID=63.

Office of Minority Health. (2016c). *Heart Disease and Hispanic Americans*. http://minorityhealth.hhs.gov/omh/browse.aspx?lvl=4&lvlID=64.

Ornelas, I. J., Lapham, G. T., Salgado, H., Williams, E. C., Gotman, N., Womack, V., et al. (2016). Binge drinking and perceived ethnic discrimination among Hispanics/Latinos: Results from the Hispanic community health study/study of Latinos sociocultural ancillary study. *Journal of Ethnicity in Substance Abuse, 15*(3), 223–239. https://doi.org/10.1080/15332640.2015.1024374.

Palta, P., McMurray, R. G., Gouskova, N. A., Sotres-Alvarez, D., Davis, S. M., Carnethon, M., et al. (2016). Self-reported and accelerometer-measured physical activity by body mass index in US Hispanic/Latino adults: HCHS/SOL. *Preventive Medicine Reports, 2*, 824–828. https://doi.org/10.1016/j.pmedr.2015.09.006.

Parra-Medina, D., Liang, Y., Yin, Z., Esparza, L., & Lopez, L. (2015). Weight outcomes of Latino adults and children participating in the Y Living Program, a family-focused lifestyle intervention,

San Antonio, 2012–2013. *Preventing Chronic Disease, 12,* E219. https://doi.org/10.5888/pcd12.150219.

Penedo, F., Yanez, B., Castañeda, S., Gallo, L., Wortman, K., Gouskova, N., ... Ramirez, A. (2016). Self-reported cancer prevalence among Hispanics in the US: Results from the Hispanic Community Health Study/Study of Latinos. *PLoS One, 11*(1).

Perez, L. G., Arredondo, E. M., Elder, J. P., Barquera, S., Nagle, B., & Holub, C. K. (2013). Evidence-based obesity treatment interventions for Latino adults in the U.S.: A systematic review. *American Journal of Preventive Medicine, 44*(5), 550. https://doi.org/10.1016/j.amepre.2013.01.016.

Pinheiro, P. S., Callahan, K. E., Siegel, R. L., Jin, H., Morris, C. R., Trapido, E. J., et al. (2017). Cancer mortality in Hispanic ethnic groups. *Cancer Epidemiology and Prevention Biomarkers, 26*(3), 376–382.

Ramirez, A. G., & McAlister, A. L. (1988). Mass media campaign—A su salud. *Preventive Medicine, 17*(5), 608–621.

Rhodes, S. D., Foley, K. L., Zomea, C. S., & Bloom, F. R. (2008). Lay health advisor interventions among Hispanics/Latinos: A qualitative systematic review. *American Journal of Preventive Medicine, 33*(6), 418.

Rosser, F. J., Forno, E., Cooper, P. J., & Celedón, J. C. (2014). Asthma in Hispanics. An 8-year update. *American Journal of Respiratory and Critical Care Medicine, 189*(11), 1316–1327.

Rowe, A. K., Rowe, S. Y., Peters, D. H., Holloway, K. A., Chalker, J., & Ross-Degnan, D. (2018). Effectiveness of strategies to improve health-care provider practices in low-income and middle-income countries: a systematic review. *The Lancet Global Health*.

Sanchez-Vaznaugh, E. V., Kawachi, I., Subramanian, S. V., Sanchez, B. N., & Acevedo-Garcia, D. (2008). Differential effect of birthplace and length of residence on body mass index (BMI) by education, gender and race/ethnicity. *Social Science and Medicine, 67*(8), 1300–1310. https://doi.org/10.1016/j.socscimed.2008.06.015.

Sanchez-Vaznaugh, E. V., Kawachi, I., Subramanian, S. V., Sanchez, B. N., & Acevedo-Garcia, D. (2009). Do socioeconomic gradients in body mass index vary by race/ethnicity, gender, and birthplace? *American Journal of Epidemiology, 169*(9), 1102–1112. https://doi.org/10.1093/aje/kwp027.

Schneiderman, N., Llabre, M., Cowie, C. C., Barnhart, J., Carnethon, M., Gallo, L. C., et al. (2014). Prevalence of diabetes among Hispanics/Latinos from diverse backgrounds: The Hispanic Community Health Study/Study of Latinos (HCHS/SOL). *Diabetes Care, 37*(8), 2233.

Siega-Riz, A. M., Sotres-Alvarez, D., Ayala, G. X., Ginsberg, M., Himes, J. H., Liu, K., ... & Gellman, M. D. (2014). Food-group and nutrient-density intakes by Hispanic and Latino backgrounds in the Hispanic Community Health Study/Study of Latinos. https://doi.org/10.3945/ajcn.113.082685.

Siegel, R. L., Fedewa, S. A., Miller, K. D., Goding-Sauer, A., Pinheiro, P. S., Martinez-Tyson, D., et al. (2015). Cancer statistics for Hispanics/Latinos, 2015. *Cancer Journal for Clinicians, 65*(6), 457–480.

Staten, L. K., Cutshaw, C. A., Davidson, C., Reinschmidt, K., Stewart, R., & Roe, D. J. (2012). Effectiveness of the Pasos Adelante chronic disease prevention and control program in a US-Mexico border community, 2005–2008. *Preventing Chronic Disease, 9,* E08.

Stellefson, M., Dipnarine, K., & Stopka, C. (2013). Peer reviewed: The chronic care model and diabetes management in US primary care settings: A systematic review. *Preventing Chronic Disease, 10*.

Stern, M., Fejerman, L., Das, R., Setiawan, V., Cruz-Correa, M., Perez-Stable, E., et al. (2016). Variability in cancer risk and outcomes within US Latinos by national origin and genetic ancestry. *Current Epidemiology Reports, 3,* 181–190.

Stoklos, D., Allen, J., & Bellingham, R. (1996). The social ecology of health promotion; Implications for research and practice. *American Journal of Health Promotion, 10*(4), 247–251.

Sundquist, J., & Winkleby, M. A. (1999). Cardiovascular risk factors in Mexican American adults: A transcultural analysis of NHANES III, 1988–1994. *American Journal of Public Health, 89*(5), 723–730.

Thomson, M. D., & Hoffman-Goetz, L. (2009). Defining and measuring acculturation: A systematic review of public health studies with Hispanic populations in the United States. *Social Science and Medicine, 69*(7), 983–991. https://doi.org/10.1016/j.socscimed.2009.05.011.

Trust for America's Health, & Robert Wood Johnson Foundation. (2014). *The state of obesity: Racial and ethnic disparities in obesity.* https://stateofobesity.org/disparities/latinos/.

Wang, Y., & Beydoun, M. A. (2007). The obesity epidemic in the United States–gender, age, socioeconomic, racial/ethnic, and geographic characteristics: A systematic review and meta-regression analysis. *Epidemioogicl Reviews, 29,* 6–28. https://doi.org/10.1093/epirev/mxm007.

Chapter 3
Mental Health Issues Within Latinx Populations: Evaluating the State of the Field

Esther J. Calzada, Lauren E. Gulbas, Carolina Hausmann-Stabile, Su Yeong Kim and Jodi Berger Cardoso

Abstract Despite chronic exposure to social stressors that are known to undermine health, the Latinx population within the USA is healthier than the non-Latinx White population on most indicators of mental health. However, Latinx children and youth who were born and/or raised in the USA amid a culture of anti-immigrant sentiment, racial/ethnic discrimination, and socioeconomic disadvantage are in a context that increases the risk for depression and maladaptive behaviors. In this chapter, we examine mental health within the Latinx population by summarizing extant epidemiologic data and highlighting theoretical models that are applied to the study of Latinx mental health. We also explore how culture shapes mental health outcomes and mental health disparities related to national origin and immigrant status. We conclude with a discussion of a key mental health issue, adolescent depression, through a systems dynamics approach to illustrate potential future directions.

Keywords Latinx adults · Latinx children and adolescents · Culture · Mental health epidemiology · Systems dynamics theory

Mental health disorders represent one of the costliest public health problems worldwide and in the USA. An estimated one in two adults in the USA will experience a mental health disorder in their lifetime, and nearly one in four experience problems at any given point in time (Reeves et al., 2011). Risk for mental health problems may be even higher in minority groups such as the Latinx population, who are disproportionately affected by environmental stressors that, according to social determinants

---

E. J. Calzada (✉) · L. E. Gulbas
Steve Hicks School of Social Work, University of Texas-Austin, Austin, TX, USA
e-mail: esther.calzada@austin.utexas.edu

S. Y. Kim
Department of Human Development and Family Sciences, University of Texas-Austin, Austin, TX, USA

C. Hausmann-Stabile
Graduate School of Social Work and Social Research, Bryn Mawr College, Bryn Mawr, PA, USA

J. Berger Cardoso
University of Houston, Houston, TX, USA

© Springer Nature Switzerland AG 2020
A. D. Martínez and S. D. Rhodes (eds.), *New and Emerging Issues in Latinx Health*, https://doi.org/10.1007/978-3-030-24043-1_3

of health theory, undermining well-being (Marmot, 2005). Additionally, striking and persistent disparities exist in access to mental health services, resulting in limited opportunities for treatment that could decrease impairment and improve quality of life among Latinx persons affected by mental illness (Alegría et al., 2002; Wang et al., 2005). In light of these findings, minority health and mental health disparities are now emphasized in the strategic plans of multiple Institutes of the National Institute of Health (NIH). Furthermore, the National Institute on Minority Health and Health Disparities was established as an NIH Center in 2000 to lead research to improve minority health and reduce health disparities.

In the USA, the Latinx population has grown 43% within the past decade, currently numbers about 57 million, and continues to grow (more than 17% of the general population) (Passel, Cohn, & Lopez, 2011). This chapter examines mental health within the US Latinx population by summarizing the extant epidemiologic literature and highlighting current theoretical models that may be applied to the study of Latinx mental health through a cultural lens. Because mental health is invariably affected by differences related to national origin and immigrant status (Arellano-Morales, Elder, Sosa, Baquero, & Alcántara, 2016), we direct attention to the immigrant paradox and how culture, broadly speaking, shapes mental health outcomes. We conclude with an in-depth discussion of a key mental health issue, adolescent depression, as an illustrative case for potential future directions.

Mental Health Within the Latinx Population

Research in mental health disparities began in earnest in the 1980s, when the first psychiatric epidemiologic study that included Latinx persons, the Epidemiological Catchment Area Study, was conducted (Regier et al., 1988). Since then, a number of regional or national studies on mental health, about half with adults and half with children and youth, have been conducted with Latinx participants (see Table 3.1 for 20 highlighted studies). For the most part, these studies have focused on the more common disorders (i.e., anxiety, mood, and substance use) to examine (a) prevalence rates based on a widely used psychiatric diagnostic system (i.e., the Diagnostic and Statistical Manual of Mental Disorders [DSM]) (American Psychiatric Association, 2000); (b) mental health functioning using behavior rating scales; and (c) engagement in risk behaviors that are indicative of mental health problems. Of the highlighted studies, 14 (70%) have been interethnic studies that allow for comparisons among subgroups to inform knowledge of racial/ethnic mental health disparities. The remaining six studies have focused on Mexican American adults (two studies), Mexican American children (one study), Puerto Rican adults (two studies), and Puerto Rican children (one study), facilitating an examination of variations within a specific Latinx subgroup to inform cultural theories of mental health.

Overall, this body of research has greatly advanced the field of Latinx mental health in significant ways. However, this research has relied almost exclusively on Westernized conceptualizations of psychopathology that ignore cultural variations

3 Mental Health Issues Within Latinx Populations: Evaluating ...

Table 3.1 Landmark epidemiological studies including Latinx participants (adult and pediatric samples)

Study	Years	Design[a]	Sample size	Percentage of Latinx participants	Main goal
Adults (18 years or older)					
Epidemiological Catchment Area	1980–1985	2[b]	$N = 18,571$	7.8%	Assess the prevalence and incidence of mental disorders (DSM III criteria), and on the use of and need for services by the mentally ill
Mexican American Prevalence and Service Survey	1980s	1	$N = 3012$	100% (Mexican American)	Assess the prevalence of mental health disorders (DSM-III-R criteria)
South Florida Refugee Study	1980s	1	$N = 952$	47% (Cuban)	Assess the prevalence of mental health symptoms and functioning
Hispanic Health and Nutrition Examination Survey	1982–1984	1	$N = 3118$	100% (Mexican American)	Assess the presence and one-week persistence of depressive symptoms
Healthcare for Communities Study	1996–1997	2[b]	$N = 9585$	6%	Examine ethnic group differences in unmet need for alcoholism, drug abuse, and mental health treatment
National Epidemiological Survey of Alcohol and Related Conditions	2001–2006	2[b]	$N = 43,093$ $N = 34,653$	Not reported	Assess the 12-month and lifetime prevalence, correlates, and comorbidity of major depressive disorder (DSM-IV criteria)

(continued)

Table 3.1 (continued)

Study	Years	Design[a]	Sample size	Percentage of Latinx participants	Main goal
National Latino and Asian American Study	2002–2003	1	$N = 4649$	55% (Mexican origin: 19%; Cuban: 12%; Puerto Rican: 10%; Other Latinx: 13%)	Assess the prevalence of mental health disorders and rates of mental health service utilization by Latinx and Asian individuals
Need Assessment Study of Mental Health and Substance Use Disorders and Service Utilization among Adult Population of Puerto Rico	2014–2016	1	$N = 3062$	100% (Puerto Rican)	Assess the prevalence rates of serious mental health and substance use disorders, service utilization, and barriers to treatment
Adults and children					
Puerto Rico Epidemiological Catchment Area Study	1984	1	$N = 1513$	100% (Puerto Rican)	Assess the six-month and lifetime prevalence rates of several mental health disorders (DSM III criteria) among participants between the ages of 17 and 74
National Surveys on Drug Use and Health	Annually since 1988	1	Varies by year: in 2001–2003 $N = 134,875$	Varies by year; includes Mexican Americans and Mexican immigrants, Puerto Rican, Central or South American, and other Hispanic/Latinx	Describe national and state-level data on the use of tobacco, alcohol, illicit drugs (including non-medical use of prescription drugs) and mental health of individuals 12 years of age and older

(continued)

Table 3.1 (continued)

Study	Years	Design[a]	Sample size	Percentage of Latinx participants	Main goal
National Comorbidity Study; National Comorbidity Survey Replication Study	1990–1992; 2001–2002	2[b]	N = 8098	9.7%	Assess the prevalence and correlates of mental health disorders (DSM-III-R criteria) among participants 15–54 years of age
Children and adolescents					
Monitoring the Future	1975–present	3	>50,000 per year since 1975	Varies by year	Assess behaviors (including substance and alcohol use), attitudes, and values, among adolescents (8th, 10th, and 12th graders)
Youth Risk Behaviors Surveillance System	1990–present	3	N = 15,425 (2011)	20% Latinx in 2011 (varies by wave)	Assess prevalence of risk behaviors among youth in high school
Methods for the Epidemiology of Child and Adolescent Mental Disorders Study	1991–1992	1	N = 1285	28% Latinx	Assess prevalence rates of mental health disorders among youth 9–17 years of age
The Great Smoky Mountains Study	1992–2003	2	N = 1073	Not reported; Latinx children were "oversampled"	Assess prevalence and persistence of emotional and behavioral disorders, risk factors, and use of services, among children and youth 9–16 years of age

(continued)

Table 3.1 (continued)

Study	Years	Design[a]	Sample size	Percentage of Latinx participants	Main goal
National Longitudinal Study of Adolescent Health	1994–1995	2[b]	N = 90,118	Varies by wave. Wave I (1995) included 1500 Mexican origin, 450 Cubans, 437 Puerto Ricans, and "significant" numbers of Nicaraguans	Study the transition from adolescence to adulthood
Boricua Youth Study	2000–present	2	N = 2491	100% (Puerto Rican)	Assess prevalence rates of mental health disorders among 5–13-year-old children followed up longitudinally
National Comorbidity Survey Replication—Adolescent Supplement	2001–2006	1	N = 10,123	14.4%	Assess lifetime prevalence of mental health disorders (DSM-IV criteria) among youth 13 to 18 years of age
National Survey of Children's Health	2003–2017	3	N = 91,000–102,000 (depending on year)	23.7% (in 2011–2012)	Assess health, mental health, and well-being of children and youth 0–17 years of age
Latino Adolescent Migration, Health, and Adaptation	2004–2006	1	N = 250 (adolescents and their caregivers)	85% born in Mexico, 15% "other Latinx"	Assess mental health functioning of Latinx immigrant youth 12–18 years of age

[a]1 = cross-sectional; 2 = longitudinal; 3 = ongoing cross-sectional
[b]Multiple waves

in lived experiences (Arellano-Morales et al., 2016). Indeed, the most commonly used nosology, outlined in the DSM, has been widely critiqued for its potential to pathologize normative behaviors and beliefs and ignore significant environmental stressors (e.g., discrimination and segregation) experienced by minority populations (Canino & Alegría, 2008). Moving forward, we urge researchers in the field to critically evaluate the validity of DSM diagnoses in persons in Latinx and other minority populations.

Mental Health in Latinx Adults

The Substance Abuse and Mental Health Services Administration (SAMHSA) estimates past-year mental illness among Latinx adults at 14.5% (Center for Behavioral Health Statistics and Quality, 2016); this rate is consistent with that in epidemiological studies, in which prevalence rates for the Latinx population is similar to or lower than that for most other racial/ethnic groups. Specifically, rates of anxiety, mood, and substance use disorders among Latinx adults appear to be lower than among non-Latinx Whites (Kessler et al., 1994) and comparable to those of non-Latinx Blacks (Kessler et al., 2005). These findings, however, must be interpreted within the context of a relatively robust literature documenting considerable differences within the Latinx population based on nativity (e.g., foreign- or US-born) (Canino et al., 1987; Hasin, Goodwin, Stinson, & Grant, 2005; Vega et al., 2004). For example, in the Mexican American Prevalence and Service Survey (MAPSS), the rates of anxiety disorders were higher for US-born Mexican adults than for Mexican immigrants (23.2% vs. 13%). Across disorders, one in every two US-born Mexican adults reported experiencing a mental health disorder in his or her lifetime, a 2.5-fold increase over Mexican immigrants (Vega et al., 1998).

This pattern, in which later generations of Latinx persons are more likely to experience mental health problems than Latinx immigrants, despite relatively better socioeconomic circumstances, is collectively referred to as the immigrant paradox (Alegría et al., 2008). Although not well understood, numerous hypotheses have been offered to explain the paradox, including the selective migration hypothesis (in which only the most resilient individuals immigrate), the salmon bias (in which immigrants return to their countries of origin when they experience health problems), and methodological limitations of past studies. Suppositions about the paradox must be tempered with the recognition of likely but understudied within-group differences based on country of origin, age at time of migration, gender, documentation status, and insurance status, as well as mental health disorder (Teruya & Bazargan-Hejazi, 2013). For example, a number of studies suggest that within the immigrant population, the prevalence rate of mental health disorders differs depending on age at arrival in the country, with the risk for psychopathology lower for immigrants who spend more years of residence—and in particular, their childhood years—in their country of origin (Alderete, Vega, Kolody, & Aguilar-Gaxiola, 2000; Alegría, Scribney, Woo, Torres, & Guarnaccia, 2007). Data from MAPSS indicate that arrival before the age of 24 was associated with an increased prevalence of substance use, and that arrival before the age of 16 was associated with more anxiety and mood disorders as well as substance use (Vega, Sribney, Aguilar-Gaxiola, & Kolody, 2004). The National Latino and Asian American Study found no evidence of the immigrant paradox for Latinx persons who arrived in the USA before age of six (Alegría et al., 2004; Alegría, Mulvaney-Day, et al., 2007).

Mental Health in Latinx Children and Adolescents

The pediatric literature includes documentation of disproportionately high rates of mental health problems among Latinx youth—the vast majority of whom were born in the USA. For example, findings from the Youth Risk Behaviors Surveillance System (YRBSS) (Kann et al., 2016) have consistently shown greater risk for Latinx adolescents on a number of indicators of disruptive behavior disorders, including carrying a weapon at school, being injured in a fight, and being threatened or injured with a weapon. Latinx adolescents initiate smoking and drinking at earlier ages, and report more use of cocaine (11%) than non-Latinx White (7%) and Black (2%) youth (Kann et al., 2016). In addition, the rate of feeling sad or hopeless is higher for Latinx adolescents (35.3%) than for adolescents from other minority groups (25.2–28.6%), as are the rates of suicide ideation, plans, and attempts. Disparities are even more striking for Latinx girls; in 2015, nearly 50% reported symptoms of depression, 25% reported suicidal ideation, and 15% reported a suicide attempt (Kann et al., 2016).

Similar to the situation with adults, mixed findings point to significant heterogeneity within Latinx child and youth populations. In the Boricua Youth Study, researchers found higher rates of disruptive behavior disorders and conduct disorders among Puerto Rican children in New York City compared with children in Puerto Rico (Bird et al., 2007). Likewise, research suggests higher alcohol and substance use in later-generation compared with immigrant Latinx youth (Gfroerer & Tan, 2003; Perreira & Ornelas, 2011). On the other hand, time spent in the USA was found to be protective against anxiety and depression among first-generation Latinx adolescents in the Latinx Adolescent Migration, Health, and Adaptation study (Potochnick & Perreira, 2010). It may be that the immigrant paradox does not manifest for immigrant adolescents who directly experience migration-related stressors (e.g., separation from parents, or robbery or assault during migration).

Future Directions

Data on prevalence rates of mental health disorders among the Latinx population and its subgroups remain relatively scarce (Vega & Alegría, 2001). To pinpoint the most vexing mental health problems, rigorous studies are needed with all segments of the Latinx population, especially Latinx persons from Central America, unaccompanied and undocumented youth, and child and older adult populations. Moreover, a lifespan perspective is essential because mental health symptoms increase in severity and impairment the longer they go untreated (Wang et al., 2005). Understanding mental health problems as they emerge and manifest over time can inform the development of interventions that target symptoms before they become complex, and often comorbid, psychiatric diagnoses. Furthermore, there is a crucial need for data based on culturally congruent nosology and comprehensive assessment procedures that are standardized with Latinx populations in both English and Spanish. Currently, national studies of children and youth tend to rely on problem-behavior checklists, and for children younger than 11 years old, assessments are almost exclusively based on parent report (Harris & Udry, 2012). Behavior ratings are vulnerable to "reporter biases," including social desirability among parents and cultural misunderstandings and prejudices among clinicians (Youngstrom, Meyers, Youngstrom, Calabrese, & Findling, 2006). Given the growing body of evidence that points to the ways in which cultural factors shape prevalence rates, etiology, and assessment of mental illness, research that attends to culture is vital (Arellano-Morales et al., 2016).

Cultural Theories of Latinx Mental Health

Concerted attention to the role of culture in mental illness emerged in the 1970s as a growing number of researchers became interested in the perceived uniqueness of specific illness experiences within cultural groups, and thus, analyses were directed more broadly toward understanding how the experiential nature of distress was interpreted through the lens of culture (Zayas & Gulbas, 2012). Within this framework, the interplay among psychophysiologic processes, social interaction, and broader sociocultural structures is hypothesized to produce a flow of experience that is both culturally shared and idiosyncratic in its expression. As Kleinman (2008) argued, "the peculiar expression of misery as depression, anxiety, backache, or fear of being possessed results from the particular cultural apparatus of language, perceptual schema, and symbolic categories which constitute distress in one or other mode" (p. 70).

Through its attention to the cultural meanings of mental illness, this framework has been conceptually useful for investigating cultural factors that shape individual responses to distress. For example, Laria and Lewis-Fernández (2001) studied the links between sociocultural contexts and dissociative and somatic experiences often found among Latinx persons who have experienced trauma. Dissociation operates as a protective mechanism, blocking an individual's conscious awareness of the stressful event that caused emotional distress. Somatization converts emotions into somatic symptoms, displacing the expression of emotional distress. In describing the role that sociocultural factors play in these experiences, some researchers point to well-documented cross-cultural variations in the process of perception, assessment, and behavioral and symptomatologic response to stressful events. "*Ataque de nervios*," an idiom of distress in Latinx persons, is an excellent example of how cultural scripts offer meaning systems that shape the expression of intense emotionality and uncontrolled behaviors in response to stressful disrupted social relations (Guarnaccia, Lewis-Fernández, & Marano, 2003). The emergence of research on the cultural expression of mental illness has stimulated extensive debate about the universality of psychiatric disorders, diagnoses, and symptoms (Canino & Alegría, 2008).

Cultural explanations for mental health outcomes within the Latinx population have also shown that rates of mental health outcomes, the expression of symptoms, and the associated risk and protective factors vary across other dimensions of social identity such as gender, immigration status, national and ethnic heritage, age, and sexual orientation (Chu, Goldblum, Floyd, & Bongar, 2010; Viruell-Fuentes, Miranda, & Abdulrahim, 2012). In light of this evidence, researchers have increasingly called for more intersectional approaches that avoid conceptualizing Latinx populations as a monolithic whole (Brown, Donato, Laske, & Duncan, 2013). Intersectional theory emphasizes that mental health disparities are best understood through an examination of the ways in which social identities interrelate to differentially shape life experiences and put individuals at risk (Crenshaw, 1994; Warner, 2008). Similarly, minority stress theory suggests that experiences of discrimination among minority populations shape risk for mental health (Meyer, 2003). Each of these theoretical approaches has been used to show differences in mental health outcomes among individuals who identify as Latinx and lesbian, gay, bisexual, or transgender (Bauermeister, Morales, Seda, & González-Rivera, 2007; Bostwick et al., 2014; Díaz, Ayala, Bein, Henne, & Marin, 2001; Sutter & Perrin, 2016). Risk for anxiety, depression, and suicide attempts is higher in sexual minority groups (Choi, Paul, Ayala, Boylan, & Gregorich 2013; Rhodes et al., 2013), showcasing disparities that shed light on the complex dynamics associated with having multiple oppressed identities. For example, in their study of the mental health of sexual minority Latinx adults, Velez, Moradi, and DeBlaere (2015) showed that when individuals experienced discrimination based on one identity (e.g., sexual orientation), the individuals who were able to reframe their experiences on the basis of the positive appraisal of another identity (e.g., Latinx) experienced better mental health outcomes. Future research should consider the ways in which intersectional identities confer differential risk and contribute to different mental health profiles, particularly across the lifespan.

Although deep knowledge of the underlying psychological and sociocultural processes that give rise to differences in the prevalence of mental illness remains unknown, advances in theoretical and conceptual understandings of acculturation have helped to elucidate potential pathways to health in the pan-Latinx population (Lopez & Guarnaccia, 2000). Acculturation is broadly conceptualized as a multidimensional process of cultural change produced through cross-cultural engagement (Berry, 1997; Guarnaccia & Hausmann-Stabile, 2016). Research suggests that acculturation serves as a risk factor for Latinx persons on at least some outcomes, even as it is necessary, inevitable, and in some ways beneficial (e.g., by providing opportunities for employment) (Lara, Gamboa, Kahramanian, Morales, & Bautista, 2005).

Acculturation and mental health: The cultural buffers hypothesis. There is consensus that, despite tremendous diversity, members of the Latinx population share common characteristics reflective of a collectivistic culture. Although empirical evidence is limited and we must avoid a reductionist view of the population, the literature describes a number of Latinx cultural values such as *familismo* (the mutual support and obligation among family members), *personalismo* (the value placed on personal relationships), and *respeto* (respect for and deference to authority figures) that emphasize interdependence. Acculturation may lead to the erosion of these core cultural characteristics, which then, according to the cultural buffers hypothesis, increases risk for mental health problems. In contrast, Latinx persons who retain these characteristics are at lower risk for negative outcomes, even in the face of adverse circumstances stemming from poverty and discrimination.

Supporting the cultural buffers hypothesis, a robust literature shows that a strong ethnic identity, or sense of commitment and belonging to one's culture of origin, attenuates risk for mental health problems, possibly by fostering a high self-esteem (Smith & Silva, 2011). Relatedly, adherence to cultural values such as *familismo*, with its emphasis on the extended family unit as a source of instrumental and emotional support, has been described as inherently protective and has been found to promote numerous positive outcomes (Calzada, Tamis-LeMonda & Yoshikawa, 2013). Some researchers have called into question whether cultural buffers, including ethnic identity and *familismo*, uniformly promote health and well-being and, based on recent evidence, emphasize the need to further understand for which individuals, contexts, and outcomes they may be protective (Calzada et al., 2013; Smith & Silva, 2011). Despite these uncertainties, cultural buffers are widely considered key explanatory mechanisms between acculturation and psychopathology.

Acculturation and mental health: The parent–child acculturation gap. Children and adolescents have been shown to acculturate faster (e.g., learn English and embrace Americanized norms related to preferences for food and clothes) than their parents (Birman & Trickett, 2001), resulting in so-called acculturation gaps (Kwak, 2003) that appear to increase parent–child conflict (Coatsworth, Pantin, & Szapocznik, 2002), and culture- and language-brokerage responsibilities among children and youth (McQuillan & Tse, 1995). Acculturation gaps influence youth internalizing problems and self-esteem via these family dynamics (Portes & Zady, 2002; Smokowski & Bacallao, 2007). Parenting practices appear to be one of the strongest mediators in the relationship between acculturation and adolescents' mental health outcomes. For example, Martinez (2006) found that the negative effects of differential acculturation on teen substance use were decreased through effective parenting. At the same time, effective parenting practices were decreased by differential acculturation. Such studies illustrate the need to understand how universal family processes (e.g., parenting) interact with processes unique to immigrant and minority families (e.g., acculturation) to shape mental health (Liang, Matheson, & Douglas, 2016).

Future Directions

Acculturation theory has taken a spotlight in the study of Latinx mental health, but knowledge of how acculturation influences the pathogenesis of mental illness remains limited for several reasons. First, acculturation theory has evolved to outpace the methodological approaches that are typically applied to its study. One leading researcher (Bornstein, 2017) emphasizes that acculturation "is actually a much more subtle and differentiated process moderated by multiple factors, disabusing us of typological notions or broad generalities" (p. 5). Most research, however, relies on simplistic linear models to describe the association between acculturation and psychiatric symptomatology. Second, acculturation is influenced by pre-migration factors, including individual personality factors that are rarely considered in Latinx mental health research (Boneva & Frieze, 2001). Third, acculturation unfolds over time and across generations, but most research has used cross-sectional methods with no follow-up of individuals as they undergo the dynamic process of acculturation (Calzada, Huang, Covas, Ramirez, & Brotman, 2016). Lastly, the study of acculturation *per se* may be less germane to Latinx mental health than the study of acculturative stress that arises from intercultural contact. Stressors such as experiences of discrimination, social and linguistic isolation, economic stress, and family conflict related to acculturation gaps appear to increase risk for depression and anxiety but are relatively understudied (Finch & Vega, 2003). For instance, although we highlighted the parent–child acculturation gap, acculturation gaps exist between other family members (e.g., spouses and older adults and their adult children) and outside of the family context (e.g., between peers or neighbors). These gaps have thus far been neglected in research. Future work is necessary to elucidate these acculturative stress processes and the ways in which Latinx persons are able or unable to successfully manage them.

A New Conceptual Approach to the Study of Latinx Mental Health: System Dynamics Theory

Latinx persons must function within a context characterized by multiple, complex societal factors (e.g., anti-immigrant sentiment, segregation, community poverty, disorganization and crime) that may potentially undermine mental health functioning, although there are related factors that may also be protective (e.g., ethnic enclaves). Distal factors influence and interact with proximal factors such as cultural socialization in the family and peer interactions and ethnic identity, to influence vulnerability and resilience among Latinx persons. How these dynamics and mechanisms play out, however, is likely a function of a plethora of individual characteristics like country of origin, nativity, and documentation status.

To date, theories and methods that guide Latinx mental health research have fallen short of capturing the complexities and nuances in the lived experiences of Latinx persons in the USA. However, this may not be unique; to varying extents, similar concerns apply to all populations. To address such shortcomings, the mental health field is moving toward more comprehensive and dynamic models of psychopathology that account for the active, reactive, and interactive nature of individuals within their environmental contexts (Granic & Hollenstein, 2003; Wittenborn, Rahmandad, Rick, & Hosseinichimeh, 2015).

System dynamics theory conceptualizes human development as an open system that is composed of multiple, mutual, and continuous interactions between an individual and his or her ecologic context, like overlapping spheres that change shape as they move through time. Within the system, microlevel and macrolevel variables may relate to each other in any number of nonlinear ways, reflecting the complexities of human development. Because each sphere transforms as it moves through time, development may be seen as an ever-evolving system in which each new state is dependent on its previous state and informs its future state. That is, behavior is always context- and time-dependent, reflecting the unique convergence of individual and contextual components at a given point in time.

Despite this fluidity, the system is driven by self-organization or a pattern that emerges from the interaction of its components. With repetition, behavioral patterns settle into predictable states, and the system develops an affinity for these states of relative stability. In other words, beginning in childhood, individuals develop characteristic ways of thinking and feeling and, as these cognitions and emotions become coupled through feedback loops (i.e., causal relationships between variables that have self-reinforcing or self-correcting effects), behavioral tendencies become more probable across situations and over time. Development, then, may be viewed as a fluid process that nonetheless tends toward stability and predictability in the absence of perturbations or disturbances to the system.

Systems are disrupted, and subsequently "unequilibriated," during the normative (e.g., moving to a new community) and non-normative (e.g., parental divorce) transitions that occur throughout the lifespan. In the face of a perturbation, individuals must reorganize by drawing on their existing resources to meet the new challenge. Importantly, any given factor within the system may serve as either an advantage or disadvantage in meeting a specific challenge, depending on its interaction with other elements of the system (Hendry & Kloep, 2002). Individuals with the sufficient number of the needed resources are able to successfully navigate a challenge, although the system will become temporarily unbalanced before stabilizing with higher-order skills; this represents developmental growth. If, however, individuals do not have the resources to meet the challenge, the system may remain in equilibrium, with no developmental growth. When the demands of the challenge overwhelm the system, developmental may be compromised; this may occur when resources are insufficient and/or a poor "fit" for the demands of the challenge and may lead to psychopathology, including depression (Wittenborn et al., 2015).

Latinx Youth Depression

System dynamics holds great promise for capturing the complexities of developmental psychopathology in a population, such as Latinx youth, that is subject to powerful and unstable ecological challenges (e.g., non-normative transitions). With time spent in the USA (whether within or across generations) and amid shifting and often negative immigrant policies and sentiments, adolescents face challenges individually and within their family and peer networks related to migration, documentation status, deportation, new language acquisition, loss of native language, conflicting identities, acculturation gaps, social isolation, racism, and discrimination. In the absence of socioeconomic resources (30% of all Latinx children and 40% of children with an immigrant parent live in poverty) (Passel et al., 2011), adolescents must garner considerable individual resources (e.g., active coping skills and pride in their ethnic identity) to face these challenges. The application of system dynamics could illustrate how variables interact to reinforce or disrupt associations between underlying cognitive, behavioral, and mood symptoms of depression and identify which of these variables act as crucial leverage points for intervention. For instance, it may be that for Latinx youth, hopelessness, which increases depressed mood, is itself increased by experiences of discrimination and fear of deportation but decreased by ethnic identity and strong parent-child relationships. The lever (i.e., that controls the degree of hopelessness experienced by youth) may be parent–child relationships, such that strengthening the parent–child relationship through interventions would serve to attenuate the influence of discrimination, fear, and ethnic identity.

Currently, the field relies on interventions for depression that were developed for non-Latinx White populations with little consideration of other ethnic cultures. Rigorous studies of these evidence-based treatments (e.g., cognitive behavioral therapy and interpersonal therapy) with Latinx individuals are scarce, despite compelling evidence of disparities on these outcomes (Garcia, Skay, Sieving, Naughton, & Bearinger, 2008; Siegel, Aneshensel, Taub, Cantwell, & Driscoll, 1998; Saluja et al., 2004). A small number of randomized control trials to evaluate depression interventions in adolescents have included Latinx youth (e.g., Rosselló & Bernal, 1999). Some efforts toward cultural adaptations, or changes based on culture and context, of evidence-based interventions have been made, including the use of parent–child modalities to supplement the traditional reliance on individual treatment modalities (Duarté-Vélez, Bernal, & Bonilla, 2010). Results from these trials are promising, but more investment in prevention and treatment programs that target underlying cultural mechanisms related to Latinx youth depression is clearly warranted.

Summary

In aggregate, the Latinx population in the USA is healthier than the non-Latinx White population on most indicators of mental health, despite chronic exposure to significant social stressors that are known to undermine health. However, for many Latinx persons, negative experiences (e.g., discrimination and isolation) in the USA have had a documented impact on their mental health. For example, Latinx children and youth who were born and/or raised in the USA amid a culture of socioeconomic disadvantage in which aggression, delinquency, substance use, early sexual activity, and school dropout are normative outcomes are at higher risk for depression. Furthermore, as disadvantaged youth reach childbearing age and become parents themselves, they may be less likely to have the resources needed to create an optimal home environment for their children; thus, the risk for mental illness advances progressively across generations (Vega & Scribney, 2011). It is incumbent on Latinx mental health researchers to disrupt this pattern of cascading disadvantage within and across Latinx generations by pushing for innovative theory (e.g., lifespan and system dynamics perspectives) and methodologies (e.g., sampling and measurement) that capture the complexities of culture and mental health.

References

Alderete, E., Vega, W. A., Kolody, B., & Aguilar-Gaxiola, S. (2000). Lifetime prevalence of and risk factors for psychiatric disorders among Mexican migrant farmworkers in California. *American Journal of Public Health, 90*(4), 608.

Alegría, M., Canino, G., Ríos, R., Vera, M., Calderón, J., Rusch, D., et al. (2002). Inequalities in use of specialty mental health services among Latinos, African Americans, and non-Latino whites. *Psychiatric Services, 53*(12), 1547–1555.

Alegría, M., Canino, G., Shrout, P. E., Woo, M., Duan, N. ... Meng, X. L. (2008). Prevalence of mental illness in immigrant and non-immigrant US Latino groups. *American Journal of Psychiatry, 165*(3), 356–369.

Alegría, M., Mulvaney-Day, N., Woo, M., Torres, M., Gao, S., & Oddo, V. (2007a). Correlates of past-year mental health service use among Latinos: Results from the National Latino and Asian American Study. *American Journal of Public Health, 97*(1), 76–83.

Alegría, M., Sribney, W., Woo, M., Torres, M., & Guarnaccia, P. (2007b). Looking beyond nativity: The relation of age of immigration, length of residence, and birth cohorts to the risk of onset of psychiatric disorders for Latinos. *Research in Human Development, 4*(1–2), 19–47.

Alegría, M., Takeuchi, D., Canino, G., Duan, N., Shrout, P., Meng, X. L., ... Vera, M. (2004). Considering context, place and culture: The National Latino and Asian American Study. *International Journal of Methods in Psychiatric Research, 13*(4), 208–220.

American Psychiatric Association. (2000). *Diagnostic and statistical manual of mental disorders* (4th ed., text rev.). Washington, DC: American Psychiatric Association.

Arellano-Morales, L., Elder, J. P., Sosa, E. T., Baquero, B., & Alcántara, C. (2016). Health promotion among Latino adults: Conceptual frameworks, relevant pathways, and future directions. *Journal of Latina/o Psychology, 4*(2), 83.

Bauermeister, J., Morales, M., Seda, G., & González-Rivera, M. (2007). Sexual prejudice among Puerto Rican young adults. *Journal of Homosexuality, 53*(4), 135–161.

Behavioral Sciences Research Institute. (2016). Need assessment study of mental health and substance use disorders and service utilization among adult population of Puerto Rico. San Juan, Puerto Rico: Behavioral Sciences Research Institute, University of Puerto Rico. http://www.assmca.pr.gov/BibliotecaVirtual/Estudios/Need%20Assessment%20Study%20of%20Mental%20Health%20and%20Substance%20of%20Puerto%20Rico%202016.pdf.

Berry, J. W. (1997). Immigration, acculturation, and adaptation. *Applied Psychology: An International Review, 46*(1), 5–43.

Bird, H., Shrout, P., Davies, M., Canino, G., Duarte, C., Shen, S., et al. (2007). Longitudinal development of antisocial behaviors in young and early adolescent Puerto Rican children at two sites. *Journal of American Academy of Child & Adolescent Psychiatry, 46*(1), 5–14.

Birman, D., & Trickett, E. J. (2001). Cultural transitions in first-generation immigrants. Acculturation of Soviet Jewish refugee adolescents and parents. *Journal of Cross-Cultural Psychology, 32*(4), 456–477.

Boneva, B. S., & Frieze, I. H. (2001). Toward a concept of a migrant personality. *Journal of Social Issues, 57*(3), 477–491.

Bornstein, M. (2017). The specificity principle in acculturation science. *Perspectives on Psychological Sciences, 12*(1), 3–45.

Bostwick, W. B., Meyer, I., Aranda, F., Russell, S., Hughes, T., Birkett, M., et al. (2014). Mental health and suicidality among racially/ethnically diverse sexual minority youths. *American Journal of Public Health, 104*(6), 1129–1136.

Brown, T. N., Donato, K. M., Laske, M. T., & Duncan, E. M. (2013). Race, nativity, ethnicity, and cultural influences in the sociology of mental health. In C. S. Aneshensel, J. C. Phelan, & A. Bierman (Eds.), *Handbook of the sociology of mental health* (2nd ed., pp. 255–276). New York: Springer.

Calzada, E. J., Huang, K., Covas, M., Ramirez, D., & Brotman, L. (2016). A longitudinal study of cultural adaptation among Mexican and Dominican immigrant women. *Journal of International Migration & Integration, 17*(4), 1049–1063.

Calzada, E., Tamis-LeMonda, C., & Yoshikawa, H. (2013). Familismo in Mexican and Dominican families from low-income, urban communities. *Journal of Family Issues, 34*(12), 1696–1724.

Canino, G., & Alegría, M. (2008). Psychiatric diagnosis–is it universal or relative to culture? *Journal of Child Psychology and Psychiatry, 49*(3), 237–250.

Canino, G. J., Bird, H. R., Shrout, P. E., Rubio-Stipec, M., Bravo, M., Martinez, R., … Guevara, L. M. (1987). The prevalence of specific psychiatric disorders in Puerto Rico. *Archives of General Psychiatry, 44*(8), 727–735.

Center for Behavioral Health Statistics and Quality. (2016). Key substance use and mental health indicators in the United States: Results from the 2015 National Survey on Drug Use and Health (HHS Publication No. SMA 16-4984, NSDUH Series H-51). http://www.samhsa.gov/data/.

Choi, K., Paul, J., Ayala, G., Boylan, R., & Gregorich, S. E. (2013). Experiences of discrimination and their impact on the mental health among African American, Asian and Pacific Islander, and Latino men who have sex with men. *American Journal of Public Health, 103*(5), 868–874. https://doi.org/10.2105/ajph.2012.301052.

Chu, J. P., Goldblum, P., Floyd, R., & Bongar, B. (2010). The cultural theory and model of suicide. *Applied and Preventive Psychology, 14*(1–4), 25–40.

Coatsworth, J. D., Pantin, H., & Szapocznik, J. (2002). Familias Unidas: A family-centered ecodevelopmental intervention to reduce risk for problem behaviors among Hispanic adolescents. *Clinical Child and Family Psychology Review, 5*(2), 113–132.

Crenshaw, K. W. (1994). Mapping the margins: Intersectionality, identity politics, and violence against women of color. In M. A. Fineman & R. Mykitiuk (Eds.), *The public nature of Private violence* (pp. 93–118). New York: Routledge.

Díaz, R. M., Ayala, G., Bein, E., Henne, J., & Marin, B. V. (2001). The impact of homophobia, poverty, and racism on the mental health of gay and bisexual Latino men: Findings from three US cities. *American Journal of Public Health, 91*(6), 927–932.

Duarté-Vélez, Y., Bernal, G., & Bonilla, K. (2010). Culturally adapted cognitive-behavior therapy: integrating sexual, spiritual, and family identities in an evidence-based treatment of a depressed Latino adolescent. *Journal of Consulting Psychology, 66*(8), 895–906.

Finch, B. K., & Vega, W. A. (2003). Acculturation stress, social support, and self-rated health among Latinos in California. *Journal of Immigrant Health, 5*(3), 109–117.

Garcia, C., Skay, C., Sieving, R., Naughton, S., & Bearinger, L. (2008). Family and racial factors associated with suicide and emotional distress among Latino students. *Journal of School Health, 78*(9), 487–495.

Gfroerer, J. C., & Tan, L. L. (2003). Substance use among foreign-born youths in the United States: Does the length of residence matter? *American Journal of Public Health, 93*(11), 1892–1895.

Granic, I., & Hollenstein, T. P. (2003). Dynamic systems methods for models of developmental psychopathology. *Development and Psychopathology, 15*(3), 641–669.

Guarnaccia, P. J., & Hausmann-Stabile, C. (2016). Acculturation and its discontents: A case for bringing anthropology back into the conversation. *Sociology and Anthropology, 4*(2), 114.

Guarnaccia, P. J., Lewis-Fernández, R., & Marano, M. R. (2003). Toward a Puerto Rican popular nosology: *Nervios* and *ataque de nervios*. *Culture, Medicine and Psychiatry, 27*(3), 339–366.

Harris, K. M., & Udry, J. R. (2012). *National longitudinal study of adolescent health, 1994–2008*. Ann Arbor, MI: Inter-university Consortium for Political and Social Research.

Hasin, D. S., Goodwin, R. D., Stinson, F. S., & Grant, B. F. (2005). Epidemiology of major depressive disorder: Results from the National Epidemiologic Survey on Alcoholism and Related Conditions. *Archives of General Psychiatry, 62*(10), 1097–1106.

Hendry, L., & Kloep, M. (2002). *Lifespan development: Resources, challenges and risks*. London: Thomson.

Kann, L., McManus, T., Harris, W. A., Shanklin, S. L., Flint, K. H., Hawkins, J., ... Zaza, S. (2016). Youth risk behavior surveillance—United States, 2015. *Morbidity and Mortality Weekly Report Surveillance Summaries, 65*(6), 1–174.

Kessler, R. C., Berglund, P., Demler, O., Jin, R., Merikangas, K. R., & Walters, E. E. (2005). Lifetime prevalence and age-of-onset distributions of DSM-IV disorders in the National Comorbidity Survey Replication. *Archives of General Psychiatry, 62*(6), 593–602.

Kessler, R. C., McGonagle, K. A., Zhao, S., Nelson, C. B., Hughes, M., Eshleman, S., ... Kendler, K. S. (1994). Lifetime and 12-month prevalence of DSM-III-R psychiatric disorders in the United States: Results from the National Comorbidity Survey. *Archives of General Psychiatry, 51*(1), 8–19.

Kleinman, A. (2008). *Rethinking psychiatry*. New York: Simon and Schuster.

Kwak, K. (2003). Adolescents and their parents: A review of intergenerational family relations for immigrant and non-immigrant families. *Human Development, 46*(2–3), 15–136.

Lara, M., Gamboa, C., Kahramanian, M. I., Morales, L., & Bautista, D. (2005). Acculturation and Latino health in the United States: A review of the literature and its sociopolitical context. *Annual Review of Public Health, 26*, 367–397.

Laria, A. J., & Lewis-Fernández, R. (2001). The professional fragmentation of experience in the study of dissociation, somatization, and culture. *Journal of Trauma & Dissociation, 2*(3), 17–46.

Liang, J., Matheson, B., & Douglas, J. M. (2016). Mental health diagnostic considerations in racial/ethnic minority youth. *Journal of Child and Family Studies, 25*(6), 1926–1940.

Lopez, S. R., & Guarnaccia, P. J. (2000). Cultural psychopathology: Uncovering the social world of mental illness. *Annual Review of Psychology, 51*(1), 571–598.

Marmot, M. (2005). Social determinants of health inequalities. *The Lancet, 365*(9464), 1099–1104.

Martinez, C. R. (2006). Effects of differential family acculturation on Latino adolescent substance use. *Family Relations, 55*(3), 306–317.

McQuillan, J., & Tse, L. (1995). Child language brokering in linguistic minority communities: Effects on cultural interaction, cognition, and literacy. *Language and Education, 9*(3), 195–215.

Meyer, I. H. (2003). Prejudice, social stress, and mental health in lesbian, gay, and bisexual populations: Conceptual issues and research evidence. *Psychological Bulletin, 129*(5), 674–697.

Passel, J., Cohn, D., & Lopez, M. (2011). *Census 2010: 50 million Latinos Hispanics account for more than half of nation's growth in past decade*. Washington, DC: Pew Hispanic Center.

Perreira, K. M., & Ornelas, I. J. (2011). The physical and psychological well-being of immigrant children. *The Future of Children, 21*, 195–218.

Portes, P. R., & Zady, M. F. (2002). Self-esteem in the adaptation of Spanish-speaking adolescents: The role of immigration, family conflict and depression. *Hispanic Journal of Behavioral Sciences, 24*(3), 296–318.

Potochnick, S. R., & Perreira, K. M. (2010). Depression and anxiety among first-generation immigrant Latino youth: Key correlates and implications for future research. *Journal of Nervous and Mental Disease, 198*(7), 470–477.

Reeves, W., Strine, T., Pratt, L., Thompson, W., Ahluwalia, I., Dhingra, S., ... Safran, M. (2011). *Mental illness surveillance among adults in the United States*. https://www.cdc.gov/mmwr/preview/mmwrhtml/su6003a1.htm?s_cid=su6003a1_w.

Regier, D. A., Boyd, J. H., Burke, J. D., Rae, D. S., Myers, J. K., Kramer, M., ... Locke, B. Z. (1988). One-month prevalence of mental disorders in the United States based on five Epidemiologic Catchment Area sites. *Archives of General Psychiatry, 45*(11), 977–986.

Rhodes, S. D., Martinez, O., Song, E., Daniel, J., Alonzo, J., Eng, E., et al. (2013). Depressive symptoms among immigrant Latino sexual minorities. *American Journal of Health Behavior, 37*(3), 404–413. https://doi.org/10.5993/ajhb.37.3.13.

Robins, L. N., & Regier, D. A. (Eds.). (1991). *Psychiatric disorders in America: The epidemiologic catchment area study*. New York: The Free Press.

Rosselló, J., & Bernal, G. (1999). The efficacy of cognitive-behavioral and interpersonal treatments for depression in Puerto Rican adolescents. *Journal of Consulting and Clinical Psychology, 67*(5), 734–745.

Saluja, G., Iachan, R., Scheidt, P. C., Overpeck, M. D., Sun, W., & Giedd, J. N. (2004). Prevalence of and risk factors for depressive symptoms among young adolescents. *Archives of Pediatrics and Adolescent Medicine, 158*(8), 760–765.

Siegel, J., Aneshensel, C., Taub, B., Cantwell, D., & Driscoll, A. (1998). Adolescent depressed mood in a multiethnic sample. *Journal of Youth and Adolescence, 27*(4), 413–427.

Smith, T. B., & Silva, L. (2011). Ethnic identity and personal well-being of people of color: A meta-analysis. *Journal of Counseling Psychology, 58*(1), 42–60.

Smokowski, P. R., & Bacallao, M. L. (2007). Acculturation, internalizing mental health symptoms, and self-esteem: Cultural experiences of Latino adolescents in North Carolina. *Child Psychiatry and Human Development, 37*(3), 273–292.

Sutter, M., & Perrin, P. B. (2016). Discrimination, mental health, and suicidal ideation among LGBTQ people of color. *Journal of Counseling Psychology, 63*(1), 1, 98.

Teruya, A., & Bazargan-Hejazi, S. (2013). The immigrant and Hispanic paradoxes: A systematic review of their predictions and effects. *Hispanic Journal of Behavioral Sciences, 35*(4), 486–509.

Vega, W., & Alegría, M. (2001). Latino mental health and treatment in the United States. In M. Aguirre-Molina, C. W. Molina, & R. E. Zambrana (Eds.), *Health issues in the Latino community* (pp. 179–208). San Francisco: Jossey-Bass.

Vega, W. A., Kolody, B., Aguilar-Gaxiola, S., Alderete, E., Catalano, R., & Caraveo-Anduaga, J. (1998). Lifetime prevalence of DSM-III-R psychiatric disorders among urban and rural Mexican Americans in California. *Archives of General Psychiatry, 55*(9), 771–778.

Vega, W., Sribney, W., Aguilar-Gaxiola, S., & Kolody, B. (2004). 12-Month prevalence of DSM-III-R psychiatric disorders among Mexican Americans: Nativity, social assimilation, and age determinants. *Journal of Nervous & Mental Disease, 192*(8), 532–541.

Vega, W. A., & Sribney, W. M. (2011). Understanding the Hispanic health paradox through a multi-generation lens: A focus on behaviour disorders. In C. Gustavo, L. J. Crockett, & M. A. Carranza (Eds.), *Health disparities in youth and families: Research and applications* (pp. 151–168). New York: Springer Science + Business Media.

Velez, B. L., Moradi, B., & DeBlaere, C. (2015). Multiple oppressions and the mental health of sexual minority Latina/o individuals. *The Counseling Psychologist, 43*(1), 7–38.

Viruell-Fuentes, E. A., Miranda, P. Y., & Abdulrahim, S. (2012). More than culture: Structural racism, intersectionality theory, and immigrant health. *Social Science and Medicine, 75*(12), 2099–2106.

Wang, P. S., Berglund, P., Olfson, M., Pincus, H. A., Wells, K. B., & Kessler, R. C. (2005). Failure and delay in initial treatment contact after first onset of mental disorders in the National Comorbidity Survey Replication. *Archives of General Psychiatry, 62*(6), 603–613.

Warner, L. R. (2008). A best practices guide to intersectional approaches in psychological research. *Sex Roles, 59*(5–6), 454–463.

Wittenborn, A., Rahmandad, H., Rick, J., & Hosseinichimeh, N. (2015). Depression as a systemic syndrome: Mapping the feedback loops of major depressive disorder. *Psychological Medicine, 46*(3), 551–562.

Youngstrom, E., Meyers, O., Youngstrom, J., Calabrese, J., & Findling, R. (2006). Diagnostic and measurement issues in the assessment of pediatric bipolar disorder: Implications for understanding mood disorder across the life cycle. *Development and Psychopathology, 18*(4), 989–1021.

Zayas, L. H., & Gulbas, L. E. (2012). Are suicide attempts by young Latinas a cultural idiom of distress? *Transcultural Psychiatry, 49*(5), 718–734.

Chapter 4
Latinx Child Health: Challenges and Opportunities to Build a Healthy Future

Julie M. Linton and J. Raul Gutierrez

Abstract Latinx children represent the most rapidly growing pediatric population and the nation's youngest major racial/ethnic group. The health of Latinx children represents a critical indicator of the future health of our nation. However, inequities in access to and quality of care and disparities in health outcomes continue to threaten the health of many Latinx children. In this chapter, we briefly outline what is known about the health of Latinx children in the USA; describe some challenges to their health and well-being, highlighting both critical social determinants of health and community-level protective factors; and propose opportunities at individual, local, and policy levels to promote the health and well-being of Latinx children in the USA.

Keywords Child health · Latinx · Adolescent · Social determinants of health · Well-being · Discrimination

Latinx children represent the most rapidly growing racial/ethnic pediatric population in the USA and the nation's youngest major racial/ethnic group (Patten, 2016). The health of our nation depends on the health of this diverse, potentially vulnerable, and deeply resilient population. The health of Latinx children is optimized when access to comprehensive health services is recognized as a human right, delivered as part of a broader system of public services, and valued as a means to achieve collective prosperity. In this chapter, we briefly outline what is known about the health of Latinx children in the USA; describe some of the main challenges to their health and well-being, highlighting both critical social determinants of health and community-level protective factors; and propose opportunities at individual, local, and policy levels to improve the health and well-being of Latinx children.

J. M. Linton (✉)
University of South Carolina School of Medicine, Greenville, USA
e-mail: julie.linton@prismahealth.org

Department of Pediatrics, Prisma Health Children's Hospital-Upstate, Greenville, SC, USA

J. R. Gutierrez
Department of Pediatrics, Zuckerberg San Francisco General Children's Health Center, University of California, San Francisco, CA, USA
e-mail: juan.gutierrez@ucsf.edu

© Springer Nature Switzerland AG 2020
A. D. Martínez and S. D. Rhodes (eds.), *New and Emerging Issues in Latinx Health*, https://doi.org/10.1007/978-3-030-24043-1_4

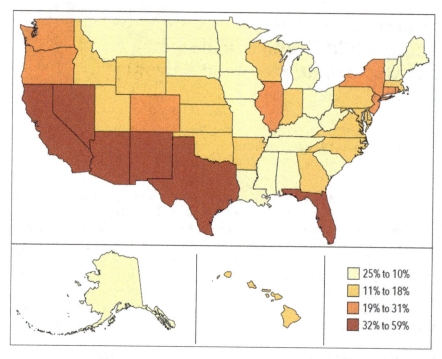

Fig. 4.1 Percent of the total population of the Latinx population by US State. *Source* Adapted from Annie E. Casey Foundation (2017)

Nearly one-third of the nation's entire Latinx population and nearly half of US-born Latinx persons are younger than 18 years of age (Patten, 2016). By 2060, it is predicted that one-third of children in the USA will be Latinx (Colby & Ortman, 2015). Although Latinx families traditionally immigrated to and/or resided in particular regions of the USA, Latinx children live in all 50 states. The states with the largest Latinx populations include California, Texas, Florida, New York, and Illinois, but the South currently leads the nation in Latinx population growth (Stepler & Lopez, 2016) (Fig. 4.1). States in the South are often referred to as "new destination states" or "nontraditional settlement states" (Gilbert, Barrington, Rhodes, & Eng, 2016; Painter, 2008).

Given the cultural, linguistic, and generational diversity within Latinx populations, it is essential to define key terms as they relate to Latinx child health (Table 4.1). Although definitions vary, for the purposes of this chapter, the term "immigrant children" specifically refers to children born outside of the USA, and "children in immigrant families" are those who are either US- or foreign-born with at least one foreign-born parent. Children are defined as those who are younger than 18 years of age, adolescents include those aged 10–19 years, and youth include those aged 15–24. Generational status (Table 4.1) as it relates to immigration is also critical to consider given the influence on children's development, family dynamics, and health disparities.

Table 4.1 Definitions and legal statuses

Children in immigrant families	Children born outside of the USA or who are US born and have at least one foreign-born parent
Immigrant children	Children born outside of the USA
First generation	A person born outside of the USA
Second generation	A person born in the USA with at least one foreign-born parent
Third generation or higher	A person born in the USA with US-born parents
Refugee	A person outside his or her country of nationality who is unable or unwilling to return to that country because of persecution or a well-founded fear of persecution based on the person's race, religion, nationality, membership in a particular social group, or political opinion
Asylee	A foreign national in the USA or at a port of entry who is unable or unwilling to return to his or her country of nationality, or to seek the protection of that country because of persecution or a well-founded fear of persecution based on religion, nationality, membership in a particular social group, or political opinion
T visa (T Nonimmigrant Status)	Provides immigration protection to victims of human trafficking
U visa (U Nonimmigrant Status)	Provides immigration protection to crime victims who have suffered substantial mental or physical abuse as a result of the crime
Special Immigrant Juvenile Status (SIJS)	Provides immigration status to foreign children in the USA who have been abused, abandoned, or neglected by at least one parent
Deferred action	Prosecutorial discretion that allows an individual to remain in the USA for a set period of time, determined on case-by-case basis and only establishes lawful presence but does not provide immigration status or benefits of any kind

Legal definitions adapted from US Citizenship and Immigration Services (USCIS), available at: https://www.uscis.gov

Among children in immigrant families, a number of different immigration statuses may apply to the child and their parents. US-born children are constitutionally citizens, and those who are not US-born may be US citizens, have other legal statuses, or be undocumented. Many Latinx children live in mixed-status families, such as those in which a child may be a US citizen, but at least one of the parents is undocumented. The legal status of the parent and the child can affect access to public services for the child and entire family and may affect developmental and psychosocial experiences of each family member (Suro, Suárez-Orozco, & Canizales, 2016; Yoshikawa & Kholoptseva, 2013).

The Health of Latinx Children in the USA: A Brief Introduction

The health of Latinx children should not be generalized by Latinx identity alone. However, Latinx children as a group face particular health risks. More than one in five Latinx children aged 10–17 is obese, and more than one in six is overweight (Murphey, Guzman, & Torres, 2014). While diet is an important factor, physical activity also contributes; only about one in four Latinx males and just over one in six Latinx females get the recommended amount of daily exercise. This may be exacerbated by higher rates of television watching, which may also interrupt regular sleep schedules. Overall, 8% of Latinx children have asthma, and the vast majority of these children are Puerto Rican (Isasi, Rastogi, & Molina, 2016; Lara, Morgenstern, Duan, & Brook, 1999; US Environmental Protection Agency, 2014). Latinx children are also twice as likely to be hospitalized for asthma-related complications (US Environmental Protection Agency, 2014). Additionally, Latinx children have higher rates of early childhood dental disease. While the rates of caries are similar when they have permanent teeth, rates of those who go untreated are higher among Latinx than White children, and the burden of dental disease is higher for migrant and rural Latinx children (Flores et al., 2002; Kaste, Drury, Horowitz, & Beltran, 1999; US Department of Health and Human Services, 2000).

Latinx children in the USA are at high risk for mental health conditions, the most common of which are depression and anxiety (Caballero et al., 2016). Latinx youth also have disproportionate rates of tobacco smoking and other substance use (El-Toukhy, Sabado, & Choi, 2016; Estrada et al., 2016; Johnston, O'Malley, Miech, Bachman, & Schulenberg, 2016).

Challenges and Opportunities in Latinx Child Health

Social Determinants of Health

Social determinants of health are "the economic and social conditions that shape the health of individuals and communities" (Gorski, Kuo, & American Academy of Pediatrics Council on Community Pediatrics, 2013). Recognizing the importance of social determinants of health is critical in both understanding Latinx children's state of health and identifying relevant resources to promote their health. Latinx children are affected by multiple social determinants of health, including those based on race, ethnicity, family immigration status, family income and poverty status, parental educational attainment, gender identity, and sexual orientation, as examples. These determinants and where they intersect profoundly influence the health and well-being of Latinx children.

Although two-thirds of Latinx children have at least one parent with steady, full-time employment, many Latinx families struggle to meet basic needs. Sixty-two percent live in low-income families (incomes less than twice the federal poverty level), and one-third live in poverty (Murphey et al., 2014). Additionally, approximately one-third of Latinx children live in neighborhoods of concentrated poverty, with 23% of parents characterizing their neighborhoods as "never safe" (Murphey et al., 2014). Latinx children tend to live in environments with substandard housing, lower-quality schools, and increased community violence. Such environments may increase the risk of poor health, lower school performance, and promote maladaptive coping behavior. Prolonged exposure to serious stress, known as toxic stress, can negatively impact brain development and threaten short- and long-term health (Garner et al., 2012).

First- and second-generation Latinx children and children from families with US-born parents have appreciable differences in some social determinants of health. For example, immigrant Latinx children are more likely to live in a multigenerational household and one headed by a married couple. However, US-born Latinx children are more likely to live in a household in which one parent finished high school or is fluent in English.

Social determinants affect health-related outcomes for children in complex ways. Consider, for instance, the high prevalence of obesity among Latinx children compared to other racial/ethnic groups (Isasi et al., 2016; Murphey et al., 2014; Ogden, Carroll, Fryar, & Flegal, 2015). Less expensive (affordable) food choices are often lower in nutritional quality; calorie-dense; low in fiber; and high in fat, sodium, and carbohydrates. Latinx children also tend to consume higher amounts of sugar-sweetened beverages than other children (The State of Obesity, 2014). Other factors contributing to obesity among Latinx children may include lack of access to grocery stores, unhealthy foods at school, limited actual or perceived access to public assistance programs, and lack of safe spaces to play.

Food insecurity—lack of consistent access to nutritious food—also disproportionately affects Latinx children. Risk factors for food insecurity include poverty, unemployment and underemployment, living in an immigrant family, large families, families headed by single women, families with less educational attainment, and families experiencing parental separation (Schwartzenberg et al., 2015). Although the relationship between food insecurity and obesity is complex, stress associated with food insecurity may also contribute to obesity (Institute of Medicine, 2011). Further, the potential impact of stress related to anti-immigration and anti-Latinx sentiment cannot be underestimated as a potential factor contributing to obesity among Latinx persons.

Racial and ethnic discrimination Race and ethnicity are recognized social determinants of health that lead to profound disparities and inequities, particularly in terms of the environments and the discrimination to which Latinx children are exposed. Institutional and policy decisions have and continue to affect the health of Latinx persons in the USA, reducing their potential for healthy and rewarding lives (Sanders-Phillips, Settles-Reaves, Walker, & Brownlow, 2009). For instance, in 2010, Arizona passed Senate Bill 1070: *Support Our Law Enforcement and Safe Neighborhoods Act* (SB 1070), which made it a misdemeanor for immigrants not to carry immigration documentation and allowed law enforcement to determine individuals' status based on mere suspicion of unauthorized status. SB 1070 has been perceived as racial profiling and discriminatory and has led to fear of separation among Latinx families. It also was identified as being detrimental to social ties between mothers and their children's teachers, among others, and affecting parent-child ties negatively, as mothers have reported increased family stress and financial hardship and decreased parental availability (Valdez, Padilla, & Valentine, 2013). Latinx mothers also have reported decreased use of public assistance, decreased likelihood of taking their children to a provider when needed, and being less likely to use preventive health care as a result of SB 1070. Simply, mothers reported being afraid to get the help they and their children needed (Toomey et al., 2014).

There is a growing body of evidence to suggest a link between racial discrimination and health and well-being, including associations between discrimination and a number of negative outcomes such as depression, anxiety, self-esteem, behavioral problems, and reduced general well-being (Paradies et al., 2015). The development of racial prejudice or feelings of inferiority can be reliably assessed as early as age three (Wilson, 1978). At this age, children can already distinguish racial differences (Sangrigoli & De Schonen, 2004; Vogel, Monesson, & Scott, 2012; Xiao et al., 2017). The process of identifying as Latinx and how children perceive themselves starts early and may be defined by how society views Latinx and immigrant communities. Even grade-school children may perceive discrimination based on race and ethnicity. Latinx children who both perceive and report discrimination in school are more likely to have symptoms of depression, attention deficit hyperactivity disorder, oppositional defiant disorder, and conduct disorder (Coker et al., 2009). Latinx adolescents also commonly perceive discrimination, and their experiences of discrimination are associated with poor mental health (Fischer, Wallace, & Fenton, 2000; Romero & Roberts, 2003; Szalacha et al., 2003).

In addition to racial and ethnic discrimination, Latinx children face other challenges, such as bullying, harassment, stress related to acculturation, and institutionalized exclusion. Up to 19% of Latinx students report some manner of bullying at school (Zhang, Musu-Gillette, & Oudekerk, 2016). Moreover, bias-based harassment may have a particularly strong and negative effect on health outcomes (Rosenthal et al., 2015; Russell, Sinclair, Poteat, & Koenig, 2012). Acculturative stress may also play a role for both US- and foreign-born Latinx children and may involve feelings of anxiety, marginalization, and identity confusion as they attempt to resolve cultural differences. Latinx children may also experience institutionalized exclusion at school, limiting their participation by linguistic barriers, inadequate support systems, and stigmatization (Kuperminc, Wilkins, Roche, & Alvarez-Jimenez, 2009).

Additionally, emerging studies demonstrate that the length of time Latinx persons are in the USA does not affect the perceived risk of discrimination, social exclusion, threat to family, or children's vulnerability. In fact, longer time periods in the USA have been associated with increased reported discrimination (Daniel-Ulloa et al., 2014). Identifying as Latinx or being identified as Latinx carries vulnerabilities that are not buffered by years of residence alone, giving exclusionary policies, such as immigration and policing policies, the potential to affect Latinx persons in multiple harmful ways (Ayón, Valencia-Garcia, & Kim, 2017; Rhodes et al., 2015; Viruell-Fuentes, Miranda, & Abdulrahim, 2012). In sum, discrimination based on race and ethnicity by means of sociocultural barriers, micro- and macro-aggressions, and marginalization can lead to social isolation and negatively affect the health and well-being of entire Latinx communities (Rhodes et al., 2015).

Language The impact of family language preference on the healthcare delivery is a critical consideration for Latinx families. Among Latinx persons aged five or older in the USA, 68% speak English proficiently, and 73% speak Spanish at home (Krogstad, Stepler, & Lopez, 2015). Just as Latinx children are diverse in their nationality, immigration history, and family composition, their language preference and proficiency can also be quite layered and diverse. For instance, some Latinx children may learn English as a third language; Spanish is their second language, and their primary language is an indigenous language (Reigelhaupt, Carrasco, & Brandt, 2003). Guatemala, for example, has more than 20 distinct languages, including K'icke', Q'eqchi', Kaqchikel, Mam, and Tz'utujil.

Knowing the child's nationality, immigrant generational history, and language spoken at home is critical to understand a family's preferred language for discussing health topics and the proficiencies of members of the family. Language preferences and proficiencies may differ between members in a family and by generation. Among foreign-born Latinx persons, English proficiency is attained at higher rate for children than adults overall (Krogstad et al., 2015). The age of immigration also contributes to English proficiency. From the time of immigration to the USA, children become more proficient over time compared to adults, with 84% of children reaching proficiency after 11–15 years of age, compared to 28% for adults (Krogstad et al., 2015).

English proficiency and the availability of skilled interpreters can be a barrier for many Latinx families attempting to access the US healthcare system and obtain the services they need. Children depend on caregivers to navigate the healthcare system. In some instances, language barriers can be the most impactful variable in healthcare access (Flores, Abreu, Olivar, & Kastner, 1998). The lack of Spanish-speaking staff and inadequate interpreter services may lead to relying on family members to translate, a burden that all too often falls on children. In fact, more than half of pediatricians in the USA continue to rely on family members to communicate with patients and families with limited English proficiency (DeCamp, Kuo, Flores, O'Connor, & Minkovitz, 2013). The lack of adequate Spanish-language resources can result in unintended medical errors, miscommunication, or suboptimal counseling and discussion of care-related risks and benefits. Additionally, some studies suggest that the use of children for language interpretation and "cultural brokering," which is the act of bridging, linking, or mediating between groups or persons of different cultural backgrounds, may have adverse effects when it becomes a burden for children. Children who interpret and broker on behalf of family members experience family-based acculturative stress that may lead to maladaptive coping behavior (Kam & Lazarevic, 2014). Challenges relating to health literacy, defined as the capacity to "obtain, process, and understand basic health information and services needed to make appropriate health decisions" (US Department of Health and Human Services, 2000) can also complicate decision-making for Latinx families.

Rather than placing Latinx children into situations that can threaten their health and well-being, both provider- and systems-level efforts are needed to acknowledge and accommodate linguistic diversity within the healthcare setting. The lack of healthcare provision within the context of family language preferences and proficiency can inhibit access to care and limit the quality of care for Latinx children.

Education The education of Latinx children not only has an impact on social and economic development at the individual and family levels, but may also influence health outcomes on community and population levels. Research consistently identifies educational status as a major predictor of health outcomes (Zimmerman, Woolf, & Haley, 2015). In the USA, education is also a pathway to economic mobility, and potentially, ending the cycle of poverty.

The Latinx population in the USA tends to place a high value in education. For example, nearly nine out of ten Latinx persons aged 16–25 report that college is important (Lopez, 2009). This appreciation of education is demonstrated in more young children enrolling in early education programs; these children tend to have a decreased dropout rate and an increase in post-secondary education enrollment (Murphey et al., 2014). However, Latinx persons still tend to lag in academic performance compared to other groups (Bell & Bautsch, 2011; Hernandez & Napierala, 2013). Looking within the Latinx population, there is variation among subgroups with respect to national origin, immigration and generation status, and family language preference (American Psychological Association, 2012; Hernandez & Napierala, 2013). Educational attainment for Latinx parents, particularly those of Mexican descent, is lower than for non-Hispanic White and African-American/Black parents (Child Trends, 2015b). Yet, intergenerational educational transmission is weaker among immigrant families than in native families and varies by national origin (Luthra & Soehl, 2015). Higher levels of parent educational attainment are associated with certain positive health outcomes, such as decreased incidence of smoking and binge drinking (Child Trends, 2015a, 2015b, 2016). However, research exploring and linking the impact of parental education to Latinx children's health outcomes is limited, and further research is needed.

It is well established that early childhood education sets the stage for future success. While enrollment in early care and education programs has increased (Murphey et al., 2014), many Latinx families may still opt for home-based care with a parent or relative, and Latinx children are significantly less likely than other children to be enrolled in prekindergarten programs (Hernandez & Napierala, 2013). Proposed reasons for these differences include lack of awareness regarding early childhood education programs, transportation barriers, and cultural preferences. Participation in learning activities at home prior to kindergarten appears to be similar to other groups; however, Latinx children are less academically ready for kindergarten when measuring skills such as recognizing letters of the alphabet or counting numbers. Conversely, Latinx children have well-developed social-emotional skills such as self-control and positive interpersonal communication (Crosby, Medez, Guzman, & Lopez, 2016; Murphey et al., 2014). This may reflect cultural differences in socialization versus academic skills and may be at odds with a school environment that holds academic skills paramount. Latinx children have seen improvements in national assessments, but the achievement gap compared to White students continues to exist and widens as educational attainment increases (Murphey et al., 2014), and although the graduation rate has improved, Latinx students have the highest high school dropout rate (Fry, 2014). Of course, like most rates used to describe and characterize the US Latinx population, the rates of achievement and dropout differ across subgroups of the population.

It is important to note that school instruction is often unresponsive to language differences and needs (Kuperminc et al., 2009; President's Advisory Commission on Educational Excellence for Hispanics, 2000). Approximately 76% of all English language learners (ELL) in the USA prefer Spanish, and most were born in the USA. However, only about 2.5% of teachers who instruct these students are adequately trained in English as a second language (ESL) or bilingual education (Nachazel, 2016).

The support or lack of support of Latinx children and students, particularly those of immigrant families, may frame how they view themselves and their relationship to society. Discrimination may be expressed as negative interactions with school staff and peers, narrow learning experiences, low educational expectations, and/or devaluation of primary languages. Structural discrimination may manifest itself as segregation (by language, ethnicity, or income), lack of high-quality educational resources, low engagement of parents, and misdiagnosis of special education needs (Adair, 2015). These types of negative interactions in school may ultimately affect academic achievement, graduation, and economic advancement. Gaps in support for compensating inequities, navigating the school system, and establishing strong relationships with teachers accumulate over the years resulting in Latinx persons being the most uneducated group in the USA (Schneider, Martinez, & Ownes, 2006).

College represents yet another frontier for many Latinx youth. Latinx persons now represent the largest minority group on college campuses, with many first-generation attendees (Murphey et al., 2014); yet, the achievement gap between Latinx and White students continues to exist in higher education. Among Latinx youth aged 18–25, less than 29% of immigrants plan to get a bachelor's degree compared to 60% of their US-born Latinx peers. The vast majority (74%) of Latinx youth 16–25 who did not pursue higher education reported that supporting their family was the reason they did not pursue higher education (Lopez, 2009). Immigrant Latinx youth are more likely than US-born Latinx youth to send remittances to family members in their country of origin, and immigrant Latinx young women are more likely to be mothers than US-born counterparts (Lopez, 2009); thus, they may lack the time and the funding to pursue educational goals. The obligation to work to send money home to their families and extended families and provide for their children may take priority over higher education.

Achievement gaps exist for Latinx children, but progress is indeed being made. It is crucial to understand how social determinants and other barriers converge and affect the educational experiences and opportunities for Latinx children. Advocating for policy that ameliorates such barriers and embraces the value placed on education, parental involvement, language diversity, and strong family values may be advantageous for Latinx children in narrowing the achievement gap.

Disparities

Health disparities are differences that exist in health outcomes when comparing groups of peoples, particularly adversely affecting marginalized groups. Although these differences are multifactorial, many health disparities and inequities occur at the population level, resulting in differences in health that are avoidable, unfair, and unjust and are affected by social, economic, and environmental conditions (Health Equity Institute, 2017; Office of Disease Prevention and Health Promotion, 2017).

The Latino immigrant paradox or the epidemiological paradox While the US Latinx population is diverse in terms of country of origin, culture, generational status, and socioeconomic status, Latinx immigrant families, in particular, are among the most resource poor, particularly with respect to income, education, insurance, and access to health care. Despite this, immigrant and second-generation Latinx children have better outcomes than might be expected in some instances. This phenomenon of low-socioeconomic status, better than expected health and mortality outcomes compared to their US-born peers, and worsening outcomes as acculturation to US culture increases over time and across generations has been termed the Latino Immigrant Paradox or the Epidemiological Paradox (Adam, McGuire, Walsh, Basta, & LeCroy, 2005; Chen, Ng, & Wilkins, 1996; Franzini, Ribble, & Keddie, 2001; Garcia Coll & Marks, 2012; Markides & Coreil, 1986).

US-born Latinx infants tend to begin with a healthy weight at birth and have high rates of breastfeeding, and for the most part, the US Latinx population has low infant mortality. However, infant mortality is high among Puerto Ricans. Latinx parents also tend to rate their children's health as good, very good, or excellent more than 90% of the time, and Latinx families tend not to be as food insecure as other groups (Murphey et al., 2014). Immigrant children tend to do well after receiving appropriate care for health problems such as stunting from malnutrition, untreated infectious diseases, dental problems, and serious mental health problems related to their immigration (Mendoza & Dixon, 1999; Nelson, Schneider, Wells, & Moore, 2004; Schumacher, Pawson, & Kretchmer, 1987). Furthermore, first-generation Latinx adolescents are less likely to report fair or poor health. In addition, they tend not to miss school because of health or emotional problems; experience learning difficulties; have obesity or asthma; or engage in health-compromising risk behaviors (Harris, 1999).

Certainly it appears that first- and second-generation Latinx children are at an advantage in the USA, despite their frequently poorer socioeconomic conditions.

Specifically, it has been suggested that less acculturation in Latinx children and their parents may be associated with lower infant and post-neonatal mortality, decreased low birth weight rates, better immunization coverage, a healthier diet, possibly a lower prevalence of asthma and allergies, less sexual activity in adolescents, fewer suicide attempts, and decreased use of tobacco, alcohol, and other drugs (Flores & Brotanek, 2005).

However, the Latino immigrant paradox is much more complex and likely to be multifactorial in nature and social in origin. Variations in characteristics such as age, gender, ethnicity and race, and acculturation influence the Latino immigration paradox and health outcomes. Furthermore, the operational definitions that are used to measure the paradox are inconsistent, and methodological approaches to measurement vary (Marks, Ejesi, & García Coll, 2014). Moreover, while some studies focusing on generational status conclude that childhood obesity follows the same paradox pattern (Perreira & Ornelas, 2011; Popkin & Udry, 1998), for example, others have found that children of US-born mothers were less likely to be obese than otherwise similar children of foreign-born mothers and children of the least-acculturated immigrant mothers were the most likely to be obese (Baker, Rendall, & Weden, 2015). Thus, it is important to be critical of the Latino immigrant paradox, its application, its generalizability, and the shifting evidence describing the phenomenon.

Acculturation Acculturation (also see Chap. 15) refers to psychological and cultural changes that occur when interacting with culturally dissimilar people, groups, and social influences and generally is studied among persons living in countries or regions outside of their place of birth (Berry, 1980, 2006; Gibson, 2001). The health of Latinx children is particularly affected by the family's immigration history and the dynamics surrounding their intersecting identifies. For example, having closer ties to one's native culture may serve as a protective factor. It is suggested that the closer one is to first-generation status, the more connected he or she is to protective factors of native cultures and less assimilated he or she is to the health-compromising lifestyle practices of US-born cohorts (Lara, Gamboa, Kahramanian, Morales, & Bautista, 2005; Rumbaut, 1997). This is contrary to assimilation paradigms that posited that acculturation to the American way of life (increased use of English, adoption of American values and traditions, and loss of culture from the country of origin) would result in thriving immigrant children and adolescents (Alba, 1997; Marks et al., 2014).

It is important to note that over 90% of Latinx children currently in the USA were born in the USA, but more than half of them have a foreign-born parent (Murphey et al., 2014). The process of acculturation, and how well one adapts as a result, has psychological and sociocultural implications that influence health and well-being (Berry, Phinney, Sam, & Vedder, 2006). The context of acculturation may include circumstances of migration, the groups or countries from which Latinx persons originate, social determinants, the receptiveness of local community in which immigrants settle, language proficiency, ethnicity and race, the degree of difference between cultures, and discrimination (Schwartz, Unger, Zamboanga, & Szapocznik, 2010).

Uninsured Opportunities for prevention and early care and treatment are missed, as Latinx children are least likely of racial/ethnic populations to get regular wellness child checks. This can partially be explained by lack of health insurance. The Affordable Care Act (ACA; described in Chap. 11) resulted in widespread coverage gains for Latinx children, and for all children across age, income, race, and ethnicity. However, Latinx children continue to have the highest rates of being uninsured, and the majority of these children are eligible for public insurance (Alker & Chester, 2016; Schwartz, Chester, Lopez, & Vargas Poppe, 2016).

Study challenges to understanding Latinx children's health Generally, research instrumentation may not gain an accurate understanding of the state of health among Latinx children. Many instruments are not culturally or linguistically congruent or lack evidence of validity within different Latinx subgroups. The paucity of informative, unbiased, validated research may also be due to study design. Many studies arbitrarily exclude non-English speakers, only enroll and compare White versus Black participants when investigating disparities, or categorize all Latinx persons in one group or as other (Flores et al., 2002). Although these studies offer some insight into general health trends, they offer limited information when trying to understand disparities and evidence-based interventions within the Latinx populations.

Regional differences Health disparities for Latinx children vary across states and regions because of policy discrepancies at state and local levels. Nationally, Latinx children are less likely to have health insurance than their non-Hispanic White and Black peers, and regionally, rates of uninsured children are generally highest in states that did not expand Medicaid (Annie E. Casey Foundation, 2017). The South has the largest share of the nation's uninsured Latinx children and the highest rate of uninsured Latinx children (S Schwartz et al., 2016). Additionally, only six states (i.e., New York, Massachusetts, Illinois, Washington, Oregon, and California) and the District of Columbia provide health coverage to all children, regardless of immigration status. Immigration status also impacts eligibility to be issued driver's licenses, and only a minority of states permit immigrants without legal status to obtain a driver's license (National Immigration Law Center (NILC), 2018). In the setting of the legal risk of driving without a license, transporting children to medical appointments, in addition to travel to work, meeting basic needs, and engaging in any "non-essential" travel can become significant barriers for undocumented parents and their children.

The threat of immigration enforcement, which varies across states, can compromise children's health directly by impeding access to care or indirectly by limiting parents' comfort in providing developmentally enriching opportunities outside of the home (Rhodes et al., 2015). Parental perceptions of state immigration policies also have been associated with parental report of their children's physical health (Vargas & Ybarra, 2017), which may exacerbate regional differences. In many states, in-state tuition is disparately available for state's high school graduates depending on immigration status (National Immigration Law Center (NILC), 2014). The cumulative impact of these regional policy differences may be indicative of, or contribute to, regional differences in risk for exposure to racism or discrimination of Latinx children.

Exposure to trauma and mental health Latinx children in the USA face a high risk for mental health conditions and may also face barriers in accessing mental health care when needed. The most common conditions faced by Latinx children are depression and anxiety (Caballero et al., 2016). Exposure to trauma, including adverse childhood experiences (ACES), may compound mental health risks for Latinx children.

Across the general population, ACES are common and increase the risk of poor health-related outcomes, including chronic illness, mental health conditions, and substance use (Mersky, Topitzes, & Reynolds, 2013). Toxic stress occurs when individuals experience a disruptive physiologic response in the setting of significant adversity in the absence or insufficiency of protective relationships (Garner et al., 2012), and has been connected with prolonged exposure to ACES. Although data evaluating ACES specifically among Latinx persons is still emerging (Allem, Soto, Baezconde-Garbanati, & Unger, 2015), Latinx children may face particular risks for ACES and toxic stress given the potential for exposure to immigration-related trauma, acculturative stress, and health disparities.

As adolescents mature, they may perceive the potential impacts of race, ethnicity, and family immigration status on their future. Mental health difficulties may emerge, and Latinx adolescents may be at increased risk for health-compromising behaviors (e.g., early and unsafe sexual activity and substance use). Discrimination in the setting of poor self-esteem and family dysfunction may heighten risks for depressive symptoms (Caballero et al., 2016). Although screening for mental health issues is part of routine health care for all children, the limited data on Latinx children and limited number and validity of Spanish-language screening tools may make early identification of mental health issues particularly difficult (Caballero et al., 2016). Furthermore, even when identified, treatment can be challenging because of the lack of providers and the absence of culturally and linguistically congruent models, frameworks, and tools for treating mental health issues among Latinx persons.

Access to mental health services can be challenging for Latinx children. Barriers to accessing mental health services may include competing family demands, transportation, communication, language, and culture (Caballero et al., 2016). Integrated mental health services, within a medical home, can facilitate enhanced access and improve care coordination. School-based mental health services also facilitate access for children, but creative solutions are needed to engage parents when mental health services are provided in school-based settings. For children who have experienced trauma, trauma-informed cognitive behavioral therapy has been shown to be effective. However, further research is needed to evaluate strategies to meet the unique needs of Latinx children who have experienced trauma.

Resilience

Despite the challenges facing some Latinx children, protective factors and remarkable resilience exist. Family strengths and cultural dynamics may contribute to positive adaptive processes that are protective. A Latinx child's identity formation is informed by context and is a reflection of environment, including the neighborhoods in which they live, adult role models to whom they are exposed, the schools they attend, and the expectations placed on them. Similarly, cultural beliefs and values may influence how Latinx youth navigate and experience their environment and ultimately shape their development and how they meet challenges (Kuperminc et al., 2009).

Protective factors common among ethnic minorities, particularly among Latinx populations in the USA, include religious involvement, culturally rooted family values, attitudes, and behaviors, as well as in the processes negotiating a bicultural identity. *Familismo* refers to an emphasis on family relationships that may include extended family members and are defined by warmth, affection, cohesion, commitment, loyalty, obedience, and emotional support for one another (Calzada, Tamis-LeMonda, & Yoshikawa, 2013). *Familismo* can be particularly protective via shared daily activities, childrearing, and social support related to emotional and financial networks related to immigration (Calzada et al., 2013). However, *familismo* is complex and may also be a source of stress when considering length of time in the USA, financial strain, interfamilial conflict, or social isolation (Calzada et al., 2013; Stein, Gonzalez, Cupito, Kiang, & Supple, 2015). While *familismo* may hold families and communities together and protect from adversity, Latinx persons who live in environments with restrictive policies and poor social capital may still experience extreme stress (Ayón, Marsiglia, & Bermudez-Parsai, 2010; Ayón et al., 2017).

Establishment of self-identity is a core task of adolescence, and ethnic identity is a component of self-identity that may act as a protective factor (Crocker & Major, 1989; Phinney, 2003). Having a well-established sense of self may strengthen self-esteem and offer resilience and psychological well-being, particularly in the face of discrimination (Phinney, 2003; Umana-Taylor, 2004). Furthermore, orientation toward their own culture may promote well-being (Gonzales, Knight, Morgan-Lopez, Saenz, & Sirolli, 2002). In a study of Latinx adolescents, higher self-esteem was associated with higher levels of ethnic identity. Among boys with low levels of Latinx cultural orientation, perceived discrimination was associated with depressive symptoms and lower self-esteem. However, among boys who reported high levels of Latinx cultural orientation, there was no association with perceived discrimination, depressive symptoms, or self-esteem (Umaña-Taylor & Updegraff, 2007). Additionally, supportive relationships in the family, peer group, school, and neighborhood are necessary and must be interconnected in establishing a sense of self while fostering community.

High-quality, organized, community-based, and out-of-school activities provide Latinx adolescents safe environments for positive development (Fredricks & Simpkins, 2012). Latinx parents often perceive organized activities as beneficial (Lin, Simpkins, Gaskin, & Menjívar, 2016) and rooting these organized activities in cultural heritage and identity formation may be protective for Latinx children.

However, barriers exist for participation of Latinx youth in out-of-school activities. Barriers may include obligations related to home, school, or work and lack of money and/or transportation (Borden, Perkins, Villarruel, & Stone, 2005). Some communities, particularly those with immigrant families, find their networks compromised by restrictive policies, fear of deportation and the stigma of being undocumented, or disruptions due to relocation and find it challenging to provide assistance or maintain these networks (Ayón, 2017; Ayón & Ghosn, 2013; Ayón et al., 2017). However, given the buffering effect that strong support networks can have on the well-being of Latinx populations, it is essential to invest in programs and policies that foster and strengthen Latinx networks, are inclusive, and allow for gains in social capital.

Higher educational attainment and self-efficacy have also been identified as protective factors. Higher education is associated with less perceived social exclusion and may serve as a marker for higher income, stable employment, and resultant increase in elements of social capital and civic participation (Ayón et al., 2017; Valencia-Garcia, Simoni, Alegría, & Takeuchi, 2012). Such attainment of social capital and participation in society could make navigating systems easier with better access to support services and opportunities to self-advocate. Self-efficacy, or the belief in one's ability to obtain a desired outcome through a successfully executed course of action (Bandura, 2004), may also help predict health outcomes for Latinx communities. In particular, high parental self-efficacy may indicate better problem-solving abilities, accessing more resources, and having more confidence to navigate challenges (Ayón et al., 2017). Parents with high self-efficacy may also be more aware of children's vulnerabilities as self-efficacy has also been associated with parental warmth (Izzo, Weiss, Shanahan, & Rodriguez-Brown, 2000). Supporting pathways to higher education and providing opportunities that boost self-efficacy through, for example, parenting classes could prove fruitful for Latinx families, communities, and future generations. For instance, mothers enrolled in the Deferred Action for Childhood Arrivals (DACA) program significantly decreased adjustment and anxiety disorder diagnoses among their children (Hainmueller et al., 2017).

In an effort to harness the continued resilience of Latinx communities, approaching children and families from a strengths-based perspective and promoting cultural wealth and integration in society could be instrumental for achieving health equity.

Special Populations

In this next section, we describe real—albeit brief—case scenarios from our own practice to illustrate the challenges facing Latinx youth in the USA. We highlight the experiences of undocumented youth; immigrant children seeking a safe haven in the USA; pregnant and parenting teens; Latinx children living along the US-Mexico border; children of migrant farmworkers; and lesbian, gay, bisexual, and transgender (LGBT) youth. Although these cases are far from comprehensive, they humanize and contextualize discussion regarding special populations of Latinx youth.

Case Example 1: Undocumented Children

Sara (pseudonym) presents to her pediatrician complaining of headaches and difficulty sleeping. Sara is a 16-year-old undocumented girl who was born in Mexico and moved to North Carolina when she was 11 years old to reunify with her parents, who are also undocumented, and younger sisters (who were born in the USA). Sara wants to be a doctor, but she recently learned that she does not qualify for in-state tuition for college, and her parents have told her that unless she can get a scholarship, they cannot afford to pay for college.

Immigration status is not only directly connected to access to services but also impacts each phase of development for undocumented children. Undocumented children may have limited understanding of the details of their immigration status, but they may perceive stress from familial uncertainty. Undocumented children face conscious uncertainty that can compromise normative identity development and threaten decision-making regarding their behavior. On a societal level, anti-immigrant rhetoric may be particularly disruptive to their health and well-being. Emerging literature continues to elucidate the direct and indirect impact of immigration status as a social determinant of health for Latinx children.

Case Example 2: Immigrant Children Seeking Safe Haven

Benito is a 7-year-old boy who presents to the local free clinic with fever and cough. Benito and his mother recently immigrated from Honduras, after his mother witnessed the murder of her husband, Benito's father. She was threatened by the local gang that she, too, would be murdered. After being apprehended at the Mexico-Texas border, Benito and his mother were detained in a family detention center for two weeks. They were recently released into the community to reunite with family friends pending immigration proceedings. Benito has never been seen by a doctor, and his mother hopes that he can enroll in the local school.

Among the most vulnerable Latinx children are those who flee their countries of origin to seek safe haven in the USA without pre-established immigration status. The detention of unaccompanied children and family units who are apprehended on the southwest border of the USA is a humanitarian crisis that threatens the health and well-being of tens of thousands of Latinx children each year. Numbers of these children, unaccompanied and in family units, have dramatically increased beginning 2014, with the largest numbers from the Northern Triangle countries of Central America (El Salvador, Guatemala, and Honduras) (Chisti & Hipsman, 2016). In 2016, 56,692 unaccompanied children and 77,674 family units were apprehended on the southwest border of the USA (US Customs and Border Protection, 2016).

Reasons for migration to the USA are often complex and may include not only the promise of family reunification and economic opportunity, but also escape from armed conflict, gang violence, abject poverty, political victimization, and/or discrimination based on group identity (i.e., gender identity, ethnicity, religious affiliation, and/or sexual identity). Pre-migration experiences may continue to affect the health of children and families, particularly as they face new stressors. During migration, many families face further threats. For instance, families may rely on "coyotes" (smugglers) to transport them during the journey. In addition, children and families who are apprehended at the US border face a complex algorithm of processing, detention, and community release proceedings (Linton, Griffin, & Shapiro, 2017). Extensive evaluation by human rights organizations, eyewitness accounts, and research from across the globe has demonstrated the negative impact of detention on physical and mental health. Even after release into communities, mental health may be further threatened complex social risks, including poverty, lack of access to care, uncertainty, acculturative stress, untreated traumatic stress, and discrimination.

For children seeking safe haven, many are eligible for legal relief upon entry into the USA. The most common forms of immigration status available for children seeking safe haven are asylum, T visa, U visa, and Special Immigrant Juvenile Status (SIJS) (Table 4.1). However, resources for legal representation, particularly those at no cost to the child, are extremely limited in many regions of the USA. Subsequently, many children and families are forced to represent themselves in court, which jeopardizes their chance of a successful legal outcome.

Children and families in deportation proceedings face not only the cumulative stress of pre-migration trauma, difficulties experienced during the journey, and acculturation, but they face added turmoil surrounding deportation proceedings. In order to help families to cope with trauma and seek community integration, they need appropriate medical evaluation and care for newly arrived immigrant children (American Academy of Pediatrics Council on Community Pediatrics, 2015), referral for legal services, and enrollment in local public education for school-age children.

Case Example 3: Pregnant and Parenting Teens

Esperanza is a 17-year-old girl who goes to see her school nurse with nausea and vomiting during class one morning. A pregnancy test is positive. Esperanza's mother delivered Esperanza at age fifteen, and she had told Esperanza not to have sex so that Esperanza "wouldn't end up like her."

Despite significant declines in racial/ethnic disparities in the teen birth rate in the USA over the past decade, Latinx teens continue to face higher birth rates (39.8/1,000) than non-Hispanic Black (37/1,000) and White (18/1,000) teens (Romero et al., 2016). Complex reasons underlying this disparity may include barriers to access to care, language barriers, cultural differences (including teen pregnancy as a "cultural rite of passage" within some communities), and educational barriers regarding contraception. Culturally congruent approaches to teach reproductive life planning to teens can facilitate prevention of unplanned pregnancy and sexually transmitted infections [e.g., ¡*Cuidate*! (Villarruel, Jemmott, & Jemmott, 2006)]. For pregnant and parenting teens, evidence-based strategies to support healthy pregnancy and positive parenting across generations include group prenatal care models [e.g., Centering Pregnancy (Centering Healthcare Institute, 2017)] and evidence-based home visiting programs (e.g., Nurse Family Partnership (Olds, 2006) and Parents as Teachers (Parents as Teachers, 2017).

Case Example 4: Latinx Children Living Along the US-Mexico Border

Denice is a 5-year-old girl who has an appointment for her kindergarten physical. Her family lives on the Texas-Mexico border in the Rio Grande Valley. This is her first appointment in three years, and she has severe caries and is obese. In developing a plan of care, it is noted that she lacks insurance and lives in a nearby "colonia" (community).

Geographically, the US-Mexico border area extends 1,954 miles from the Gulf of Mexico to the Pacific Ocean, and the total population is estimated at 15 million people. The US side of the border is comprised of 32 counties within the four states of Texas, New Mexico, Arizona, and California and is among the poorest regions in the USA. In 2012, 55% of the US border population was Latinx, compared to 17% nationally (US-México Border Health Commission, 2014a, 2015). Persons under the age of 19 comprise approximately 31% of the population. In pockets of concentrated poverty, particularly in the deep south of Texas, more than 90% of children are Latinx, and nearly 40% of Latinx children live in poverty (Annie E. Casey Foundation, 2005; US-México Border Health Commission, 2014a). Generally, border populations face challenges of high unemployment rates, high poverty rates with 37% of children living in poverty (compared to 20% nationally), high rates of uninsured status, and high rates of chronic disease, specifically obesity and diabetes (US-México Border Health Commission, 2014a). Particularly impoverished *colonias* (communities) exist along the border. In Texas, there are more than 2,000 *colonias*, with approximately 400,000 residents with 85% of the children being born in the USA (Texas Secretary of State Office). These unincorporated communities or subdivisions present environmental factors that can be harmful to health including inadequate water, sanitation service, lack of electricity, and unpaved roads (Esparza & Donelson, 2008; Korc & Ford, 2013; McDonald & Grineski, 2012).

The border region represents a dynamic binational and bicultural experience for children, some living in Mexico but attending school in the USA or vice versa, or having family ties on both sides of the border. In combination with poor access to healthcare coverage, this dynamic leads children and families to seek medical care, advice, or medications in Mexico. Further investigation is needed to understand how this binational and bicultural relationship affects health and well-being in children and how that may differ on either side of the border. Further information about the Border Health and collaborations, including programming and initiatives, can be found with the US-Mexico Border Health Commission. This commission focuses

4 Latinx Child Health: Challenges and Opportunities …

on the binational region comprised of two sovereign nations; four US states (Arizona, California, New Mexico, and Texas); six Mexican states (Baja California, Chihuahua, Coahuila, Nuevo León, Sonora, and Tamaulipas); and 26 US federally recognized indigenous tribes (US-México Border Health Commission, 2014b).

Access to health care and health outcomes vary greatly along the border, depending on the state or municipality's policies, attitudes toward immigration, and social networks. However, there are some general trends in health outcomes. The rates of obesity in this region are particularly high, with up to 22.4% of fourth graders being obese (US-Mexico Border Health Commission, 2010). In Arizona, the border counties have higher rates of dental caries than the state and national average with as much as 68% prevalence of dental caries in 6- to 8-year-old children. Among low-income Latinx households' water sources, none had enough fluoride for optimal dental health. Access to fluoride varnish or education around fluoride sources could be instrumental in these regions (Victory et al., 2017). Within the *colonias*, in some cases, up to 55% of households reported being "water insecure" (Jepson, 2014).

Case Example 5: Children of Migrant and Seasonal Farmworkers

Jorge is a 14-year-old male presenting to an urgent care clinic with back pain and fatigue. He and his family live in a housing compound near a farm where his parents pick vegetables. He helps the family by working the fields before school and will sometimes work after school during high season. You also notice old scars on his hands and arms. He mentions he is often sleepy and is not doing well in school, but he shares that his family really needs the money for the winter.

The community of migrant and seasonal farmworkers is one of the most marginalized communities in the USA (see Chap. 8 for a discussion on Latinx migrant workers). Approximately 80% of US farmworkers are Latinx; a majority are born in Mexico, and about a quarter born in the USA. Slightly more than half have authorization to work as US citizens or are legal permanent residents. Only 1% are working through a visa program, and less than 5% of the hired crop labor force arrived within the past year. Most seasonal farmworkers have been in the USA for more than 15 years and are settled seasonal workers. Migrant farmworkers have the lowest annual family incomes of any US wage and salary workers, leaving many families to include children in the work. More than half of the workers in the USA have children with an average of two minor children living in their households (US Department of Labor, 2016). Federal labor laws allow children as young as 12 to legally work with their parent's permission, as long as it is not during school hours. For particularly dangerous work, the minimum age is 16 in agriculture, but 18 in all other industries. Children may work up to 30 h per week, often during the school year (Hess, 2007). It is estimated that there are over 500,000 farmworkers under 18, and 70% of all working children in the USA work in agriculture. The majority are Latinx children (Flores et al., 2002).

These children may work long, laborious hours and be exposed to harsh weather, dangerous equipment, and toxic pesticides. Such working conditions predispose children to physical trauma, skin conditions, pulmonary symptoms, and heat-related conditions (Hess, 2007). Being a migrant worker, being undocumented, or season of the year are also associated with increased vulnerability within this community (Ip et al., 2015). Food insecurity and access to high-quality food are also challenges commonly faced by farmworkers (Borre, Ertle, & Graff, 2010; Grzywacz, Arcury, Trejo, & Quandt, 2016; Quandt, Arcury, Early, Tapia, & Davis, 2004). Moreover, hazardous conditions and remoteness of rural areas may serve as barriers to physical activity, food choices, and resources, which can limit capacity when addressing obesity (Grzywacz et al., 2016; Quandt, Grzywacz, Trejo, & Arcury, 2014).

The vast majority of children are US citizens, but very few use public assistance programs. Of public assistance used, the most commonly used is Medicaid (37%) followed by WIC (18%), food stamps (16%), and public health clinics (10%) (US Department of Labor, 2016).

Although most farmworker families do have housing, up to 18% live in employer-provided housing, only 13% received it free of charge, and 31% live in crowded dwellings (US Department of Labor, 2016). In many instances, housing may be substandard, unsanitary, and a source of environmental exposures (Arcury et al., 2012; Vallejos, Quandt, & Arcury, 2009). As can be expected, an increase in asthma and other respiratory symptoms and ailments may be found in such conditions (Kearney et al., 2014).

Children migrate with their families, causing instability and interruptions in schooling and healthcare access. Only 55% of farmworker children graduate from high school. Children receive inadequate preventive care, experience high rates of infectious diseases, have increased risks of pesticide exposures and injuries, and are at risk for nutritional disorders (Butler-Dawson, Galvin, Thorne, & Rohlman, 2016; Flores et al., 2002). Among workers with children under 18 years of age, 89% say report that all or some of their children have health insurance with the majority being provided by government programs (US Department of Labor, 2016). However, up to half of children in some areas are reported to have an unmet need (Weathers, Minkovitz, O'Campo, & Diener-West, 2003).

Case Example 6: Lesbian, Gay, Bisexual, and Transgender (LGBT) Children

José is a 15 year old who was assigned female at birth, but identifies as male. Upon puberty, José became distressed when his female body parts further developed, and he ultimately attempted suicide. Since his psychiatric hospitalization, he has begun his transition. His parents want the best for José, but struggle to understand his "behavior."

About 4% of adult Latinx consider themselves LGBT, similar to the general population. Within the LGBT Latinx community, about 146,000 live in same-sex couple households and 29% of them are raising children (Kastanis & Gates, 2013) (see Chap. 10 for more discussion about Latinx LGBT communities). The critical factors related to health and well-being among Latinx LGBT youth include rejection and acceptance (Russell & Fish, 2016; Ryan, Huebner, Diaz, & Sanchez, 2009; Ryan, Russell, Huebner, Diaz, & Sanchez, 2010). Maintaining community and facing fears of rejection are common struggles for Latinx LGBT youth. Compared to their non-LGBT Latinx peers, LGBT Latinx youth are more likely to face harassment and violence in the community, less likely to participate in a variety of community activities, twice as likely to say they do not "fit in" in the communities where they live, and less likely to have an adult in their family they can turn to for support. Only 17% said they are "out" to their medical providers. However, slightly more than half are out to their immediate family, and 60% report that their family is accepting of LGBT persons (Kane, Nicoll, Kahn, & Groves, 2012).

Family rejection is associated with higher rates of attempted suicide, depression, illegal drug use, and unprotected sex (Ryan et al., 2009). Studies show that Latinx, immigrant, religious, and low-socioeconomic status families appear to be less accepting of LGBT orientations and identities; however, family acceptance can serve as protective factor (Ryan et al., 2010).

Concluding Thoughts: Advocacy and Policy Implications

All children deserve access to health care, including basic medical care, mental health services, and dental care. Health care for children is not only a human right, but providing comprehensive preventive services protects intellectual and social capital for our nation's future. Policy priorities must address barriers to health coverage, access to health care, and equitable opportunities for Latinx children.

Insurance

Among Latinx children, in 2015, 54% were covered by public insurance, 35% had private coverage, and 4% had a combination of public and private coverage (Annie E. Casey Foundation, 2017). Public insurance is comprised of Medicaid, a joint federal and state program that provides health coverage to low-income individuals, and the Children's Health Insurance Program (CHIP), which provides federal matching funds to states to offer coverage to children who do not qualify for Medicaid but cannot afford private insurance. Private insurance includes plans provided by employers, coverage purchased through the marketplace via the ACA, and other private plans. The ACA included provisions that required states to maintain eligibility levels for public insurance, including Medicaid and CHIP (Schwartz et al., 2016). Despite coverage gains, 39% of all children who are uninsured are Latinx, many of whom are eligible for public insurance (Schwartz et al., 2016). Efforts within communities and at regional and national levels are needed to enhance enrollment of eligible children.

Medical Interpretation

It is well established that medical interpretation with trained interpreters is critical to provide high quality care to patients and families who prefer languages other than English. Federal expectations for language access based on Title VI of the Civil Rights Act and explicit national standards for Culturally and Linguistically Appropriate Services in Health Care (CLAS Standards) imply that healthcare organizations receiving federal funding must provide meaningful access to language services for patients with limited English proficiency. However, 57.1% of pediatricians use family members to communicate with patients and families with limited English proficiency (DeCamp et al., 2013). Insurance coverage and/or reimbursement for medical interpretation would allow medical providers to more successfully comply with this expectation.

Parental Immigration Status and Driver's Licenses

Efforts must be made to limit the impact of parental immigration status on the health and well-being of Latinx children. Specifically, in order to facilitate access to medical care and to promote developmentally and socially normative experiences for all Latinx children, drivers' license eligibility should not be contingent on immigration status.

Newly Arrived Immigrant Children Seeking Safe Haven

The majority of children and families apprehended at the southwest border are of Latinx origin. The American Academy of Pediatrics has endorsed policy recommendations to mitigate harm and promote health and well-being for immigrant children seeking safe haven in the USA (Linton et al., 2017). First and foremost, throughout the immigration pathway, all children should be treated with dignity and respect in effort to support their health and well-being. Specifically, no child should ever be separated from a parent or caregiver unless there are safety concerns for the child at the hands of the parent/caregiver. Children should never be exposed to conditions that perpetuate trauma, and children should always be offered access to adequate healthcare services, year-round public education, and opportunities to freely play.

All children and families should have access to no- or low-cost legal counsel, and no child should ever have to represent themselves in court.

Immigration Reform: DREAM Act, DACA, and DAPA

To stay physically and mentally healthy, children need the security of supportive relationships with parents or other caregivers and the opportunity to reach their potential. Over the past decade, promising immigration proposals have attempted to mitigate barriers for young undocumented immigrants who were brought to the USA as young children and/or to ameliorate stress of potential separation of children from their parents. The DREAM Act (Development, Relief, and Education for Alien Minors Act) was introduced as a bipartisan bill, most recently in 2011, to offer undocumented students an opportunity to obtain legal residency. The group of youth that would benefit from its provisions have been referred to as "DREAMers."

In the setting of difficulties with immigration reform, including stagnancy in DREAM Act initiatives, President Obama created "deferred action" programs to provide relief from deportation for those who qualified. These deferred action programs allow recipients to pursue employment and higher education, but do not offer a pathway to lawful permanent resident (LPR) status or US citizenship. In 2012, President Obama implemented a program entitled Deferred Action for Childhood Arrivals (DACA), which allowed youth and young adults meeting specific criteria to apply for this program. In June 2013, a bipartisan comprehensive immigration reform bill (S. 744), which incorporated key elements from the DREAM Act, passed the Senate, but the House did not pursue the legislation. Subsequently, in November 2014, President Obama proposed the Deferred Action for Parents of Americans and Lawful Permanent residents (DAPA) program, which would have offered similar benefits to certain parents of US citizens and lawful permanent residents, as well as an expanded version of the DACA program. Unfortunately, the DAPA and expanded DACA programs were blocked after a series of court rulings. Most recently, in September 2017, DACA was rescinded by President Trump. At the time that this chapter was written, the fate of the DACA program, and ultimately, of the DREAMers was unclear.

Public Services

Since the election of Donald Trump in November 2016, uncertainty in the immigrant community has escalated, and a series of Executive Orders early in the presidency substantiated concerns. Healthcare providers and advocates must prioritize the potential of all children, including those seeking safe haven and hoping for better lives, to lead healthy lives and to ultimately achieve their fullest potential. Assistance in the form of public services can be of potential benefit to the health of Latinx children. Accessing such programs as Supplemental Nutrition Assistance Program (SNAP),

Medicaid, Supplemental Security Income (SSI), and Temporary Assistance to Needy Families (TANF) is largely dictated by the Personal Responsibility and Work Opportunity Reconciliation Act of 1996 (PRWORA, 1996) or the "welfare reform bill." PRWORA 1996 largely affected the access to public services for the immigrant community and US-born children of immigrants. Confusion exists about eligibility to participate in different programs and whether participating in these programs will affect one's immigration status or increase one's risk of deportation. Additionally, certain policies that incorporate concepts such as "deeming" and "public charges" can create actual or perceived barriers to access for immigrant families (National Immigration Law Center (NILC), 2017b). Among those of Mexican heritage, first- and second- generation children were less likely to use public assistance programs than White families. However, third-generation children, along with Puerto Rican children, are more likely to use all forms of assistance. Children of Cuban heritage begin accessing such programs immediately, which likely reflects their eligibility to enter as refugees, and use declines among third-generation Cuban children (Hofferth, 1999). Further research is needed to understand the patterns of use among Latinx subpopulations and how these patterns relate to future socioeconomic status, health, and well-being.

Health care must partner with community and government organizations to assist the Latinx persons in accessing public services for which they are eligible. It is critical be that the healthcare community understand barriers and help dispel myths around eligibility. However, proposed changes in the definition of a "public charge" have created unrest within the healthcare sector and communities. Traditionally, the scope of "public charge," a determination made upon entry into the USA or when applying for legal permanent residency, has been limited to use of cash benefits or long-term institutionalization with federal funding. Efforts are currently underway to broaden the definition of public charge to include non-cash benefits (e.g., Medicaid, SNAP, and housing assistance) as well as incorporate income requirements. Broadening this definition would likely impact utilization of critical services by immigrant families (Artiga, Damico, & Garfield, 2018; Batalova, Fix, & Greenberg, 2018).

Although language presents itself as a significant barrier in some communities, particularly those areas where Spanish-speaking government employees and translators are sparse. Families with limited English proficiency do, however, have a right to request such services. The Supreme Court in *Lau v. Nichols* affirmed that under Title VI of the Civil Rights Act of 1964, recipients of federal financial assistance have a duty to provide limited English-proficient persons with a meaningful opportunity to participate in public programs. Medical legal partnerships may be useful in empowering Latinx communities with information about their rights.

Multiple policy and legislative initiatives at the federal and state level have increased the enrollment of Latinx youth in college. Among them are Hispanic-Serving Institutions (HSIs), in-state tuition to undocumented students, banning the use of race-sensitive criteria in college admission decisions, and percent plans, which guarantee admission to one or more state universities to a fixed percentage of the graduating class of each high school in the state. HSIs include about half of the Latinx students enrolled in higher education, enrolling 25% or more full-time Latinx students. However, these institutions have less total revenues and spend less on instruction, academic support functions, and student services compared to other colleges and universities. The DREAM Act was introduced several times in Congress as a pathway to legal status (and eligibility for in-state tuition) particularly for those entering college, but did not pass. Several states passed similar legislation enacting policies for tuition equity for undocumented students. As of 2017, 20 states offer in-state tuition to undocumented immigrant students, 16 by state legislative action and four by state university systems (Mendoza & Shaikh, 2015; National Immigration Law Center (NILC), 2017a).

Conclusion

As the fastest growing segment of our population, the health of Latinx children represents a critical indicator for future health of our communities and overall US population. All children deserve the opportunity to achieve optimal health and well-being and to reach their maximum potential. Healthcare providers must be aware of the unique needs of each child and family and the overarching risks and strengths of this diverse population. Future research should include efforts to understand the interplay between social determinants of health and health status of Latinx children as a whole as well as the unique ethnic groups and special populations within this diverse population. Policy efforts should prioritize elimination of structural inequity, optimization of preventive health, and investment in opportunities to mitigate risk and build resilience among Latinx children and their families.

Acknowledgements The authors would like to recognize Daniel P. Krowchuk, MD, FAAP for his critical review of this manuscript.

References

Adair, J. (2015). *The impact of discrimination on the early schooling experiences of children from immigrant families*. Retrieved from https://www.migrationpolicy.org/sites/default/files/publications/FCD-Adair.pdf.

Adam, M., McGuire, J., Walsh, M., Basta, J., & LeCroy, C. (2005). Acculturation as a predictor of the onset of sexual intercourse among Hispanic and white teens. *Archives of Pediatric and Adolescent Medicine, 15*(9), 261–265.

Alba, R. (1997). Rethinking assimilation theory for a new era of immigration. *International Migration Review, 31*, 826–874.

Alker, J., & Chester, A. (2016). *Children's health coverage rate now at historic high of 95 percent*. Retrieved from Washington, DC: https://ccf.georgetown.edu/wp-content/uploads/2016/11/Kids-ACS-update-11-02-1.odf.

Allem, J., Soto, D., Baezconde-Garbanati, L., & Unger, J. (2015). Adverse childhood experiences and substance use among Hispanic emerging adults in Southern California. *Addictive Behaviors, 50*, 199–204.

American Academy of Pediatrics Council on Community Pediatrics (Producer). (2015, July 30, 2018). *Immigrant child health toolkit*. Retrieved from http://bit.ly/1y6HR1D.

American Psychological Association, P. T. F. o. E. D. (2012). *Ethnic and racial disparities in education: Psychology's contributions to understanding and reducing disparities*. Retrieved from http://www.apa.org/ed/resources/racial-disparities.aspx.

Annie E. Casey Foundation. (2005). *Border kids count pocket guide: A snapshot of children living on the southwest border*.

Annie E. Casey Foundation. (2017). *Kids Count Data Center*. Retrieved from http://datacenter.kidscount.org/.

Arcury, T., Weir, M., Summers, P., Chen, H., Bailey, M., Wiggins, M., et al. (2012). Safety, security, hygiene and privacy in migrant farmworker housing. *New Solutions: A Journal of Environmental and Occupational Health Policy, 22*(2), 153–173.

Artiga, S., Damico, A., & Garfield, R. (2018). *Potential effects of public charge changes on health coverage for citizen children*. The Henry J. Kaiser Family Foundation, Issue Brief.

Ayón, C. (2017). Vivimos en jaula de oro: The impact of state level legislation on immigrant Latino families. *Journal of Immigration and Refugee Studies, 16*(4), 351–371.

Ayón, C., & Ghosn, M. (2013). Latino immigrant families' social support networks: Strengths and limitations during a time of stringent immigration legislation and economic insecurity. *Journal of Community Psychology, 41*(3), 359–377.

Ayón, C., Marsiglia, F., & Bermudez-Parsai, M. (2010). Latino family mental health: Exploring the role of discrimination and familismo. *Journal of Community Psychology, 38*(6), 742–756.

Ayón, C., Valencia-Garcia, D., & Kim, S. (2017). Latino immigrant families and restrictive immigration climate: Perceived experiences with discrimination, threat to family, social exclusion, children's vulnerability, and related factors. *Race and Social Problems, 9*, 300–312.

Baker, E., Rendall, M., & Weden, M. (2015). Epidemiological paradox or immigrant vulnerability? Obesity among young children of immigrants. *Demography, 52*(4), 1295–1320.

Bandura, A. (2004). Health promotion by social cognitive means. *Health Education & Behavior, 31*, 143–164.

Batalova, J., Fix, M., & Greenberg, M. (2018). *Chilling effects: The expected public charge rule and its impact on legal immigrant families' public benefit use*. Washington, DC. Retrieved from https://www.migrationpolicy.org/research/chilling-effects-expected-public-charge-rule-impact-legal-immigrant-families.

Bell, J., & Bautsch, B. (2011). *Improving Latino college completion: What state legislators should know*. Retrieved from http://www.ncsl.org/research/education/improving-latino-college-completion-what-state-1.aspx.

Berry, J. (1980). Acculturation as varieties of adaptation. In A. Padilla (Ed.), *Acculturation: Theory, models, and some new findings* (pp. 9–25). Boulder, CO: Westview Publishing.

Berry, J. (2006). Contexts of acculturation. In D. Sam & J. Berry (Eds.), *Cambridge handbook of acculturation psychology* (pp. 27–42). New York, NJ: Cambridge University Press.

Berry, J., Phinney, J., Sam, D., & Vedder, P. (2006). Immigrant youth: Acculturation, identity, and adaptation. *Applied Psychology: An International Review, 55*(3), 303–332.

Borden, L., Perkins, D., Villarruel, F., & Stone, M. (2005). To participate or not to participate: That is the question. *New Directions for Youth Development, 105*, 33–49.

Borre, K., Ertle, L., & Graff, M. (2010). Working to eat: Vulnerability, food insecurity, and obesity among migrant and seasonal farmworker families. *American Journal of Industrial Medicine, 53*, 443–462.

Butler-Dawson, J., Galvin, K., Thorne, P., & Rohlman, D. (2016). Organophosphorus pesticide exposure and neurobehavioral performance in Latino children living in an orchard community. *Neurotoxicology, 53*, 165–172.

Caballero, T., DeCamp, L., Platt, R., Shah, H., Johnson, S., Sibinga, E., et al. (2016). Addressing the mental health needs of Latino children in immigrant families. *Clinical Pediatrics, 56*(7), 648–658.

Calzada, E., Tamis-LeMonda, C., & Yoshikawa, H. (2013). Familismo in Mexican and Dominican families from low income, urban communities. *Journal of Family Issues, 34*(12), 1696–1724.

Centering Healthcare Institute. (2017). *Centering pregnancy.* Retrieved from https://www.centeringhealthcare.org/what-we-do/centering-pregnancy.

Chen, J., Ng, E., & Wilkins, R. (1996). The health of Canada's immigrants in 1994–95. *Health Reports-Statistics Canada, 7*(4), 33–46.

Child Trends. (2015a). *High school dropout rates.* Retrieved from https://www.childtrends.org/indicators/high-school-dropout-rates.

Child Trends. (2015b). *Parental education.* Retrieved from https://www.childtrends.org/wp-content/uploads/2015/12/67-Parental_Education.pdf.

Child Trends. (2016). *Binge drinking.* Retrieved from http://www.childtrends.org/?indicators=binge-drinking.

Chisti, M., & Hipsman, F. (2016). *Increased Central American migration to the United States may provide an enduring phenomenon.* http://www.migrationpolicy.org/article/increased-central-american-migration-united-states-may-prove-enduring-phenomenon.

Coker, T., Elliott, M., Kanouse, D., Grunbaum, J., Schwebel, D., Gilliland, M. ... Schuster, M. (2009). Perceived racial/ethnic discrimination among fifth-grade students and its association with mental health. *American Journal of Public Health, 99*(5), 878–884.

Colby, S., & Ortman, J. (2015). *Projections of the size and composition of the US Population: 2014 to 2060, Current Population Reports, P25-1143.* Retrieved from http://www.census.gov/content/dam/Census/library/publications/2015/demo/p25-1143.pdf.

Crocker, J., & Major, B. (1989). Social stigma and self-esteem: The self-protective properties of stigma. *Psychological Review, 96*, 608–630.

Crosby, D., Medez, J., Guzman, L., & Lopez, M. (2016). *Hispanic children's participation in early care and education: Type of care by household nativity status, race/ethnicity, and child age.* National Research Center on Hispanic Children & Families.

Daniel-Ulloa, J., Reboussin, B. A., Gilbert, P. A., Mann, L., Alonzo, J., Downs, M., et al. (2014). Predictors of heavy episodic drinking and weekly drunkenness among immigrant Latinos in North Carolina. *American Journal of Men's Health, 22*(8), 339–348. https://doi.org/10.1177/1557988313519670.

DeCamp, L., Kuo, D., Flores, G., O'Connor, K., & Minkovitz, C. (2013). Changes in language services use by US pediatricians. *Pediatrics, 132*(2), e396–e406.

El-Toukhy, S., Sabado, M., & Choi, K. (2016). Trends in susceptibility to smoking by race and ethnicity. *Pediatrics, 138*(5).

Esparza, A., & Donelson, A. (2008). *Colonias in Arizona and New Mexico: US–Mexico Border poverty and community development solutions.* Tucson: University of Arizona.

Estrada, Y., Lee, T., Huang, S., Tapia, M., Velázquez, M., Martinez, M., ... Prado, G. (2016). Patient-centered prevention of risky behaviors among Hispanic youths in Florida. *American Journal of Public Health, 107*, 607–613.

Fischer, C., Wallace, S., & Fenton, R. (2000). Discrimination distress during adolescence. *Journal of Youth and Adolescence, 29*, 679–695.

Flores, G., Abreu, M., Olivar, M., & Kastner, B. (1998). Access barriers to health care for Latino children. *Archives of Pediatric & Adolescent Medicine, 152*, 1119–1125.

Flores, G., & Brotanek, J. (2005). The healthy immigrant effect: A greater understanding might help us improve the health of all children. *Archives of Pediatrics and Adolescent Medicine, 105*, 295–297.

Flores, G., Fuentes-Afflick, E., Barbot, O., Carter-Pokras, O., Claudio, L., Lara, M., et al. (2002). The health of Latino children: Urgent priorities, unanswered questions, and a research agenda. *Journal of the American Medical Association, 288*(1), 82–90.

Franzini, L., Ribble, J., & Keddie, A. (2001). Understanding the Hispanic paradox. *Ethnicity and Disease, 11*, 496–518.

Fredricks, J., & Simpkins, S. (2012). Promoting positive youth development through organized after-school activities: Taking a closer look at participation of ethnic minority youth. *Child Development Perspectives, 6,* 280–287.

Fry, R. (2014). *US high school dropout rate reaches record low, driven by improvements among Hispanics, blacks.* Retrieved from Washington, D.C.: http://www.pewresearch.org/fact-tank/2014/10/02/u-s-high-school-dropout-rate-reaches-record-low-driven-by-improvements-among-hispanics-blacks/.

Garcia Coll, C., & Marks, A. E. (2012). *The immigrant paradox in children and adolescents: Is becoming American a developmental risk?.* Washington, DC: American Psychological Association.

Garner, A. S., Shonkoff, J. P., & Committee on Psychosocial Aspects of Child and Family Health, Committee on Early Childhood, Adoption, and Dependent Care, and Section on Developmental and Behavioral Pediatrics. (2012). Early childhood adversity, toxic stress, and the role of the pediatrician: Translating developmental science into lifelong health. *Pediatrics, 129*(1), e224–e231.

Gibson, M. (2001). Immigrant adaptation and patterns of acculturation. *Human Development, 44,* 19–23.

Gilbert, P. A., Barrington, C., Rhodes, S. D., & Eng, E. (2016). Saliendo Adelante: Stressors and coping strategies among immigrant Latino men who have sex with men in a nontraditional settlement state. *American Journal of Mens Health, 10*(6), 515–525.

Gonzales, N., Knight, G., Morgan-Lopez, A., Saenz, D., & Sirolli, A. (2002). Acculturation and the mental health of Latino youths: An integration and critique of the literature. In J. Contreras, K. Kerns, & A. Neal-Barnett (Eds.), *Latino children and families in the United States* (pp. 45–74). Westport, CT: Praeger Press.

Gorski, P., Kuo, A., & American Academy of Pediatrics Council on Community Pediatrics. (2013). Community pediatrics: Navigating the intersection of medicine, public health, and social determinants of children's health. *Pediatrics, 131,* 623–628.

Grzywacz, J., Arcury, T., Trejo, G., & Quandt, S. (2016). Latino mothers in farmworker families' beliefs about preschool children's physical activity and play. *Journal of Immigrant and Minority Health/Center for Minority Public Health, 18*(1), 234–242.

Hainmueller, J., Lawrence, D., Martén, L., Black, B., Figueroa, L., Hotard, M., …, Laitin, D. (2017). Protecting unauthorized immigrant mothers improves their children's mental health. *Science, 357*(6355), 1041–1044.

Harris, K. (1999). The health status and risk behaviors of adolescents in immigrant families. In D. Hernandez (Ed.), *Children of immigrants: Health, adjustment, and public assistance* (pp. 286–347). Washington, D.C.: National Academies Press.

Health Equity Institute. (2017). Retrieved from https://healthequity.sfsu.edu/content/infographic.

Hernandez, D., & Napierala, J. (2013). *Diverse children: Race, ethnicity, and immigration in America's new non-majority generation.* Retrieved from New York, NY: https://www.fcd-us.org/assets/2016/04/DiverseChildren-Full-Report.pdf.

Hess, B. (2007). *Children in the fields: An American problem.* Washington, DC: Association of Farmworker Opportunity Programs.

Hofferth. (1999). Receipt of public assistance by Mexican American and Cuban American children in native and immigrant families. In D. Hernandez (Ed.), *Children of immigrants: Health, adjustment, and public assistance.* Washington, DC: National Academies Press.

Institute of Medicine. (2011). *Hunger and obesity: Understanding a food insecurity paradigm: Workshop summary.* Washington, DC. National Academies Press.

Ip, E., Saldana, S., Arcury, T., Grzywacz, J., Trejo, G., & Quandt, S. (2015). Profiles of food security for US farmworker households and factors related to dynamic of change. *American Journal of Public Health, 105*(10), e42–e47.

Isasi, C., Rastogi, D., & Molina, K. (2016). Health issues in Hispanic/Latino youth. *Journal of Latina/o Psychology, 4*(2), 67–82.

Izzo, C., Weiss, L., Shanahan, T., & Rodriguez-Brown, F. (2000). Parental self-efficacy and social support as predictors of parenting practices and children's socioemotional adjustment in Mexican immigrant families. *Journal of Prevention & Intervention in the Community, 20*(1–2), 197–213.

Jepson, W. (2014). Measuring 'no-win' waterscapes: Experience-based scales and classification approaches to assess household water security in colonias on the US–Mexico border. *Geoforum, 51,* 107–120.

Johnston, L., O'Malley, P., Miech, R., Bachman, J., & Schulenberg, J. (2016). *Monitoring the future national survey results on drug use, 1975–2015: Overview, key findings on adolescent drug use.* Ann Arbor, Michigan: National Academies Press. Retrieved from: http://www.monitoringthefuture.org/pubs/monographs/mtf-overview2015.pdf.

Kam, J., & Lazarevic, V. (2014). The stressful (and not so stressful) nature of language brokering: Identifying when brokering functions as a cultural stressor for Latino immigrant children in early adolescence. *Journal of Youth and Adolescence, 43*(12), 1994–2011.

Kane, R., Nicoll, A., Kahn, E., & Groves, S. (2012). *Supporting and caring for our Latino youth.* Retrieved from https://www.aamc.org/initiatives/diversity/449830/hrc5.html.

Kastanis, A., & Gates, G. J. (2013). *LGBT Latino/a individuals and Latino/a same-sex couples.* Retrieved from https://williamsinstitute.law.ucla.edu/research/census-lgbt-demographics-studies/lgbt-latino-oct-2013/.

Kaste, L., Drury, T., Horowitz, A., & Beltran, E. (1999). An evaluation of NHANES III estimates of early childhood caries. *Journal of Public Health Dentistry, 59*(3), 198–200.

Kearney, G., Chatterjee, A., Talton, J., Chen, H., Quandt, S., Summers, P., et al. (2014). The association of respiratory symptoms and indoor housing conditions among migrant farmworkers in eastern North Carolina. *Journal of Agromedicine, 19*(4), 395–405.

Korc, M., & Ford, P. (2013). Application of the water poverty index in border colonias of west Texas. *Water Policy, 15*(1), 79–97.

Krogstad, J., Stepler, R., & Lopez, M. (2015). *English proficiency on the rise among Latinos; US born driving language changes.* Retrieved from http://www.pewhispanic.org/2015/05/12/english-proficiency-on-the-rise-among-latinos/.

Kuperminc, G., Wilkins, N., Roche, C., & Alvarez-Jimenez, A. (2009). Risk, resilience, and positive development among Latino youth. In F. Villarruel, G. Carlo, J. Grau, M. Azmitia, N. Cabrera, & T. Chahin (Eds.), *Handbook of US Latino psychology.* SAGE: Los Angelos, CA.

Lara, M., Gamboa, C., Kahramanian, M., Morales, L., & Bautista, D. (2005). Acculturation and Latino health in the United States: A review of the literature and its sociopolitical context. *Annual Review of Public Health, 26,* 367–397.

Lara, M., Morgenstern, H., Duan, N., & Brook, R. (1999). Elevated asthma morbidity in Puerto Rican children. *Western Journal of Medicine, 170*(2), 75.

Lin, A., Simpkins, S., Gaskin, E., & Menjívar, C. (2016). Cultural values and other perceived benefits of organized activities: A qualitative analysis of Mexican-origin parents' perspectives in Arizona. *Applied Developmental Science, 22*(2), 89–109.

Linton, J., Griffin, M., & Shapiro, A. (2017). Detention of immigrant children. *Pediatrics, 139*(5).

Lopez, M. G. (2009). *Latinos and education: Explaining the attainment gap.* Retrieved from https://www.pewhispanic.org/2009/10/07/latinos-and-education-explaining-the-attainment-gap/. Accessed June 21, 2009.

Luthra, R., & Soehl, T. (2015). From parent to child? Transmission of educational attainment within immigrant families: Methological considerations. *Demography, 52,* 543–567.

Markides, K., & Coreil, J. (1986). The health of Hispanics in the southwestern United States: An epidemiologic paradox. *Public Health Reports, 101,* 253–265.

Marks, A., Ejesi, K., & García Coll, C. (2014). Understanding the US immigrant paradox in childhood and adolescence. *Child Development Perspectives, 8*(2), 59–64.

McDonald, Y., & Grineski, S. (2012). Disparities in access to residential plumbing: A binational comparison of environmental injustice in El Paso and Ciudad Juárez. *Population and Environment, 34*(2), 194–216.

Mendoza, F., & Dixon, L. (1999). The health and nutritional status of immigrant Hispanic children. In D. Hernandez (Ed.), *Children of immigrants: Health adjustment and public assistance* (pp. 187–224). Washingotn, D.C.: National Academies Press.

Mendoza, G., & Shaikh, N. (2015). *Tuition benefits for immigrants*. Retrieved from http://www.ncsl.org/research/immigration/tuition-benefits-for-immigrants.aspx.

Mersky, J., Topitzes, J., & Reynolds, A. (2013). Impacts of adverse childhood experiences on health, mental health, and substance use in early adulthood: A cohort study of an urban, minority sample in the US. *Child Abuse and Neglect, 37*(11), 917–925.

Murphey, D., Guzman, L., & Torres, A. (2014). *America's Hispanic children: Gaining ground, looking forward*. Retrieved from https://www.childtrends.org/wp-content/uploads/2014/09/2014-38AmericaHispanicChildren.pdf.

Nachazel, T. (2016). *The condition of education 2016*. Retrieved from https://nces.ed.gov/pubs2016/2016144.pdf.

National Immigration Law Center (NILC). (2014). *Basic facts about in-state tuition for undocumented immigrant students*. Retrieved from https://www.nilc.org/issues/education/basic-facts-instate/.

National Immigration Law Center (NILC). (2017a). *Laws & policies improving access to higher education for immigrants*. Retrieved from https://www.nilc.org/wp-content/uploads/2017/10/table-access-to-ed-toolkit.pdf.

National Immigration Law Center (NILC). (2017b). *Trump's executive orders and immigrants' access to health, food, and other public programs: Things to keep in mind when talking with immigrants*. Retrieved from https://www.nilc.org/issues/health-care/exec-orders-and-access-to-public-programs/.

National Immigration Law Center (NILC). (2018). *Health coverage maps*. Retrieved from https://www.nilc.org/issues/health-care/healthcoveragemaps/.

Nelson, L., Schneider, E., Wells, C., & Moore, M. (2004). Epidemiology of tuberculosis in the United State, 1993–2001: The need for continued vigilance. *Pediatrics, 114*(2), 333–341.

Office of Disease Prevention and Health Promotion. (2017). *Healthy people 2020: Disparities*. Retrieved from https://www.healthypeople.gov/2020/about/foundation-health-measures/Disparities.

Ogden, C., Carroll, M., Fryar, C., & Flegal, K. (2015). Prevalence of obesity among adults and youth: United States, 2011–2014. *NCHS Data Brief, 219*.

Olds, D. (2006). The nurse-family partnership: An evidence-based preventive intervention. *Infant Mental Health Journal, 27*(1), 5–25.

Painter, T. M. (2008). Connecting the dots: When the risks of HIV/STD infection appear high but the burden of infection is not known—The case of male Latino migrants in the Southern United States. *AIDS and Behavior, 12*(2), 213–226.

Paradies, Y., Ben, J., Denson, N., Elias, A., Priest, N., Pieterse, A. … Gee, G. (2015). Racism as a determinant of health: A systematic review and meta-analysis. *PLoS One, 10*(9).

Parents as Teachers. (2017). *Home page*. Retrieved from http://www.parentsasteachers.org.

Patten, E. (2016). *The nation's Latino population is defined by its youth*. Retrieved from http://www.pewhispanic.org/files/2016/04/PH_2016-04-20_LatinoYouth-Final.pdf.

The Personal responsibility and work opportunity reconciliation act (PRWORA). (1996). Retrieved from https://aspe.hhs.gov/report/personal-responsibility-and-work-opportunity-reconciliation-act-1996. Accessed June 21, 2019.

Perreira, K., & Ornelas, I. (2011). The physical and psychological well-being of immigrant children. *Future of Children, 21,* 195–218.

Phinney, J. (2003). Ethnic identity and acculturation. In K. Chun, P. Organista, & G. Marin (Eds.), *Acculturation: Advances in theory, measurement and applied research* (pp. 63–82). Washington, DC: American Psychological Association.

Popkin, B., & Udry, J. (1998). Adolescent obesity increases significantly in second and third generation US Immigrants: The National Longitudinal Study of Adolescent Health. *Journal of Nutrition, 128,* 701–706.

President's Advisory Commission on Educational Excellence for Hispanics. (2000). *Creating the will: Hispanics achieving educational excellence*. Retrieved from Washington, DC: http://eric.ed.gov/ERICWebPortal/custom/portlets/recordDetails/detailmini.jsp?_nfpb=true&_&ERICExtSearch_SearchValue_0=ED446195&ERICExtSearch_SearchType_0=no&accno=ED446195.

Quandt, S., Arcury, T., Early, J., Tapia, J., & Davis, J. (2004). Household food security among Latino farmworkers in North Carolina. *Public Health Reports, 119*, 568–576.

Quandt, S., Grzywacz, J., Trejo, G., & Arcury, T. (2014). Nutritional strategies of Latino farmworker families with preschool children: Identifying leverage points for obesity prevention. *Social Science and Medicine, 123*, 72–81. https://doi.org/10.1016/j.socscimed.2014.10.029.

Reigelhaupt, F., Carrasco, R., & Brandt, E. (2003). *Spanish: A language of indigenous peoples of the Americas. Nurturing Native Languages*. Flagstaff, AZ: Northern Arizona University.

Rhodes, S. D., Mann, L., Simán, F. M., Song, E., Alonzo, J., Downs, M. … Hall, M. A. (2015). The impact of local immigration enforcement policies on the health of immigrant Hispanics/Latinos in the United States. *American Journal of Public Health, 105*(2), 329–337. https://doi.org/10.2105/ajph.2014.302218.

Robert Wood Johnson Foundation. Retrieved from http://stateofobesity.org/disparities/latinos/.

Romero, L., Pazol, K., Warner, L., Cox, S., Kroelinger, C., Besera, G., et al. (2016). Reduced disparities in birth rates among teens aged 15–19 Years—United States, 2006–2007 and 2013–2014. *Morbidity & Mortality Weekly Reports, 65*(16), 409–414.

Romero, A., & Roberts, R. (2003). Stress within a bicultural context for adolescents of Mexican descent. *Cultural Diversity and Ethnic Minority Psychology, 9*, 171–184.

Rosenthal, L., Earnshaw, V., Carroll-Scott, A., Henderson, K., Peters, S., McCaslin, C., et al. (2015). Weight- and race-based bullying: Health associations among urban adolescents. *Journal of Health Psychology, 20*(4), 401–412.

Rumbaut, R. (1997). Assimilation and its discontents: Between rhetoric and reality. *International Migration Review, 31*, 923–960.

Russell, S., & Fish, J. (2016). Mental health in lesbian, gay, bisexual, and transgender (LGBT) youth. *Annual Review of Clinical Psychology, 12*, 465–487.

Russell, S., Sinclair, K., Poteat, V., & Koenig, B. (2012). Adolescent health and harassment based on discriminatory bias. *American Journal of Public Health, 102*(3), 493–495.

Ryan, C., Huebner, D., Diaz, R., & Sanchez, J. (2009). Family rejection as a predictor of negative health outcomes in white and Latino lesbian, gay, and bisexual young adults. *Pediatrics, 123*(1), 346–352.

Ryan, C., Russell, S., Huebner, D., Diaz, R., & Sanchez, J. (2010). Family acceptance in adolescence and the health of LGBT young adults. *Journal of Child and Adolescent Psychiatric Nursing, 23*(4), 205–213.

Sanders-Phillips, K., Settles-Reaves, B., Walker, D., & Brownlow, J. (2009). Social inequality and racial discrimination: Risk factors for health disparities in children of color. *Pediatrics, 124*(Suppl 3), S176–S186.

Sangrigoli, S., & De Schonen, S. (2004). Recognition of own-race and other-race faces by three-month-old infants. *Journal of Child Psychology and Psychiatry, 45*, 1219–1227.

Schneider, B., Martinez, S., & Ownes, A. (2006). Barriers to educational opportunities for Hispanics in the United States. In M. Tienda, F. Mitchell, & National Research Council (US) Panel on Hispanics in the United States (Eds.), *Hispanics and the future of America; editors*. Washington, D.C.: National Academies Press.

Schumacher, L., Pawson, I., & Kretchmer, N. (1987). Growth of immigrant children in the newcomer schools of San Francisco. *Pediatrics, 80*(6), 861–868.

Schwartz, S., Chester, A., Lopez, S., & Vargas Poppe, S. (2016). *Latino children's coverage reaches historic high, but too many remain uninsured*. Retrieved from Washington, DC: ccf.georgetown.edu/wp-content/uploads/2016/12/LatinoChildren12_15.pdf.

Schwartz, S., Unger, J., Zamboanga, B., & Szapocznik, J. (2010). Rethinking the concept of acculturation: Implications for theory and research. *The American Psychologist, 65*(4), 237–251.

Schwartzenberg, S., Kuo, A., Linton, J., Flanagan, P., Council on Community Pediatrics, & Committee on Nutrition. (2015). Promoting food security for all children: American Academy of Pediatrics Policy Statement. *Pediatrics, 136*(5), e1431–e1438.

Stein, G., Gonzalez, L., Cupito, A., Kiang, L., & Supple, A. (2015). The protective role of familism in the lives of Latino adolescents. *Journal of Family Issues, 36*(10), 1255–1273.

Stepler, R., & Lopez, M. (2016). *US Latino population growth and dispersion has slowed since onset of the great recession*. Washington, DC: Pew Research Center. (September).

Suro, R., Suárez-Orozco, M., & Canizales, S. (2016). *Removing insecurity: How American children will benefit from President Obama's executive action on immigration*. UCLA Tomás Rivera Policy Institute. Los Angeles, California. Retrieved from: http://trpi.org/pdfs/research_report.pdf.

Szalacha, L., Erkut, S., García Coll, C., Alarcón, O., Fields, J., & Ceder, I. (2003). Discrimination and Puerto Rican children's and adolescents' mental health. *Cultural Diversity and Ethnic Minority Psychology, 9*(2), 141–155.

Texas Secretary of State Office. *Colonias Program*. Retrieved from http://www.sos.state.tx.us/border/colonias/index.shtml.

The State of Obesity. (2014). *Racial and Ethnic Disparities in Obesity: Trust for America's Health*.

Toomey, R., Umaña-Taylor, A., Williams, D., Harvey-Mendoza, E., Jahromi, L., & Updegraff, K. (2014). Impact of Arizona's SB 1070 immigration law on utilization of health care and public assistance among Mexican-origin adolescent mothers and their mother figures. *American Journal of Public Health, 104*(Suppl 1), S28–S34.

Umana-Taylor, A. (2004). Ethnic identity and self-esteem: examining the role of social context. *Journal of Adolescence, 27*(2), 139–146.

Umaña-Taylor, A., & Updegraff, K. (2007). Latino adolescents' mental health: Exploring the interrelations among discrimination, ethnic identity, cultural orientation, self-esteem, and depressive symptoms. *Journal of Adolescence, 30*(4), 549–567. https://doi.org/10.1016/j.adolescence.2006.08.002.

United States Environmental Protection Agency. (2014). *Children's environmental health disparities: Hispanic and Latino American children and asthma*. Retrieved from https://www.epa.gov/sites/production/files/2014-05/documents/hd_hispanic_asthma.pdf.

United States-Mexico Border Health Commission. (2010). *Health disparities and the US-Mexico border: Challenges and opportunities: a white paper*. El Paso: United States-Mexico Border Health Commission.

United States-México Border Health Commission. (2014a). *Access to health care in the US-México border region: Challenges and opportunities: A white paper*. El Paso: United States-Mexico Border Health Commission.

United States-México Border Health Commission. (2014b). Report: Health status in the U.S.-Mexico border region. El Paso: United States-Mexico Border Health Commission.

United States-México Border Health Commission (Ed.) (2015). *Healthy border 2020: A prevention & health promotion initiative: A white paper*.

US Customs and Border Protection. (2016). *United States border patrol southwest family unit subject and unaccompanied Alien children apprehensions fiscal year 2016*. Retrieved from https://www.cbp.gov/newsroom/stats/southwest-border-unaccompanied-children/fy-2016.

US Department of Health and Human Services. (2000). *Healthy people 2010: Understanding and improving health* (2nd ed.). Washington, D.C.: US Government Printing Office.

US Department of Labor. (2016). *Findings from the National Agricultural Workers Survey (NAWS) 2013–2014*. Retrieved from https://www.doleta.gov/naws/pages/research/research-reports.cfm.

Valdez, C., Padilla, B., & Valentine, J. (2013). Consequences of Arizona's immigration policy on social capital among Mexican mothers with unauthorized immigration status. *Hispanic Journal of Behavioral Sciences, 35*(3), 303–322.

Valencia-Garcia, D., Simoni, J., Alegría, M., & Takeuchi, D. (2012). Social capital, acculturation, mental health, and perceived access to services among Mexican American women. *Journal of Consulting and Clinical Psychology, 80*(2), 77–85.

Vallejos, Q., Quandt, S., & Arcury, T. (2009). The condition of farmworker housing in the Eastern United States. In S. Quandt & T. Arcury (Eds.), *Latino Farmworkers in the Eastern United States: Health, safety, and justice* (pp. 37–69). New York: Springer.

Vargas, E., & Ybarra, V. (2017). US citizen children of undocumented parents: The link between state immigration policy and the health of Latino children. *Journal of Immigrant and Minority Health, 19*(4), 913–920.

Victory, K., Cabrera, N., Larson, D., Reynolds, K., Latura, J., Thomson, C., et al. (2017). Comparison of fluoride levels in tap and bottled water and reported use of fluoride supplementation in a United States-Mexico Border Community. *Frontiers in Public Health, 5*, 87.

Villarruel, A. M., Jemmott, J. B., 3rd, & Jemmott, L. S. (2006). A randomized controlled trial testing an HIV prevention intervention for Latino youth. *Archives of Pediatrics and Adolescent Medicine, 160*(8), 772–777.

Viruell-Fuentes, E., Miranda, P., & Abdulrahim, S. (2012). More than culture: Structural racism, intersectionality theory, and immigrant health. *Social Science and Medicine, 75*(12), 2099–2106.

Vogel, M., Monesson, A., & Scott, L. (2012). Building biases in infancy: The influence of race on face and voice emotion matching. *Developmental Science, 15*(3), 359–372.

Weathers, A., Minkovitz, C., O'Campo, P., & Diener-West, M. (2003). Health services use by children of migratory agricultural workers: exploring the role of need for care. *Pediatrics, 111*(5), 956–963.

Wilson, K. (1978). *The developmental psychology of the black child*. New York: Africana Research Publications.

Xiao, N., Quinn, P., Liu, S., Ge, L., Pascalis, O., & Lee, K. (2017). Older but not younger infants associate own-race faces with happy music and other-race faces with sad music. *Developmental Science, 21*(2), e12537.

Yoshikawa, H., & Kholoptseva, J. (2013). *Unauthorized immigrant parents and their children's development: A summary of the evidence*. Washington, DC: Migration Policy Institute.

Zhang, A., Musu-Gillette, L., & Oudekerk, B. (2016). *Indicators of school crime and safety: 2015* (NCES 2016-079/NCJ 249758). Jessup, MD: National Center for Education Statistics.

Zimmerman, E. B., Woolf, S. H., & Haley, A. (2015). Understanding the relationship between education and health: A review of the evidence and an examination of community perspectives. In *Population health: behavioral and social science insights* (pp. 347–384). AHRQ Publication (15-0002).

Chapter 5
Substance Use Among Latinx Adolescents in the USA: Scope, Theory, Interventions, and Next Steps

Flavio F. Marsiglia and Elizabeth Kiehne

Abstract Substance use and abuse among Latinx adolescents is an important public health challenge because adolescents are highly vulnerable to substance use, and substance use can have a negative impact on their overall health and well-being. In this chapter, we provide a very brief history of the growth of the Latinx population in the USA and outline the epidemiology of substance use, highlighting within-group differences, including differences by country of origin, gender, and age, and explore substance use within the framework of the immigrant paradox. We also propose the use of an ecodevelopmental approach to preventing and reducing substance use among youth and describe an innovative evidence-based intervention, known as *keepin' it REAL*, for early adolescents. We conclude with a call for action, including further research to explore the roles of culture and potential sources of data that can use used to elucidate both risk and protective factors.

Keywords Substance use · Adolescent · Evidence-based intervention · Adolescent · Culture · Latinx

Preceded only by the American Indian nations, the Latinx population has been part of the social and cultural fabric of the USA for more than 450 years. St. Augustine, Florida (1565) and Santa Fe, New Mexico (1607) are the two oldest towns continuously inhabited by Latinx communities in the country (McWilliams, 2016). While Florida and New Mexico continue today to be home to sizable Latinx communities (Rochin, 2016), Latinx communities have also thrived in other areas of the country because of a variety of historical and geopolitical factors (Massey & Pren, 2012). The Mexican-American community in the Southwest and on the West Coast, the Puerto Rican and Dominican communities in New York City, and the Cuban community in Miami are examples of large historical Latinx enclaves in the USA. There are also growing Latinx communities in every state and territory of the country (Passel, Cohn & Lopez, 2011). In fact, since the turn of the century, new Latinx settlement communities have emerged in untraditional states such as those in the South and Midwest (Painter, 2008), and the Latinx population has grown into the largest and

---

F. F. Marsiglia (✉) · E. Kiehne
School of Social Work, Phoenix, AZ, USA
e-mail: marsiglia@asu.edu

© Springer Nature Switzerland AG 2020
A. D. Martínez and S. D. Rhodes (eds.), *New and Emerging Issues in Latinx Health*, https://doi.org/10.1007/978-3-030-24043-1_5

most widely dispersed ethnic–racial group in the USA. According to the latest data, 18% of the total US population identifies as Latinx (US Census Bureau, 2017).

The terms "Latina," "Latino," and "Latinx" are umbrella terms used to identify a heterogeneous group of people with diverse backgrounds in terms of race, culture, nativity, and nationality who share a historical link to Spain, the Spanish conquest, and colonialism through their ancestors. Currently, most Latinx persons in the USA are of Mexican ancestry (63%; US Census Bureau, 2017). Puerto Ricans comprise the second largest subgroup (approximately 10%), followed by Latinx persons who migrated from or can trace their ancestry to the Caribbean, Central America, or South America. The majority of Latinx persons in the USA were born in this country (65%), with 1 in 3 having immigrated (US Census Bureau, 2017). Of those who are foreign-born, 8.5 million experience challenges related to unauthorized legal status in the USA (Zong & Batalova, 2016).

Although the Latinx population is the nation's largest ethnic–racial-minority group, there is insufficient understanding of and information about their health, and more rigorous research is needed to understand the factors influencing their health and well-being and the strategies that can be harnessed to promote their health and prevent disease. Moreover, the Latinx population in the USA is heterogeneous and even less is understood about substantial within-group health-related differences (Ruiz, Campos, & Garcia, 2016). The Latinx population in the USA is drawn from a diverse mix of countries, cultural backgrounds, and language use. The limited research available appears to indicate that, despite the psychosocial and physical risks they encounter, in the aggregate, the Latinx population in the USA has some significant objective health advantages compared with non-Latinx populations. For example, the rates of drug and alcohol use are lower among Latinx persons than in other ethnic–racial groups (Delva et al., 2005). Relative to the national average, fewer Latinx persons report tobacco use, alcohol consumption in the past month, and heavy alcohol use (i.e., five or more consecutive drinks on five or more occasions in the past month; Substance Abuse and Mental Health Services Administration [SAMHSA], 2014). The Latinx population also has one of the lowest reported illicit substance use rates of all ethnic–racial groups in the USA (SAMHSA, 2014).

Although the rates of drug and alcohol use are lower among the Latinx population as a whole, the rates are not lower in all age subgroups, particularly adolescents and young adults (Delva et al., 2005). Latinx youth in middle and high school are more prone to substance use than other youth. In fact, compared with White and Black adolescents, Latinx adolescents report the highest rates of use of illicit substances, inhalants, and alcohol (Johnston, O'Malley, Miech, Bachman, & Schulenberg, 2015).

Substance use and abuse among Latinx adolescents is an important phenomenon to consider because adolescents are highly vulnerable to substance use, and this use can have a negative impact on their overall health and well-being. For example, substance use can compromise the healthy adolescent brain and normal psychosocial development. From a neuroscientific perspective, youth who engage in substance use have a reduced capacity for complex behaviors, higher-order cognitive functioning, and communication between different regions of the brain (Bava, Jacobus, Thayer, & Tapert, 2013; Squeglia, Jacobus, & Tapert, 2009). Adolescent substance use is also associated with increased risk of psychosocial and behavioral challenges, compromised academic performance, early and risky sexual activity, delinquent behaviors, and higher rates of suicidal ideation and suicide (Fergusson, Horwood, & Swain-Campbell, 2002; Kulis, Marsiglia, & Nagoshi, 2010). Furthermore, youth who initiate substance use in adolescence, particularly early adolescence, are more likely to later engage in substance use and abuse, reaching addiction (Fergusson et al., 2002; National Center on Addiction and Substance Abuse, 2002).

Substance use and abuse among Latinx youth is especially important to understand and address because the Latinx population is the largest and most rapidly growing segment of the US population and is the youngest ethnic–racial group in the country (Patten, 2016; US Census Bureau, 2017). One in five individuals under the age of 18 identifies as Latinx (Passel et al., 2011). Substance use is a particularly crucial issue affecting Latinx adolescents' health and well-being, given the high rates of use and the adverse consequences to the individual and society.

In this chapter, we describe the epidemiology and what is currently known about Latinx substance use in the USA. The diversity within the Latinx population is emphasized to demonstrate the differential rates in the use of alcohol, tobacco, and other drugs, and insights are offered into the etiology of these differences. We then focus on substance use among Latinx adolescents and the factors leading to the increased risk for Latinx youth. We approach Latinx adolescents' health and well-being from an ecodevelopmental perspective. This perspective suggests that the health and well-being of Latinx adolescents result from the interaction of many converging factors, such as family bonds, social support, collectivism, migration, developmental factors, acculturation, and discrimination. We then discuss the importance of prevention efforts during early adolescence and emphasize the need for culturally congruent prevention interventions that impart multiple drug-resistance strategies as recommended by communication competence theory. We present a specific intervention developed with and for Latinx youth through community-engaged research as a case study. We conclude with recommendations for future research to advance our understanding of the intersection of ethnicity and gender as a pending challenge in our efforts to promote the health and well-being of all Latinx youth.

Epidemiology of Latinx Substance Use: Within-Group Differences

According to most metrics, the rates of substance use and abuse are lower for the Latinx population in the USA as a whole (Delva et al., 2005; SAMHSA, 2014). However, rates of use are elevated for subgroups of the Latinx population. Substance use and abuse vary according to immigration-related factors such as nativity, generation status, and level of acculturation, as well as developmental factors, including age. The variables outlined here are some of the most salient factors associated with the different levels of substance use and abuse in the Latinx population.

Country of Origin Differences in Latinx Substance Use

Patterns of drug use differ according to nationality and national heritage. For example, rates of substance use and disorders are higher among mainland Puerto Ricans and Mexican-Americans relative to other Latinx persons (Alegría et al., 2007; SAMHSA, 2013). The rates of binge drinking and lifetime rates of illicit drug use are also higher for these two national-origin groups than for those from Cuba and Central/South America (Alvarez, Jason, Olson, Ferrari, & Davis, 2007). Cigarette use is significantly higher among Puerto Ricans than persons from Cuba or Central/South America, and the lowest rates of tobacco use are found among persons from Mexico (CDC, 2016a). Compared with Mexican-heritage persons, those of Puerto Rican heritage are more likely to experience drug abuse or dependence, but Mexican-heritage persons are more likely to report an alcohol disorder in their lifetime (Otiniano Verissimo, Grella, Amaro, & Gee, 2014). This trend has remained stable over the years, as older epidemiologic data suggest that persons from Mexico are more prone to frequent and heavy alcohol use (Nielsen, 2000). Mexican youth are also more likely to report heavy alcohol use (Delva et al., 2005).

National origin may have some explanatory power into the existing differences in use rates. However, multiple factors affect substance use attitudes and behaviors of Latinx persons. Factors such as socioeconomic status and acculturation status provide further insight and help us avoid oversimplification (Sudhinaraset, Wigglesworth, & Takeuchi, 2016).

Latinx Substance Use and the Immigrant Paradox

Immigration-related factors also explain some of the within-group differences in rates of substance use and abuse in the Latinx population, a phenomenon the "immigrant paradox" attempts to explain. Among Latinx persons, the rates of substance use and disorders are lower among those who are foreign-born than those who are born in the USA (Borges et al., 2011; Grant et al., 2004; Lipsky & Caetano, 2009). US-born Latinx persons are roughly twice as likely as those who are foreign-born to drink heavily and use illicit substances (Lipsky & Caetano, 2009). They are also more likely to use cigarettes (Acevedo-Garcia, Pan, Jun, Osypuk, & Emmons, 2005; Centers for Disease Control and Prevention [CDC], 2015). This trend exists among Latinx youth as well; foreign-born Latinx youth tend to report less substance use than their US-born counterparts (Barger & Gallo, 2008; SAMHSA, 2011). Additionally, relative to US-born Latinx persons, those who were born in another country are less likely to experience a substance use disorder, irrespective of age at the time of immigration or number of years in the USA (Alegría et al., 2007; Otiniano Verissimo et al., 2014). Nearly 20% of US-born Latinx persons have a substance use disorder in their lifetime, compared with 6% of those who are foreign-born (Canino, Vega, Sribney, Warner, & Alegria, 2008).

Related to nativity, trends in substance use and abuse among Latinx persons also emerge by generation status and level of acculturation. Notable discrepancies in substance use disorders by generation status exist among women; relative to first-generation Latinx women, second-generation women are over nine times more likely to report a substance use disorder, and third-generation Latinx women are 18 times more likely (Alegría et al., 2007). Among adolescents, Latinx youth of the second generation or later are two to three times more likely to engage in problematic alcohol use as well as marijuana and other drug use compared with first-generation (i.e., immigrant) youth (Peña et al., 2008). Regarding acculturation status, the findings of a host of studies indicate that Latinx persons of all ages who are more acculturated are more prone to drug and alcohol use and disorders (De La Rosa, 2002; Salas-Wright, Clark, Vaughn, & Córdova, 2015). The results of future research will illuminate whether it is the loss of the culture of the origin or the gain in mainstream culture that proves more problematic for drug and alcohol use and abuse.

The immigrant paradox applies to the relationship between substance use and nativity, generation status, and level of acculturation (Vega, Alderete, Kolody, & Aguilar-Gaxiola, 1998). The immigrant paradox phenomenon is counterintuitive because immigrants often live under challenging conditions and report lower economic status than natives, but their health outcomes, including substance use, do not match their relative disadvantage (Cristini, Scacchi, Perkins, Bless, & Vieno, 2015). A number of different mechanisms may be at play in the immigrant paradox as it pertains to substance use.

According to the assimilation theory, as individuals spend more time in the USA, they learn and adopt more permissive prodrug use norms; they also increasingly abandon the values associated with their culture of origin, diminishing their more protective traditional views on substance use (Caetano & Clark, 2003; Vega et al., 1998). The assertion that more lenient drug norms typify "mainstream" American culture compared with Latin American cultures may be supported by the finding that more acculturated youth report greater normative approval of substance use (i.e., prodrug attitudes) (Kulis, Marsiglia, & Nieri, 2009; Marsiglia, Kulis, Wagstaff, Elek, & Dran, 2005). Consistently lower rates of drug and alcohol use in many Latin American nations relative to rates in the USA may present additional support for the more normative nature of substance use in this country (Caetano & Medina-Mora, 1988; Medina-Mora, Conver, Sepulveda, Otero, & De La Rosa, 1989; Warner, Canino, & Colón, 2001). These explanations must be considered with caution, however, as they may oversimplify the acculturation process, treating it as if it were a linear process with those who are more acculturated versus those who are less acculturated at higher risk.

"Natural selection" is another consideration. According to this concept, premigration selection occurs, with healthier and more adventurous and entrepreneurial individuals being more likely to migrate (Sanchez et al., 2014; Walsh, Djalovski, Boniel-Nissim, & HarelFisch, 2014). In combination with other protective factors, this selection process helps provide an explanation for the better health outcomes of recent immigrants to the USA compared with immigrants who have been in the country longer.

Acculturative stress, on the other hand, may precipitate higher drug and alcohol use among those who have been in the country longer. As suggested by acculturative stress theory, stress often accompanies the acculturation process and substance use is a maladaptive response to such stress (Buchanan & Smokowski, 2009; Kulis et al., 2009; Marsiglia et al., 2005). In the case of adolescents, the complexity of family and peer relationships appears to be instrumental in the link between acculturative stress and substance use (Buchanan & Smokowski, 2009). Similarly, protective features of the culture of origin may diminish with time in the USA and acculturation. Family closeness decreases across generations, which is problematic because this factor is associated with positive parenting practices and, thus, reduced substance use (Bacio, Mays, & Lau, 2013).

Acculturation gaps between parents and youth can also increase young people's risk of substance use. Acculturation gaps in both mainstream USA and heritage culture typically emerge because children tend to adopt the new culture more quickly than adults and sometimes shed the culture of origin more rapidly. These gaps can lead to parent–child value conflicts, ineffective communication, and erosion of protective family ties, which make young people more vulnerable to substance use (Marsiglia et al., 2005; Martinez, 2006) (The next section expands on the complex nature of the intergenerational acculturation gap and stress.).

Lastly, as youth from immigrant families become older, they access new social networks which separate them from their families and ethnic enclaves; they encounter new environments in which alcohol and other drugs are easily accessible (Marsiglia et al., 2005). Existing evidence suggests that as youth acculturate, they report having more substance-using peers (Bacio et al., 2013). Additionally, as parents acculturate, they may place less emphasis on parental authority and more on youth's independence; these parenting characteristics are then associated with less firm parental rules and parental supervision, which increase the risk of initiation of substance use (Roche et al., 2014).

Although the literature documenting the existence of the immigrant paradox is extensive, some research findings suggest the opposite trend may occur for substance use. For example, stronger identification with mainstream US culture and practices has been found to predict less heavy drinking for Latinx boys (Schwartz et al., 2014). Controlling for location or context seems to be important in sorting out some of these contradictions. Additionally, thinking about acculturation as a bidimensional process in which individuals can be more or less oriented to both their culture of origin and mainstream US culture, allowing for biculturalism, is important (Marsiglia, Kiehne, & Ayers, 2018). In supportive contexts—regardless of immigrant generation—bicultural individuals have been found to have better physical and psychologic health than those who are not bicultural (LaFromboise, Coleman, & Gerton, 1993). Thus, the immigrant paradox is less straightforward than previously thought, applying to the experience of some Latinx persons but not others, further illustrating the within-group diversity of this community.

Gender-Based Influences and Associated Latinx Cultural Values in Substance Use

Differences in substance use and abuse within the Latinx population also exist by gender. Compared with women, men are four times more likely to have an alcohol use disorder in their lifetime, roughly three times more likely to experience a drug use disorder, and over twice as likely to smoke (Canino et al., 2008; CDC, 2016b; Otiniano Verissimo et al., 2014). Women of Mexican and Puerto Rican origin are less likely than men to engage in alcohol use of any kind, including heavy drinking (Nielsen, 2000). Similar trends have been reported for male and female Latinx adolescents (Delva et al., 2005).

Gender differences in substance use result in part from cultural gender role norms. Within the Latinx community—as in most communities—social norms, gender roles, and socialization patterns have long influenced substance use attitudes and behaviors, particularly alcohol use (Kulis, Marsiglia, Ayers, Booth, & Nuño-Gutiérrez, 2012; Otiniano Verissimo et al., 2014). Historically, in Latin America, the concept of *marianismo*, based on the idea of the Virgin Mary in the Roman Catholic tradition, portrays women as docile, selfless, chaste, and pure (de la Torre, 2009). Women's primary purpose and value in life are to be a supportive wife and nurturing mother and not to work outside the home. Women traditionally existed within the private domain of the home, with men operating within the public sphere (Sanchez, Whittaker, Hamilton, & Zayas, 2016). The traditional concept of femininity once socialized women to maintain a submissive attitude, focus on the family, and be morally virtuous (Toro-Morn, 2008). This traditional set of ideas about women is changing, and alternative perspectives have emerged as a Latinx reinterpretation of feminist theory. *Hembrísmo* is one such example, a concept originally proposed as an alternative to *marianismo*; this concept emphasizes the strengths of Latinx women and promotes empowerment and social change (Comas-Diaz, 1987). Through *hembrísmo* and related perspectives, female Latinx youth are engaged in the complex task of reconciling their grandmothers' and mothers' ideas about gender roles with their own perceptions about womanhood in a globalized context (Thorin, 2003). This search for integration and change includes the emergence of new attitudes and behaviors regarding substance use.

In contrast, the notion of *machismo* portrays men as assertive, self-centered, and virile (de la Torre, 2009). Traditional *machismo* involves hypermasculinity, domination over women, and aggression (Herrera, Owens, & Mallinckrodt, 2013; Rhodes et al., 2011). Latinx men who adhere to traditional *machismo* norms display restricted emotional expression, aggression, and antisocial behavior (Arciniega, Anderson, Tovar-Blank, & Tracey, 2008). The stereotypical views of masculinity are also changing in the Latinx community and alternatives, such as *caballerismo*, have emerged. *Caballerismo* rescues the positive and prosocial traits of *machismo* and aims at overturning its negative and oppressive dimensions (Arciniega et al., 2008). *Caballerismo* is a more flexible masculine style; men are caretakers and value honor, dignity, and respect for others (Hassy, Garza, Sullivan, & Serrers, 2016). Similarly to young

Latinx women, young Latinx men find themselves having to choose between competing sets of values and expectations, which include attitudes and behaviors about substance use.

Socialization patterns based on traditional notions of femininity and masculinity put men at greater risk than women for substance use for several reasons. First, gender norms lead to culturally-grounded gender expectations related to drug and alcohol use. The archetypical "pure" woman portrayed by the concept of *marianismo* has had implications for abstinence from alcohol and other drugs among women, at least in public. Women's alcohol use has carried negative social consequences (Perea & Slater, 1999); thus, gender norms have discouraged women from using and abusing alcohol, tobacco, and other drugs (Medina-Mora & Rojas Guiot, 2003).

Conversely, for men, *machismo* normalizes substance use and abuse behaviors, as these behaviors have historically been one important dimension of the archetypical *macho*. Heavy drinking and other predominantly negative behaviors complement the notion of hypermasculinity of men (Rhodes et al., 2011; Herrera et al., 2013). During social events such as family gatherings, men have the widespread expectation to use and abuse alcohol (De La Rosa, 2002). Accordingly, among men, gender role norms have traditionally encouraged permissive attitudes toward substance use and particularly heavy drinking, by promoting hypermasculinity, aggressiveness, and impulsiveness (Alaniz, 1996; Unger et al., 2002).

Because women traditionally inhabit the private sphere, and men the public sphere (de la Torre, 2009), acculturating Latinx men in the USA develop more prodrug norms than Latinx women (Caetano, 1987; Zamboanga, Schwartz, Jarvis, & Van Tyne, 2009). Because of differences in Latinx child-rearing practices for male and female offspring, male adolescents have more freedom of movement than their sisters (Marsiglia, Kulis, Hussaini, Nieri, & Becerra, 2010). Accordingly, male adolescents have more substance-using friends and more drug offers at younger ages than do female adolescents (Marsiglia et al., 2010; National Institute on Drug Abuse [NIDA], 2003a). Conversely, Latinx women have lower exposure to prodrug norms in the USA, in part because of the traditional gender role expectation that lead them to spend more supervised time in the home doing gendered domestic tasks (Williams, Alvarez, & Andrade Hauck, 2002). Female adolescents who adhere to traditional gender role norms tend to use substances less. Higher levels of parental monitoring and less exposure to risky environments, such as unsupervised parties or bars, explain some of the lower rates of substance use among female adolescents (Benjet, Borges, Mendez, Casanova, & Medina-Mora, 2014). However, the social and cultural sheltering of Latinx women can sometimes work against them. When young women encounter risky situations, they may not possess the skills to cope with them, leading to greater vulnerability. Furthermore, in some cases, the first drug offers that young women receive are from their romantic partners or boyfriends, adding a potentially coercive power dimension to the risky situation (Marsiglia, Kulis, Rodriguez, Becerra, & Castillo, 2009).

Related to gender-role norms that lead men to have more mainstream culture socialization, discrimination also partly mediates the relationship between gender and substance use. Latinx men report higher rates of discrimination than do Latinx women, likely because of men's greater involvement in the public sphere (Mann-Jackson et al., 2018). A maladaptive stress management response to discrimination is substance use (Otiniano Verissimo et al., 2014; Pérez, Fortuna, & Alegría, 2008).

As gender norms change, the gender gap related to substance use is narrowing within the Latinx population in the USA and across Latin America (Marsiglia, Yabiku, et al., 2011; Zapata-Roblyer, Grzywacz, Cervantes, & Merten, 2016). This phenomenon has implications for prevention and intervention research, a topic that we will revisit later in this chapter.

Age Differences in Substance Use

Developmental differences affect substance use and are also important to consider within the Latinx population. Rates of substance use also vary greatly by age group and ethnicity/race. The rates of drug and alcohol use among Latinx adolescents are not as low as among older Latinx persons (Delva et al., 2005). Latinx youth in middle and high school are more prone to substance use, with the exception of cigarettes, than their White and Black peers (CDC, 2014; Johnston et al., 2015; SAMHSA, 2011). The rates of self-reported use of alcohol, marijuana, inhalants, cocaine, hallucinogens, methamphetamines, heroin, ecstasy, steroids, injected drugs, and prescription drugs used recreationally are highest among Latinx youth (CDC, 2014). Additionally, they report the most binge drinking (CDC, 2014). Among Latinx youth, the reported rates of use of a variety of substances are highest in 8th grade and decrease in later grades (Johnston et al., 2015; SAMHSA, 2011). It is worth noting, however, that this reported decline comes from school-based surveys. The dropout rate tends to be higher for adolescents who use alcohol or drugs than for other students, and the dropout rate for Latinx adolescents is one of the highest for any ethnic–racial group (Child Trends, 2014). Thus, these declines in substance use associated with age warrant cautious interpretation.

Etiology of Adolescent Substance Use

The higher rate of substance use found among adolescents is not surprising, as individuals are most vulnerable to engage in a number of risky behaviors, including substance use, during this developmental stage of life (Steinberg, 1991). Adolescents' common vulnerability to risk-taking behavior stems in part from a more sensitive socio-emotional system that leads to sensation and reward-seeking, particularly when among peers. Additionally, the cognitive control system that enables self-control and longer-term planning is weaker (Casey, Jones, & Hare, 2008; Spear, 2010; Steinberg, 2008). This heightened sensitivity to reward, coupled with proneness to impulsivity, is part of the etiology of youth's vulnerability to risk-taking behavior (Casey et al., 2008).

Genetic and biologic factors make youth universally vulnerable to drug and alcohol use (Brook et al., 1998; Hopfer, Crowley, & Hewitt, 2003). However, it is unclear why some adolescents use substances while others abstain. More than 40 theories have been developed in an attempt to answer this question (Lettieri, Sayers, & Pearson, 1980). Each theory highlights a different set of developmental, personality, interpersonal, biologic, or environmental factors that precede experimentation with and ongoing use of substances among adolescents (Petraitis, Flay, & Miller, 1995). For example, family interaction theory highlights the importance of parental affection, support, and control (Brook, Brook, Gordon, Whiteman, & Cohen, 1990). In contrast, social control theory emphasizes the roles of attachment to family, neighborhood disorganization, and social values in deviant peer relationships and, ultimately, substance use involvement (Elliott, Huizinga, & Ageton, 1985; Elliott, Huizinga, & Menard, 1989). Each theory presents an understanding of the relationships between one subset of constructs relevant to adolescent substance use while downplaying or neglecting others. Thus, we contend that the phenomenon of Latinx adolescent substance use is best considered using ecodevelopmental theory.

Ecodevelopmental Theory

Ecodevelopmental theory recognizes a multitude of protective and detrimental environmental forces that act on an individual to influence substance use (Szapocznik & Coatsworth, 1999). This theory is composed of three integrated components: (a) social-ecological theory, (b) developmental theory, and (c) social interaction theory. It identifies protective assets within youth's social ecology that contribute to abstinence and low use of substances. Accordingly, relative to other perspectives, ecodevelopmental theory presents a more complete, albeit complex, picture of the antecedents and correlates of adolescent substance use. The theory can be useful to advance knowledge about Latinx youth substance use and abuse. It integrates certain processes and factors such as those pertaining to cognition and personality. The multivariate focus of the theory has made it commonly applied to the study of adolescent risk behavior and development of prevention interventions, and it is especially relevant for ethnic–racial-minority youth for whom culture is a strength and a source of resiliency against risk factors such as substance use (Gosin, Marsiglia, & Hecht, 2003).

Through the ecodevelopmental theory, the factors, including interpersonal, social, cultural, and structural, that influence substance use can be identified, explored, better understood, and intervened upon. These critical factors may include both protective factors that improve one's ability to cope with or overcome challenging experiences, known as resiliency, and risk factors that increase the likelihood of engaging in risk-taking behavior (Bogenschneider, 1996; Marsiglia & Kulis, 2015).

An Ecodevelopmental Approach to Substance Use Among Latinx Adolescents

Ecodevelopmental theory is a contextual framework that places high importance on the study of individuals within their unique social-ecological contexts (Pantin et al., 2003; Szapocznik & Coatsworth, 1999). The model highlights youth's predispositions to and protections from substance use and the interrelations between these factors. The model derives from Bronfenbrenner's ecologic systems theory (1986, 1994), which emphasizes various environmental systems that influence adolescent development and behavior. The theory notes five nested environmental contexts that influence adolescents and their development processes, including the microsystem, mesosystem, exosystem, macrosystem, and chronosystem. Within each system, various variables and processes positively and negatively influence adolescent health, including substance use, representing sources of risk or protection. Risk factors are influences in an adolescent's life that make him or her more vulnerable to substance use, and protective factors are conditions that diminish the probability of substance use. Although many risk and protective factors are common to the youth of all ethnic–racial backgrounds, Latinx youth experience some unique ecodevelopmental aspects related to factors such as family migration experiences, sociopolitical contexts, and culturally based family influences and expectations. Many of these special considerations in the study of substance use among Latinx adolescents make up the focus of the present discussion, which is organized by the environmental system.

Microsystemic Influences

The microsystem involves contexts in which youth participate directly (Pantin et al., 2003; Szapocznik & Coatsworth, 1999). It concerns the interactions between the individual and her or his surroundings, including the peer, school, neighborhood, and family contexts. Microsystemic influences are highly important and have the largest and most direct impact on adolescents' developmental processes (Coatsworth, Pantin, & Szapocznik, 2002). Peer-related predictors of drug and alcohol use include peer substance use and other delinquent behaviors (Brook et al., 1998; Schinke, Schwim, Hopkins, & Wahlstom, 2016). Neighborhood and school influences include factors such as drug availability and levels of social disorganization within the community (Yabiku et al., 2007). Family-related predictors of substance use are posited to be the most influential (Schwartz, Pantin, Szapocznik, & Coatsworth, 2003) and include factors such as the quality of the parent–child relationship and communication, parental substance use, family conflict, and parenting behaviors such as parental monitoring and involvement (Brook et al., 1998; NIDA, 2003b). In the case of Latinx adolescents, several parenting factors are protective against substance use. For example, the parenting style for many Latinx individuals is characterized by high levels of parental involvement and monitoring and the sanctioning of parental authority and firm control over youth until an older age (Roche et al., 2014). These practices have a protective effect on children.

Mesosystemic Influences

Often, microsystemic family, peer, neighborhood, and school factors interact to influence the individual and her or his decision-making processes. The mesosystem refers to these interactions (Szapocznik & Coatsworth, 1999). For example, parents' supervision over peer activities and their involvement in adolescents' education are mesosystemic factors that reduce the risk of involvement in risky behavior (Schwartz et al., 2003). Parental involvement at school is predictive of positive school outcomes, including higher educational achievement, which is then associated with reduced rates of substance use (Marschall, 2006). However, for Latinx families, language and cultural barriers as well as low levels of education stymie parents' participation in their children's education (Nino, 2014). Structurally, unwelcoming school environments, hostile anti-immigrant sociopolitical contexts, and low representation of Latinx persons in administrative and teaching positions and on school boards also represent barriers to parental involvement in children's schooling (Ayón & Becerra, 2013; Nino, 2014; Marschall, 2006). In addition, Latinx parents tend to espouse the idea that the teacher is an unquestionable expert (Cousik, 2015). Parents often see their own authority to be limited to the confines of the home and the experts to be in charge of the classroom and the school. Such a view, although respectful toward educators, can be easily misinterpreted as disengagement by those unfamiliar with the culture. The resulting disconnect between the home and school ecosystems makes youth more vulnerable to risk-taking, including substance use.

Exosystemic Influences

The exosystem affects adolescents indirectly. This system refers to higher-order factors that influence parents, siblings, teachers, peers, and others in adolescents' microsystem, thereby influencing them. For example, the underfunding of schools places a high burden on teachers and administrators; this burden can compromise youth's educational experience and affect their use of substances. Additionally, environmental factors have a significant bearing on parents and can alter their parenting practices, which then influence adolescent substance use. Such factors include parents' social support, economic stress, acculturation stress, parent–child acculturation gaps, and federal, state, and local immigration policies.

In Latinx families with recent immigration histories, acculturation processes are highly influential. Acculturation is the bidimensional process of incorporating elements of a new culture at the same time that one keeps elements of the culture of origin. It is a process of cultural and psychologic change that occurs when two cultural groups interact (Berry, 1997). The process of acculturation can be a stressor on families (i.e., acculturation stress); this stress can negatively influence parenting practices (Ayón, Williams, Marsiglia, Ayers, & Kiehne, 2015; Schwartz et al., 2003; Varela et al., 2004). Furthermore, Latinx children often adopt US culture and sometimes shed their culture of origin more quickly than their parents, leading to parent–child acculturation gaps (Marsiglia et al., 2018). Gaps in acculturation can result in the occupation of very different cultural "spaces," impeding effective parent–child communication and parental monitoring and involvement (Marsiglia et al., 2018; Martinez, 2006; Schwartz et al., 2012). Thus, by their effect on the family, acculturation gaps contribute to youth's risk-taking behaviors, including substance use (Marsiglia et al., 2018; Schwartz et al., 2012).

In addition to acculturative stress, many Latinx families experience stressors related to precarious economic and legal situations (Ayón & Becerra, 2013). The influence of economic stress on parenting is an important exosystemic factor to consider, given that nearly one in five Latinx persons in the USA lives in poverty (US Census Bureau, 2017; Varela et al., 2004). Fear, stress, and depression also derive from hostile sociopolitical environments toward immigrants, and by extension, the Latinx population as a whole. These influences lead to changes in family functioning and stability (Ayón & Becerra, 2013), which are of particular concern for the estimated 5–5.5 million children in the USA who have at least one undocumented parent (Vargas & Ybarra, 2017; Chaudry et al., 2010).

Additionally, migration experiences of the nuclear and extended family can influence Latinx parents' social support by eroding geographic proximity to extended family. Separation from the extended family can positively or negatively influence family processes and parenting practices linked to youth outcomes, such as substance use (Izzo, Weiss, Shanahan, & Rodriguez-Brown, 2000). Due to traditional childrearing practices that include the involvement of grandparents, uncles, aunts, and neighbors, migration can create a decrease in adult supervision and monitoring, increasing the risk of substance use by youth (Voisine, Parsai, Marsiglia, Kulis, & Nieri, 2008).

Macrosystemic Influences

Many of the aforementioned exosystemic interactions between youth's microsystem and higher-order systems involve macrosystemic factors. The macrosystem refers to the social and cultural context in which adolescents exist. Social conditions that influence Latinx youth's substance use include poverty, discrimination, and social policymaking. Both immigrant and native Latinx youth report discrimination within their school contexts stemming from peers and teachers (Ayón & Becerra, 2013; Córdova & Cervantes, 2010). Discrimination is directly related to antisocial behavior (as a coping mechanism) as well as indirectly by disrupting youth's educational process (Kulis et al., 2009; Rivera et al., 2011). Policies such as marijuana legalization influence youth's perception of the social acceptability of legal and illegal substances. Media influences such as drug and alcohol advertisements are also macrosystemic social conditions that influence youth substance use (NIDA, 2003b). The discrepant allocation of funding to schools influence the quality of the education children receive, their educational aspirations, and the high dropout rates, all of which increase the risk for substance use and other negative health outcomes (Johnston et al., 2015; Maynard, Salas-Wright and Vaughn, 2015). Approximately 11% of Latinx youth drop out of high school compared with 8% of Black and 5% of White youth (National Center for Educational Statistics, 2016).

Many aspects of the Latinx culture represent assets and sources of protection that promote resiliency (Gosin et al., 2003). *Familismo*, or the social centrality of family, is a cultural factor that influences Latinx adolescents' patterns of substance use (Brook et al., 1998). *Familismo* is protective against substance use through its greater parental monitoring and involvement (Romero & Ruiz, 2007). The aforementioned culturally based gender norms and socialization patterns that are associated with gender discrepancies in substance use are also a part of youth's macrosystem and represent a source of both risk and protection.

Chronosystemic Influences

The final ecologic context influencing adolescents is the chronosystem. This system concerns life transitions and changes over the life span that influence an individual (Bronfenbrenner, 1986). For example, developmental shifts that occur as an individual matures into adolescence, such as puberty and educational transitions, affect substance use. Additionally, for many Latinx persons, the migration experience is a major life transition that restructures social interactions and cultural influences, influencing substance use risk and protection. Migration, deportations, and other life transitions can be added stressors and sources of risk for substance use and abuse (Zhang et al., 2015).

Summary of Ecosystem Influences

In summary, all of the ecosystems have the potential to influence the substance use attitudes and behaviors of Latinx youth. One ecosystem alone cannot explain the attitude and behaviors of an adolescent. Instead, the accumulation of protective and risk factors from each environmental context determines adolescent substance use. However, two adolescents exposed to the same risks and with similar protective factors may have very different substance use profiles. The impact may vary depending on the context and stage of development of each adolescent.

Based on our experience and the accumulated evidence, greater prevention benefits can be attained by intervening directly after the transition from elementary to middle school (a chronosytemic consideration). Furthermore, intervention at the individual, family, and school levels (microsystem and mesosystem) is ideal. The exosystem and macrosystem exercise an influence on youth; however, their impacts are indirect and complex. Intervening at those levels and measuring the results of such interventions is substantially more difficult. In the following section, we provide a review of one possible approach to intervention to prevent substance use among

Latinx youth. The intervention approach is tailored to both the needs and assets of Latinx youth.

Evidence-Based Approaches to Preventing Substance Use Among Latinx Adolescents

The negative social and health effects of using and abusing alcohol and other drugs affect not only youth but their families, communities, and society. Preventing the onset of substance use and abuse at or before adolescence is the most effective tool for avoiding these negative consequences and for supporting youth to live healthy, productive lives (Gottfredson et al., 2015). Evidence-based prevention interventions are effective for reducing the risk of developing behavioral health problems, including underage use of alcohol use, tobacco, and illicit drugs and misuse and abuse of prescription drugs (SAMSHA, 2016). The implementation of such interventions is also cost-effective. The findings of cost–benefit analyses suggest that, if implemented nationwide, for every $1 spent on effective school-based prevention programs, the nation would save an estimated $18 (Miller & Hendrie, 2008).

There is an urgent need to address substance use as a risk factor compromising youths' health and well-being. Prevention that targets youth in early adolescence is important because as noted earlier, developmentally, this is one of the most vulnerable times for initiation of drug and alcohol use (NIDA, 2003). During this early adolescence, youth go through major biopsychosocial transitions. Their social and academic experiences broaden; their autonomy increases; and their brain architecture and function change, leading to the expansion of risk-taking behaviors (Crone, van Duijvenvoorde, & Peper, 2016). Investing in the prevention of the onset of alcohol, tobacco, and drug use among adolescents is crucial, particularly among Latinx adolescents, because the rates of substance use are highest among them compared to other adolescents.

Adolescent substance use prevention interventions often aim to boost protective factors and minimize risk factors (Hawkins, Catalano, & Arthur, 2002). Bolstering youth's communication and drug-resistance skills are important components of drug and alcohol prevention as a means of increasing protective factors and resilience (NIDA, 2003b). Thus, communication competence theory offers a valuable foundation for the development of prevention programming for youth, particularly those from ethnic-minority groups.

Communication Competence Theory: Implications for Prevention

According to communication competence theory (Spitzberg & Cupach, 1984), individuals tailor their communication style to the situation at hand. This theory, then, can serve as the basis for the design of adolescent substance use interventions that seek to bolster youth's communication strategies as they confront negative ecodevelopmental influences. The premise behind the teaching of drug-resistance strategies is that many youth do not actually want to use substances; these youth need the right tools to do what they want and not confront risk situations without a set of efficacious and culturally-appropriate resistance techniques. Teaching multiple resistance approaches allows youth to select among a repertoire of drug-resistance strategies in accordance with the situation (Marsiglia, 2016). The assumption is that when youth learn multiple drug-resistance strategies, they are able to assess risky situations and determine which strategy is likely to be most effective and employ additional strategies as needed (Wright, Nichols, Graber, Brooks-Gunn, & Botvin, 2004).

In addition to elucidating the importance of teaching a variety of drug-resistance strategies, communication competence theory recognizes the central role of culture in determining norms of communication (Spitzberg, 1983). This central role of culture is an all-important consideration for prevention interventions for Latinx youth. The style, accessibility, and social acceptability of drug-resistance strategies vary across social and cultural contexts. Culture and values are relational in nature and are communicated through conversations (Spitzberg & Cupach, 1984). Thus, the cultural relevancy of prevention messaging for ethnic–racial minority youth is crucial (Spitzberg, 1983). Adolescents from different ethnic–racial groups may receive drug "offers" in various contexts, and prevention curricula must be responsive to these contexts (Gosin et al., 2003). As indicated by communication competence theory, cultural values influence communication, relational patterns, and norms that have implications for drug and alcohol resistance. Ethnic–racial minority adolescents will incorporate resistance strategies into their repertoire if they feel comfortable using them (Kulis, Marsiglia, Castillo, Becerra, & Nieri, 2008). If a strategy feels culturally awkward or uncomfortable, adolescents may integrate it in the short term but then drop it in the long term, reducing the overall efficacy of the intervention.

Many times, youth from the same community or cultural origin share certain values and communication styles. Those values should serve as the foundation of prevention programs for diverse youth. For example, Latinx youth tend to resist substance offers by providing an explanation rather than simply refusing to take the substance. For example, messaging that focuses on just saying "no" does not feel "right" and is not effective. An explanation instead of a simple or direct no is culturally more acceptable because it is more respectful and less confrontational (Marsiglia, Kulis, Booth, Nuño-Gutiérrez, & Robbins, 2015). Additionally, although it may be important for prevention programs to highlight the consequences of drug use on future goals, adding the impact on one's family and community may be important for Latinx youth. Given the importance of family within traditional Latinx cultures, such cultural considerations are integral to the efficacy of interventions (Gosin et al., 2003).

Despite recommendations for cultural specificity, many substance use prevention interventions for ethnically and racially diverse youth are surface adaptations or modifications of existing programs developed and tested largely with middle-class White youth (Botvin, Griffin, Diaz, & Ifill-Williams, 2001; Roosa, Dumka, Gonzales, & Knight, 2002). One exception is *keepin' it REAL* (*kiR*)—a universal and culturally congruent prevention program for Latinx youth designated as a model program by SAMHSA (2017). *kiR* is presented as a case study and an illustration of a concrete application of ecodevelopmental and communication competence theories to address unmet needs in substance use prevention for Latinx youth.

kiR: *A Model Substance Use Prevention Intervention for Early Adolescents*

kiR is a manualized efficacious school-based intervention that was developed using community-engaged research. The intervention has 10 lessons, which classroom teachers facilitate after receiving intensive training in the curriculum. To aid in the prevention of adolescent substance use, *kiR* (a) promotes drug- and alcohol-resistance skills, (b) encourages anti-substance use attitudes and norms, and (c) increases positive decision-making and communication skills (Marsiglia & Hecht, 2005). *kiR* teaches four main resistance strategies, and Latinx and other youth have reported that they effectively use these strategies to resist offers of alcohol and other drugs (Marsiglia, Kulis, Yabiku, Nieri, & Coleman, 2011). These four drug-resistance strategies are known as "REAL" strategies; each letter signifies a strategy: *Refuse, Explain, Avoid,* and *Leave* (Gosin et al., 2003). The curriculum teaches youth how to *Refuse* substance offers by simply declining the offer. They also acquire the skill of communicating their disinterest in drugs and alcohol by providing an *Explanation*. Youth learn how to *Avoid* substance use offers by physically distancing themselves from a drug-related situation or by topic shifting. Lastly, they learn that they have the option to *Leave* a situation where others are actively using or offering alcohol and other drugs (Marsiglia & Hecht, 2005).

Through the *kiR* curriculum, participants review drug-related situations in order to consider the most appropriate resistance strategy given the setting and person offering the substance (e.g., peer, stranger, or family member). Through role-playing, students practice their newly acquired drug-resistance skills. *kiR* is a highly interactive and engaging curriculum that also involves videos scripted and acted out by youth that model each of the drug-resistance strategies (Gosin et al., 2003). The interactive design of *kiR* is crucial, particularly for adolescents from ethnic and racial minorities (Tobler & Stratton, 1997; Tobler et al., 2000).

In addition to its interactive nature, the *kiR* curriculum is culturally congruent and primarily reflects Mexican-American and Mexican values. As an example, in the lesson that covers the drug-resistance strategy of refusing, students are encouraged to discuss ways in which they can say no and set firm boundaries. Reflecting the cultural value of *simpatía*, or kindness to others, students learn how to be clear in their communication, but not to embarrass or attack others. Accordingly, a refusal option presented to students and modeled in a DVD that is part of the *kiR* curriculum is, "I really like hanging out with you, but I'm not into smoking" (Harthun, Drapeau, Dustman, & Marsiglia, 2002).

Research supports the efficacy of the culturally congruent, comprehensive *kiR* curriculum in preventing adolescent substance use among Latinx adolescents. After completion of the curriculum, participants reported a host of positive effects that persisted from two to 14 months (Marsiglia et al., 2005). Positive effects were greatest for alcohol, the most commonly used substance among adolescents of this age group. The findings of subgroup analyses indicated that positive effects hold over time for participants of Mexican heritage (Kulis et al., 2005); among this group of adolescents, the program worked best for those who were more acculturated, as they were at higher risk of initiating substance use (Marsiglia et al., 2005). In addition to being efficacious, *kiR* is cost-effective; for every $1 spent on administration of the program to students, the estimated savings in future costs to taxpayers, the students, and others is nearly $12 (Washington State Institute for Public Policy, 2016).

kiR's promising results have led the US-based research team to collaborate with colleagues in Mexico to implement a series of studies to adapt it for youth in that country (Booth, Marsiglia, Nuño-Gutiérrez, & García-Pérez, 2014; Marsiglia et al., 2014, 2015). These efforts have served as the foundation for a randomized controlled trial of the culturally-adapted *kiR* and test its efficacy in Mexico. The developers of *kiR* have found that Mexico-based research also informs and strengthens prevention efforts in the USA, resulting in a mutually beneficial research partnership. For example, the Mexico adaptation and efficacy studies highlighted gender differences in the use of the REAL drug-resistance strategies, and gender differences in resistance strategies have now been explored and documented among adolescents in both the USA and Mexico (Kulis et al., 2011; Marsiglia et al., 2009). The relationship between use of REAL strategies and substance use may be stronger for male than for female adolescents, and in some cases, only significant for male adolescents (Kulis et al., 2012). Importantly, the effectiveness of using drug-resistance strategies by participants was associated with differences in their actual substance use (Kulis, Marsiglia, Castillo, et al. 2008; Kulis et al., 2012).

The Intersection of Ethnicity and Gender: A Call for Future Research

Along with the divergent rates of substance use among Latinx persons by gender, the gender-specific findings associated with *kiR* point toward the important intersection of ethnicity and gender. Gender roles and norms have a significant impact on the substance use attitudes and behaviors of male and female Latinx youth (Kulis et al., 2012). As discussed in-depth earlier, the concepts of *marianismo* and *machismo* affect the social acceptability of alcohol and drug use for men and women. These concepts also affect the strategies that persons of both genders are more prone to use to resist substances (Kulis et al., 2012). The gendered use and effectiveness of drug-resistance strategies may reflect gendered communication patterns. Future research will help elucidate these persistent gender differences and how they affect substance use.

The area of ethnicity and gender as it relates to Latinx persons' substance use is an understudied area of research. It is crucial that future research be designed to more carefully examine gender as a developmental factor influencing substance use patterns among Latinx youth. Such research has significant implications for the development and tailoring of prevention interventions to meet the unique needs of Latinx adolescents and, ultimately, realize health equity in substance use and abuse.

Another area of research warranting further attention is the way in which gender roles and norms are changing in Latin America and within Latinx communities in the USA and their effects on substance use. Feminism has contributed to the diminishing dominance of *marianismo* within Latin American society and Latinx communities in the USA (de la Torre, 2009). Macrosystemic conditions in Latin America, such as revolutions, wars, economic crises, and migration, have further altered the patriarchal system under which *marianismo* and *machismo* have historically thrived (Rankin, 2008). Women are increasingly entering the public sphere and changing the definition of what it means to be a woman in society (Rankin, 2008). Similarly, a growing proportion of young people in the USA, Mexico, and other countries in Latin America are questioning traditional gender norms and working toward gender equity (Torres, Solberg, & Carlstrom, 2002). Latinx youth in the USA are often growing up in two worlds—their parents' culture of origin and the mainstream youth culture, each of which has its own paradigms and expectations. These youth may be questioning the traditional *marianismo* and *machismo* attitudes and behaviors of their parents and siblings and reinterpreting certain societal expectations and stereotypes associated with femininity and masculinity (Torres Stone & Meyler, 2007). In this context, then, it is only natural that many contradictions emerge related to gender roles and expectations about substance use.

Although *marianismo* in its more traditional form is no longer as normative as it once was, gender inequality and oppression persist in many communities (Liang, Knauer-Turner, Molenaar and Price, 2017). Additionally, *machismo* is moving away from its most oppressive manifestation, and the efforts are underway to support the prosocial aspects of Latinx masculinity encompassed under the concept of *caballerismo* (Estrada & Arciniega, 2015). Communities no longer uncritically follow archetypal gender roles, and they are creating new notions of gender, such as *hembrismo* and *caballerismo. Hembrismo*, another concept influenced by feminist thought, now often complements *marianismo. Hembrismo*, as described earlier in this chapter, builds on the strengths of Latinx women as capable, strong, understanding, and patient; it expands on those traditional attributes by emphasizing empowerment, adaptation, and flexibility in role relationships as well as promotion of competence and commitment to social change (Comas-Diaz, 1987; Kulis et al., 2010). Additionally, within the literature on Latinx masculinities, the term *caballerismo* is part of a postcolonial reinterpretation of *machismo*. The argument behind *caballerismo* is that the original cultures of Mesoamerica were mostly matriarchal and that *machismo* and patriarchy were introduced by the colonial powers and enforced by their religion (Nuñez et al., 2016). *Caballerismo* embodies positive male behaviors of the nurturing provider who is respectful, defends the weak, and lives by an ethical code of chivalrous values (Ojeda & Piña-Watson, 2014). *Caballerismo* includes positive aspects of adjustment, such as affiliation, nurturance, family protection, responsibility, wisdom, hard work, spirituality, and avoidance of substance abuse (Arciniega et al., 2008).

Rapidly changing gender norms appear to be contributing to more gender parity in substance use among the Latinx population (Marsiglia, Yabiku, et al., 2011; Zapata-Roblyer et al., 2016). One of the byproducts of the positive developments toward gender equity is a weakening of the traditional cultural protections against substance use for young women (Kulis, Marsiglia, Castillo, et al. 2008). Thus, the health impacts of these social and cultural changes present a dilemma and opportunity for prevention research. Communities cannot return to the way things were; the cultural norms that protected young women from substance use also oppressed them in other substantial social domains. Equality, we propose, means responding to the new risks young women encounter, and in partnership with them through approaches to community-engaged research, identifying strengths that come with the new paradigms of gender equity and substance use prevention. Such research that attempts to increase the effectiveness of substance use prevention in light of changing gender roles and norms is crucial.

Additionally, changing gender norms have several other implications for future research and considerations for prevention programming. First, traditional gender norms appear to be rapidly changing in some urban communities but somehow persist in many rural communities. Thus, prevention messages may need to be tailored to specific contexts (Rhodes et al., 2012). For example, drug-resistance interventions may be most effective in some contexts when they provide male adolescents with strategies to counterbalance persistent unhealthy cultural messages about *machismo* with prosocial and healthier cultural norms. Future research will help us elucidate how to better integrate young women and men's gender-specific assets and risks on both sides of the Mexico–USA border.

Future Research

Culture provides both risk and protective factors, and both sets of influences are in need of further research in order to design efficacious substance use prevention interventions for Latinx youth. We must better define culture as it relates to diverse groups of people like the Latinx community. After we make progress conceptually, research is needed to develop or adapt existing measures to make them more appropriate for

Latinx persons in the USA. Acculturation, perceived discrimination, gender roles, and ethnic-identity formation measures grounded in the experience of Latinx youth will greatly contribute to the generation of knowledge to solve contemporary challenges. Better measurement will yield a better understanding. Better understanding will, in turn, inform the design of more appropriate prevention interventions that are able to incorporate the assets as well as the unmet needs of Latinx youth.

There is a dearth of inquiry related to the interaction between gender and substance use (Benjet et al., 2014; Kulis, Marsiglia, Lingard, et al., 2008). However, traditional gender roles as described in the literature—with their historical share of stereotypes—do not provide sufficient insight into the fast-changing gendered beliefs, norms, attitudes, and behaviors related to substance use. Changing gender norms and their impact on substance use among Latinx adolescents warrant further investigation. Substance use prevention interventions must incorporate such future findings, as interventions will become more efficacious by systematically incorporating new knowledge about the intersection of ethnicity and gender and by moving beyond dated stereotypes.

Because original research is costly and takes a long time to implement, we also suggest conducting more studies using secondary analysis of existing datasets. The following are some examples of publicly-accessible, nationally-representative datasets to consider to move the knowledge base forward.

1. The National Longitudinal Study of Adolescent to Adult Health (Add Health): http://www.cpc.unc.edu/projects/addhealth/documentation/publicdata
2. The National Latino and Asian American Study: www.icpsr.umich.edu/icpsrweb/ICPSR/studies/00191
3. Acculturation and Sexual Behavior among Latino Youth: Findings from the National Longitudinal Survey of Youth 1997–2003: http://www.thenationalcampaign.org/resources/pdf/SS/SS35_Acculturation.pdf
4. The Sexual Behavior of Young Adolescents: http://www.thenationalcampaign.org/resources/pdf/SS/SS3_YoungAdols.pdf
5. The Pew Research Center, Hispanic Trends: www.pewhispanic.org/data-and-resources

Conclusions

The Latinx population is the largest ethnic–racial minority group in the USA. This group is very diverse in terms of nativity, generational status, national origin, migration, acculturation status, socioeconomic status, region, geographic context (e.g., living in rural versus urban areas), and gender norms, among other characteristics. The overall substance use rate for the Latinx population can be misleading and allow researchers, service providers, and policy makers to overlook health risks in this population.

This chapter outlines evidence that the rate of substance use is lower in the Latinx population overall than for other ethnic–racial groups in the USA; however, this trend differs among Latinx youth. Instead, Latinx youth are highly vulnerable and further intervention research for this group is warranted. Evidence-based prevention interventions are cost-effective and can address substance use-related health disparities and their related negative health and social outcomes. Based on ecodevelopmental and communication theories, *kiR* is an exemplar of culturally-congruent prevention interventions for Latinx youth. Integrating the changing gender norms of Latinx communities warrants further research and is a vital component of a more gendered approach to prevention.

Among the many questions that need answering through research, several emerge from this chapter, including (1) How are some Latinx youth staying healthy despite vulnerabilities? (2) How can the development, implementation, evaluation, and dissemination of evidence-based interventions more effectively and efficiently support Latinx youth to stay healthy? (3) How can existing culturally-congruent practices be incorporated into new interventions to help other Latinx adolescents with higher levels of risk incorporate prosocial behaviors and achieve higher levels of well-being?

The health of Latinx youth is paramount. However, much work is needed to move the science and practice of substance use prevention forward. A robust research agenda for Latinx health is needed, particularly during this time in US history, in which anti-Latinx sentiment is especially high. Ecodevelopmental theory offers a framework that facilitates the inclusion of relevant factors to explore, understand, and intervene on risk-taking behaviors, including substance use, among Latinx youth.

References

Acevedo-Garcia, D., Pan, J., Jun, H. J., Osypuk, T. L., & Emmons, K. M. (2005). The effect of immigrant generation on smoking. *Social Science and Medicine, 61*(6), 1223–1242.

Alaniz, M. L. (1996). Husband's level of drinking and egalitarianism in Mexican-American families. *Substance Use and Misuse, 31*(6), 647–661.

Alegría, M., Mulvaney-Day, N., Torres, M., Polo, A., Cao, Z., & Canino, G. (2007). Prevalence of psychiatric disorders across Latino subgroups in the United States. *American Journal of Public Health, 97*(1), 68–75.

Alvarez, J., Jason, L. A., Olson, B. D., Ferrari, J. R., & Davis, M. I. (2007). Substance abuse prevalence and treatment among Latinos and Latinas. *Journal of Ethnicity in Substance Abuse, 6*(2), 115–141.

Arciniega, G. M., Anderson, T. C., Tovar-Blank, Z. G., & Tracey, T. J. G. (2008). Toward a fuller conception of machismo: Development of a traditional machismo and caballerismo scale. *Journal of Counseling Psychology, 55*(1), 19–33.

Ayón, C., & Becerra, D. (2013). Latino immigrant families under siege: The impact of SB1070, discrimination, and economic crisis. *Advances in Social Work, 14*, 206–228.

Ayón, C., Williams, L. R., Marsiglia, F. F., Ayers, S., & Kiehne, E. (2015). A latent profile analysis of Latino parenting: The infusion of cultural values on family conflict. *Families in Society, 96*(3), 203–210.

Bacio, G. A., Mays, V. M., & Lau, A. S. (2013). Drinking initiation and problematic drinking among Latino adolescents: Explanations of the immigrant paradox. *Psychology of Addictive Behaviors, 27*(1), 14–22.

Barger, S. D., & Gallo, L. C. (2008). Ability of ethnic self-identification to partition modifiable health risk among US residents of Mexican ancestry. *American Journal of Public Health, 98*(11), 1971–1978.

Bava, S., Jacobus, J., Thayer, R. E., & Tapert, S. F. (2013). Longitudinal changes in white matter integrity among adolescent substance users. *Alcoholism: Clinical and Experimental Research, 37*, e181–e189.

Benjet, C., Borges, G., Mendez, E., Casanova, L., & Medina-Mora, M. E. (2014). Adolescent alcohol use and alcohol use disorders in Mexico City. *Drug and Alcohol Dependence, 136,* 43–50.

Berry, J. W. (1997). Immigration, acculturation and adaptation. *Applied Psychology: An International Review, 46*(1), 5–34.

Bogenschneider, K. (1996). An ecological risk/protective theory for building prevention programs, policies, and community capacity to support youth. *Family Relations, 45,* 127–138.

Booth, J., Marsiglia, F. F., Nuño-Gutiérrez, B., & García-Pérez, H. (2014). The association between engaging in romantic relationships and Mexican adolescent substance use offers: Exploring gender differences. *Substance Use and Misuse, 49*(11), 1480–1490.

Borges, G., Breslau, J., Orozco, R., Tancredi, D. J., Anderson, H., Aguilar-Gaxiola, S., & Medina Mora, M. (2011). A cross-national study on Mexico-US migration, substance use and substance use disorders. *Drug and Alcohol Dependence, 117*(1), 16–23.

Botvin, G. J., Griffin, K. W., Diaz, T., & Ifill-Williams, M. (2001). Drug abuse prevention among minority adolescents: Posttest and one-year follow-up of a school-based preventive intervention. *Prevention Science, 2*(1), 1–13.

Bronfenbrenner, U. (1986). Ecology of the family as context for human development: Research perspectives. *Developmental Psychology, 22*(6), 723–742.

Bronfenbrenner, U. (1994). Ecological models of human development. In *International encyclopedia of education* (2nd ed., Vol. 3). Oxford: Elsevier.

Brook, J. S., Brook, D. W., De La Rosa, M., Duque, L. F., Rodriguez, E., Montoya, I. D., & Whiteman, M. (1998). Pathways to marijuana use among adolescents: Cultural/ecological, family, peer, and personality influences. *Journal of the American Academy of Child & Adolescent Psychiatry, 37*(7), 759–766.

Brook, J. S., Brook, D. W., Gordon, A. S., Whiteman, M., & Cohen, P. (1990). The psychosocial etiology of adolescent drug use: A family interactional approach. *Genetic, Social, and General Psychology Monographs, 116,* 111–267.

Buchanan, R. L., & Smokowski, P. R. (2009). Pathways from acculturation stress to substance use among Latino adolescents. *Substance Use and Misuse, 44*(5), 740–762.

Caetano, R. (1987). Acculturation and attitudes toward appropriate drinking among US Hispanics. *Alcohol and Alcoholism, 22*(4), 427–433.

Caetano, R., & Clark, C. L. (2003). Acculturation, alcohol consumption, smoking, and drug use among Hispanics. In K. M. Chun, P. Organista, & G. Marin (Eds.), *Acculturation: Advances in theory, measurement, and applied research* (pp. 223–239). Washington D.C.: American Psychological Association.

Caetano, R., & Medina-Mora, M. E. (1988). Acculturation and drinking among people of Mexican descent in Mexico and the United States. *Journal of Early Adolescence, 49*(5), 462–471.

Canino, G., Vega, W. A., Sribney, W. M., Warner, L. A., & Alegria, M. (2008). Social relationships, social assimilation, and substance use disorders among adult Latinos in the US. *Journal of Drug Issues, 38*(1), 69–101.

Casey, B. J., Jones, R. M., & Hare, T. A. (2008). The adolescent brain. *Annals of the New York Academy of Sciences, 1124,* 111–126.

Centers for Disease Control and Prevention. (2014). *Youth risk behavior surveillance—United States 2013*. Atlanta, GA.

Centers for Disease Control and Prevention. (2015). Vital signs: Leading causes of death, prevalence of diseases and risk factors, and use of health services among Hispanics in the United States—2009–2013. *Morbidity and Mortality Weekly Report, 64*(17), 469–478.

Centers for Disease Control and Prevention. (2016a). Disparities in adult cigarette smoking—United States, 2002–2005 and 2010–2013. *Morbidity and Mortality Weekly Report, 65*(30).

Centers for Disease Control and Prevention. (2016b). *Health, United States, 2015: With special feature on Racial and Ethnic Health Disparities.* Atlanta, GA.

Chaudry, A., Capps, R., Pedroza, J. M., Castañeda, R. M., Santos, R., & Scott, M. M. (2010). *Facing our future. Children in the aftermath of immigration enforcement.* Washington, D.C.: The Urban Institute.

Child Trends. (2014). High school dropout rates. Retrieved from www.childtrends.org/?indicators=high-school-dropout-rates.

Coatsworth, J., Pantin, H., & Szapocznik, J. (2002). Familias Unidas: A family-centered ecodevelopmental intervention to reduce risk for problem behavior among Hispanic adolescents. *Clinical Child and Family Psychology Review, 5*(2), 113–132.

Comas-Diaz, L. (1987). Feminist therapy with mainland Puerto Rican women. *Psychology of Women Quarterly, 11*(4), 461–474.

Córdova, D., & Cervantes, R. C. (2010). Intergroup and within-group perceived discrimination among U.S.-born and foreign-born Latino youth. *Hispanic Journal of Behavioral Sciences, 32*(2), 259–274.

Cousik, R. (2015). Cultural and functional diversity in the elementary classroom: Strategies for teachers. *Journal for Multicultural Education, 9*(2), 54–67.

Cristini, F., Scacchi, L., Perkins, D. D., Bless, K. D., & Vieno, A. (2015). Drug use among immigrant and non-immigrant adolescents: Immigrant paradox, family and peer influences. *Journal of Community & Applied Social Psychology, 25*(6), 531–548.

Crone, E. A., van Duijvenvoorde, A. C. K., & Peper, J. S. (2016). Annual research review: Neural contributions to risk-taking in adolescence—Developmental changes and individual differences. *Journal of Child Psychology and Psychiatry, 57*(3), 1469–7610.

De La Rosa, M. (2002). Acculturation and Latino adolescents' substance use: A research agenda for the future. *Substance Use and Misuse, 37*(4), 429–456.

de la Torre, M. (2009). Marianismo. In M. A. de La Torre (Ed.), *American religious cultures: Hispanic American religious cultures* (Vol. 1, pp. 346–348). Santa Barbara, CA: ABC-CLIO.

Delva, J., Wallace, J. M., Jr., O'Malley, P. M., Bachman, J. G., Johnston, L. D., & Schulenberg, J. E. (2005). The epidemiology of alcohol, marijuana, and cocaine use among Mexican American, Puerto Rican, Cuban American, and other Latin American eighth-grade students in the United States: 1991–2002. *American Journal of Public Health, 95*(4), 696–702.

Elliott, D. S., Huizinga, D., & Ageton, S. S. (1985). *Explaining delinquency and drug use.* Beverly Hills, CA: Sage.

Elliott, D. S., Huizinga, D., & Menard, S. (1989). *Multiple problem youth: Delinquency, substance use, and mental health problems.* New York: Springer.

Estrada, F., & Arciniega, G. M. (2015). Positive masculinity among Latino men and the direct and indirect effects on well-being. *Journal of Multicultural Counseling and Development, 43*(3), 191–205.

Fergusson, D. M., Horwood, L. J., & Swain-Campbell, N. (2002). Cannabis use and psychosocial adjustment in adolescence and young adulthood. *Addiction, 97*(9), 1123–1135.

Gosin, M., Marsiglia, F. F., & Hecht, M. L. (2003). Keepin' it R.E.A.L: A drug resistance curriculum tailored to the strengths and needs of preadolescents of the Southwest. *Journal of Drug Education, 33*(2), 119–142.

Gottfredson, D. C., Cook, T. D., Gardner, F. E. M., Gorman-Smith, D., Howe, G. W., Sandler, I. N., & Zafft, K. M. (2015). Standards of evidence for efficacy, effectiveness, and scale-up research in prevention science: Next generation. *Prevention Science, 16*(7), 893–926.

Grant, B. F., Stinson, F. S., Hasin, D. S., Dawson, D. A., Chou, S. P., & Anderson, K. (2004). Immigration and lifetime prevalence of DSM-IV psychiatric disorders among Mexican Americans and non-Hispanic whites in the United States: Results from the National Epidemiologic Survey on Alcohol and Related Conditions. *Archives of General Psychiatry, 61*(12), 1226–1233.

Harthun, M. L., Drapeau, A. E., Dustman, P. A., & Marsiglia, F. F. (2002). Implementing a prevention curriculum: An effective researcher-teacher partnership. *Education and Urban Society, 34*(3), 353–364.

Hassy, F., Garza, Y., Sullivan, J. M., & Serrers, S. (2016). Affluent Mexican immigrant parents' perceptions of child-parent relationship training. *International Journal of Play Therapy, 25*(3), 114–122.

Hawkins, J. D., Catalano, R. F., & Arthur, M. (2002). Promoting science-based prevention in communities. *Addictive Behaviors, 27*(6), 951–976.

Herrera, C. J., Owens, G. P., & Mallinckrodt, B. (2013). Traditional machismo and caballerismo as correlates of posttraumatic stress disorder, psychological distress, and relationship satisfaction in Hispanic veterans. *Journal of Multicultural Counseling and Development, 41*(1), 21–35.

Hopfer, C. J., Crowley, T. J., & Hewitt, J. K. (2003). Review of twin and adoption studies of adolescent substance use. *Journal of the American Academy of Child and Adolescent Psychiatry, 42*(6), 710–719.

Izzo, C., Weiss, L., Shanahan, T., & Rodriguez-Brown, F. (2000). Parental self-efficacy and social support as predictors of parenting practices and children's socio-emotional adjustment in Mexican immigrant families. *Journal of Prevention & Intervention in the Community, 20*(1–2), 197–213.

Johnston, L. D., O'Malley, P. M., Miech, R. A., Bachman, J. G., & Schulenberg, J. E. (2015). *Monitoring the Future national survey results on drug use, 1975–2015: Overview, key findings on adolescent drug use*. Ann Arbor: Institute for Social Research, The University of Michigan.

Kulis, S., Marsiglia, F. F., Ayers, S. L., Booth, J., & Nuño-Gutiérrez, B. L. (2012). Drug resistance and substance use among male and female adolescents in alternative secondary schools in Guanajuato, Mexico. *Journal of Studies on Alcohol and Drugs, 73*(1), 111–119.

Kulis, S., Marsiglia, F. F., Ayers, S. L., Calderón-Tena, C. O., & Nuño-Gutiérrez, B. L. (2011). Gender differences in drug resistance skills in youth in Guanajuato, Mexico. *Journal of Primary Prevention, 32*(2), 113–127.

Kulis, S., Marsiglia, F. F., Castillo, J., Becerra, D., & Nieri, T. A. (2008). Drug resistance strategies and substance use among adolescents in Monterrey, Mexico. *Journal of Primary Prevention, 29*(2), 167–192.

Kulis, S., Marsiglia, F. F., Elek, E., Dustman, P., Wagstaff, D. A., & Hecht, M. L. (2005). Mexican/Mexican American adolescents and keepin' it REAL: An evidence-based substance use prevention program. *Children and Schools, 27*, 133–145.

Kulis, S., Marsiglia, F. F., Lingard, E. C., Nieri, T., & Nagoshi, J. (2008). Gender identity and substance use among students in two high schools in Monterrey, Mexico. *Drug and Alcohol Dependence, 95*(3), 258–268.

Kulis, S., Marsiglia, F. F., & Nagoshi, J. L. (2010). Gender roles, externalizing behaviors, and substance use among Mexican-American adolescents. *Journal of Social Work Practice in the Addictions, 10*(3), 283–307.

Kulis, S., Marsiglia, F. F., & Nieri, T. (2009). Perceived ethnic discrimination versus acculturation stress: influences on substance use among Latino youth in the southwest. *Journal of Health and Social Behavior, 50*(4), 443–459.

LaFromboise, T., Coleman, H. L., & Gerton, J. (1993). Psychological impact of biculturalism: Evidence and theory. *Psychological Bulletin, 114*(3), 395–412.

Lettieri, D. J., Sayers, M., & Pearson, H. W. (Eds.). (1980). *Theories on drug abuse: Selected contemporary perspectives* (Research Monograph 30). Rockville, MD: National Institute of Drug Abuse.

Liang, C. T. H., Knauer-Turner, E. A., Molenaar, C. M., & Price, E. (2017). A qualitative examination of the gendered and racialized lives of Latina college students. *Gender Issues, 34*(2), 149–170.

Lipsky, S., & Caetano, R. (2009). Epidemiology of substance abuse among Latinos. *Journal of Ethnicity in Substance Abuse, 8*(3), 242–260.

Mann-Jackson, L., Song, E. Y., Tanner, A. E., Alonzo, J., Linton, J. M., & Rhodes, S. D. (2018). The health impact of experiences of discrimination, violence, and immigration enforcement among Latino men in a new settlement state. *American Journal of Men's Health, 12*(6), 1937–1947.

Marschall, M. (2006). Parent involvement and educational outcomes for Latino students. *Review of Policy Research, 23*(5), 1053–1076.

Marsiglia, F. F. (2016). Youth substance use prevention interventions: Opportunities and challenges (editorial). *Revista Internacional de Investigación en Addicciones, 2*(2), 1–2.

Marsiglia, F. F., Booth, J., Ayers, S. L., Nuño-Gutiérrez, B. L., Kulis, S., & Hoffman, S. (2014). Short-term effects on substance use of the keepin' it REAL pilot prevention program: Linguistically adapted for youth in Jalisco, Mexico. *Prevention Science, 15*(5), 694–704.

Marsiglia, F. F., & Hecht, M. L. (2005). *Keepin' it REAL: An evidence-based program.* Santa Cruz, CA: ETR Associates.

Marsiglia, F. F., Kiehne, E., & Ayers, S. L. (2018). Reexamining the acculturation gap: The relationship between the bidimensional parent-adolescent gap and risky behavior among Mexican-Heritage adolescents. *The Journal of Early Adolescence, 38*(5), 581–605.

Marsiglia, F. F., & Kulis, S. S. (2015). *Diversity, oppression, and change: Culturally grounded social work* (2nd ed.). Chicago, IL: Lyceum Books.

Marsiglia, F. F., Kulis, S., Booth, J. M., Nuño-Gutiérrez, B. L., & Robbins, D. E. (2015). Long term effects of the keepin' it REAL model program in Mexico: Substance use trajectories of Guadalajara middle school students. *Journal of Primary Prevention, 36*(2), 93–104.

Marsiglia, F. F., Kulis, S., Hussaini, S. K., Nieri, T. A., & Becerra, D. (2010). Gender differences in the effect of linguistic acculturation on substance use among Mexican-origin youth in the Southwest United States. *Journal of Ethnicity in Substance Abuse, 9*(1), 40–63.

Marsiglia, F. F., Kulis, S., Rodriguez, G. M., Becerra, D., & Castillo, J. (2009). Culturally specific youth substance abuse resistance skills: Applicability across the US-Mexico border. *Research on Social Work Practice, 19*(2), 152–164.

Marsiglia, F. F., Kulis, S., Wagstaff, D. A., Elek, E., & Dran, D. (2005). Acculturation status and substance use prevention with Mexican and Mexican American youth. *Journal of Social Work Practice in the Addictions, 5*(1–2), 85–111.

Marsiglia, F. F., Kulis, S., Yabiku, S., Nieri, T., & Coleman, E. (2011). When to intervene: Elementary school, middle school or both? Effects of keepin' it REAL on substance abuse trajectories of Mexican heritage youth. *Prevention Science, 12*(1), 48–62.

Marsiglia, F. F., Yabiku, S. T., Kulis, S., Nieri, T., Parsai, M., & Becerra, D. (2011). The influence of linguistic acculturation and gender on the initiation of substance use among Mexican heritage preadolescents in the borderlands. *Journal of Early Adolescence, 31*(2), 271–299.

Martinez, C. R. (2006). Effects of differential family acculturation on Latino adolescent substance use. *Family Relations, 55*(3), 306–317.

Massey, D. S., & Pren, K. A. (2012). Origins of the new Latino underclass. *Race and Social Problems, 4*(1), 5–17.

Maynard, B. R., Salas-Wright, C. P., & Vaughn, M. G. (2015). High school dropouts in emerging adulthood: Substance use, mental health problems, and crime. *Community Mental Health Journal, 51*(3), 289–299.

McWilliams, C. (2016). *North from Mexico: The Spanish speaking people of the United States* (3rd ed.). Santa Barbara, CA: ABC-CLIO.

Medina-Mora, M. E., Conver, R. T., Sepulveda, J., Otero, M., & De La Rosa, M. (1989). Extensión del consumo de drogas en México: Escuela Nacional de Adicciones. *Resultados nacionales. Salud Mental, 12*(2), 7–12.

Medina-Mora, M. E., & Rojas Guiot, E. (2003). Mujer, pobreza, y adicciones. *Perinatolgia y Reproducción Humana, 17*(4), 230–244.

Miller, T., & Hendrie, D. (2008). *Substance abuse prevention dollars and cents: A cost-benefit analysis*, DHHS Pub. No. (SMA) 07-4298. Rockville, MD: Center for Substance Abuse Prevention, Substance Abuse and Mental Health Services Administration.

National Center for Educational Statistics. (2016). *Fast Facts: Status dropout rates of 16- to 24-year-olds, by race/ethnicity: 1990 through 2014* (NCES 2015-144). National Center for Education Statistics.

National Center on Addiction and Substance Abuse. (2002). *Teen tipplers: America's underage drinking epidemic (CASA report)*. New York: Columbia University.

National Institute on Drug Abuse. (2003a). *Drug use among racial/ethnic minorities*. Bethesda, MD: National Institutes of Health.

National Institute on Drug Abuse. (2003b). *Preventing drug use among children and adolescents: A research-based guide for parents, educators, and community leaders* (2nd ed.). Bethesda, MD: National Institutes of Health.

Nielsen, A. L. (2000). Examining drinking patterns and problems among Hispanic groups: Results from a national survey. *Journal of Studies on Alcohol, 61*(2), 301–310.

Nino, M. D. (2014). Linguistic services and parental involvement among Latinos: A help or hindrance to involvement? *The Social Science Journal, 51*(3), 483–490.

Nuñez, A., González, P., Talavera, G. A., Sanchez-Johnsen, L., Roesch, S. C., Davis, S. M., ... & Penedo, F. J. (2016). Machismo, marianismo, and negative cognitive-emotional factors: Findings from the Hispanic Community Health Study/Study of Latinos Sociocultural Ancillary Study. *Journal of Latina/o Psychology, 4*(4), 202–217.

Ojeda, L., & Piña-Watson, B. (2014). Caballerismo may protect against the role of machismo on Mexican day laborers' self-esteem. *Psychology of Men & Masculinity, 15*(3), 288–295.

Otiniano Verissimo, A. D., Grella, C. E., Amaro, H., & Gee, G. C. (2014). Discrimination and substance use disorders among Latinos: The role of gender, nativity, and ethnicity. *American Journal of Public Health, 104*(8), 1421–1428.

Painter, T. M. (2008). Connecting the dots: When the risks of HIV/STD infection appear high but the burden of infection is not known—The case of male Latino migrants in the Southern United States. *AIDS and Behavior, 12*(2), 213–226.

Pantin, H., Coatsworth, J. D., Feaster, D. J., Newman, F. L., Briones, E., Prado, G., ... Szapocznik, J. (2003). Familias unidas: The efficacy of an intervention to promote parental investment in Hispanic immigrant families. *Prevention Science, 4*(3), 189–201.

Passel, J. S., Cohn, D., & Lopez, M. H. (2011). *Hispanics account for more than half of nation's growth in past decade*. Pew Hispanic Center. Washington, DC: Pew Research Center.

Patten, E. (2016). *The nation's Latino population is defined by its youth: Nearly half of U.S.-born Latinos are younger than 18*. Washington, DC: Pew Research Center, April.

Peña, J. B., Wyman, P. A., Brown, C. H., Matthieu, M. M., Olivares, T. E., Hartel, D., & Zayas, L. H. (2008). Immigration generation status and its association with suicide attempts, substance use, and depressive symptoms among Latino adolescents in the USA. *Prevention science, 9*(4), 299–310.

Perea, A., & Slater, M. (1999). Power distance and collectivist/individualist strategies in alcohol warnings: Effects of gender and ethnicity. *Journal of Health Communication, 4*(4), 295–310.

Pérez, D. J., Fortuna, L., & Alegría, M. (2008). Prevalence and correlates of everyday discrimination among US Latinos. *Journal of Community Psychology, 36*(4), 421–433.

Petraitis, J., Flay, B. R., & Miller, T. Q. (1995). Reviewing theories of adolescent substance use: Organizing pieces in the puzzle. *Psychological Bulletin, 117*(1), 67–86.

Rankin, M. (2008). Marianismo. In P. N. Stearns (Ed.), *The Oxford encyclopedia of the modern world* (pp. 51–52). New York, NY: Oxford University.

Rhodes, S. D., Hergenrather, K. C., Vissman, A. T., Stowers, J., Davis, A. B., Hannah, A., ... Marsiglia, F. F. (2011). Boys must be men, and men must have sex with women: A qualitative CBPR study to explore sexual risk among African American, Latino, and White gay men and MSM. *American Journal of Men's Health, 5*(2), 14–151.

Rhodes, S. D., Kelley, C., Simán, F. Cashman, R., Alonzo, J., McGuire, J., ... & Brown, M. (2012). Using community-based participatory research (CBPR) to develop a community-level HIV prevention intervention for Latinas: A local response to a global challenge. *Women's Health Issues, 22*(3), e293–e301.

Rivera, F., López, I., Guarnaccia, P., Ramirez, R., Canino, G., & Bird, H. (2011). Perceived discrimination and antisocial behaviors in Puerto Rican children. *Journal of Immigrant and Minority Health, 13*(3), 453–461.

Roche, K. M., Caughy, M. O., Schuster, M. A., Bogart, L. M., Dittus, P. J., & Franzini, L. (2014). Cultural orientations, parental beliefs and practices, and Latino adolescents' autonomy and independence. *Journal of Youth and Adolescence, 43*(8), 1389–1403.

Rochin, R. I. (2016). Latinos and Afro-Latino legacy in the United States: History, culture, and issues of identity. *Professional Agricultural Workers Journal, 3*(2), 2–22.

Romero, A. J., & Ruiz, M. (2007). Does familism lead to increased parental monitoring? Protective factors for coping with risky behaviors. *Journal of Child and Family Studies, 16*(2), 143–154.

Roosa, M. W., Dumka, L. E., Gonzales, N. A., & Knight, G. P. (2002). Cultural/ethnic issues and the prevention scientist in the 21st century. *Prevention & Treatment, 5*(1), Specified Article 5a.

Ruiz, J. M., Campos, B., & Garcia, J. J. (2016). Special issue on Latino physical health: Disparities, paradoxes, and future directions. *Journal of Latina/o Psychology, 4*(2), 61–66.

Salas-Wright, C. P., Clark, T. T., Vaughn, M. G., & Córdova, D. (2015). Profiles of acculturation among Hispanics in the United States: Links with discrimination and substance use. *Social Psychiatry and Psychiatric Epidemiology, 50*(1), 39–49.

Sanchez, M., De La Rosa, M., Blackson, T. C., Sastre, F., Rojas, P., Li, T., Dillon, F. (2014). Pre- to post-immigration alcohol use trajectories among recent Latino immigrants. *Psychology of Addictive Behaviors, 28*(4), 990–999.

Sanchez, D., Whittaker, T. A., Hamilton, E., & Zayas, L. H. (2016). Perceived discrimination and sexual precursor behaviors in Mexican American preadolescent girls: The role of psychological distress, sexual attitudes, and marianismo beliefs. *Cultural Diversity and Ethnic Minority Psychology, 22*(3), 395–407.

Schinke, S., Schwim, T., Hopkins, J., & Wahlstom, L. (2016). Drug abuse risk and protective factors among Hispanic adolescents. *Prevention Medicine Reports, 3,* 185–188.

Schwartz, S. J., Montgomery, M. J., & Briones, E. (2012). Substance use and sexual behavior among recent Hispanic immigrant adolescents: Effects of parent-adolescent differential acculturation and communication. *Drug and Alcohol Dependence, 125,* S26–S34.

Schwartz, S. J., Pantin, H., Szapocznik, J., & Coatsworth, J. D. (2003). Ecodevelopmental theory. In J. Miller, R. Lerner, & L. Schiamberg (Eds.), *The encyclopedia of human ecology* (Vol. 1). Santa Barbara, CA: ABC-CLIO.

Schwartz, S. J., Unger, J. B., Des Rosiers, S. E., Lorenzo-Blanco, E. I., Zamboanga, B. L., … Szapocznik, J. (2014). Domains of acculturation and their effects on substance use and sexual behavior in recent Hispanic immigrant adolescents. *Prevention Science, 15*(3), 385–396.

Spear, L. P. (2010). *The behavioral neuroscience of adolescence.* New York, NY: W.W. Norton.

Spitzberg, B. H. (1983). Communication competence as knowledge, skill, and impression. *Communication Education, 32*(3), 323–329.

Spitzberg, B. H., & Cupach, W. R. (1984). *Interpersonal communication competence.* Beverly Hills, CA: Sage.

Squeglia, L. M., Jacobus, J., & Tapert, S. F. (2009). The influence of substance use on adolescent brain development. *Clinical EEG Neuroscience, 40*(1), 31–38.

Steinberg, L. (1991). Adolescent transitions and alcohol and other drug use prevention. *Preventing adolescent drug use: From theory to practice* (Office of Substance Abuse Prevention Monograph 8, pp. 13–51). Washington, D.C.: US Department of Health and Human Services.

Steinberg, L. (2008). A social neuroscience perspective on adolescent risk-taking. *Developmental Review, 28*(1), 78–106.

Substance Abuse and Mental Health Services Administration. (2014). *Results from the 2013 National Survey on Drug Use and Health: Summary of national findings.* Rockville, MD: Center for Behavioral Health Statistics and Quality.

Substance Abuse and Mental Health Services Administration. (2017). *Preventing youth marijuana use: Programs and strategies.* Rockville, MD: Center for the Application of Prevention Technologies.

Substance Abuse and Mental Health Services Administration, Center for Behavioral Health Statistics and Quality. (2011, October 4). *The NSDUH report: Substance use among Hispanic adolescents*. Rockville, MD.

Sudhinaraset, M., Wigglesworth, C., & Takeuchi, D. T. (2016). Social and cultural contexts of alcohol use. *Alcohol Research, 38*(1), 35–45.

Szapocznik, J., & Coatsworth, J. D. (1999). An ecodevelopmental framework for organizing the influences on drug abuse: A developmental model of risk and protection. In D. Meyer & C. R. Hartel (Eds.), *Drug abuse: Origins and interventions* (pp. 331–366). Washington, D.C.: American Psychological Association.

Thorin, M. (2003). *The gender dimension of economic globalization*. Santiago, Chile: CEPAL.

Tobler, N. S., Roona, M. R., Ochshorn, P., Marshall, D. G., Streke, A. V., & Stackpole, K. M. (2000). School-based adolescent drug prevention programs: 1998 meta-analysis. *Journal of Primary Prevention, 20*(4), 275–336.

Tobler, N. S., & Stratton, H. H. (1997). Effectiveness of school-based drug prevention programs: A meta-analysis of the research. *Journal of Primary Prevention, 18*(1), 71–128.

Toro-Morn, M. I. (2008). Beyond gender dichotomies: Toward a new century of gendered scholarship in the Latina/o Experience. In H. Rodriguez, R. Saenz, & C. Menjivar (Eds.), *Latinas/os in the United States: Changing the face of America* (pp. 277–293). New York, NY: Springer.

Torres, J. B., Solberg, V. S. H., & Carlstrom, A. H. (2002). The myth of sameness among Latino men and their machismo. *American Journal of Orthopsychiatry, 72*(2), 163–181.

Torres Stone, R. A., & Meyler, D. (2007). Identifying potential risk and protective factors among non-metropolitan Latino youth: Cultural implications for substance use research. *Journal of Immigrant Health, 9*(2), 95–107.

Unger, J. B., Ritt-Olson, A., Teran, L., Huang, T., Hoffman, B. R., & Palmer, P. (2002). Cultural values and substance use in a multiethnic sample of California adolescents. *Addiction Research & Theory, 10*(3), 257–279.

US Census Bureau. (2017). *Facts for features: Hispanic heritage month 2017*.

Varela, R. E., Vernberg, E. M., Sanchez-Sosa, J. J., Riveros, A., Mitchell, M., & Mashunkashey, J. (2004). Parenting style of Mexican, Mexican American, and Caucasian-non-Hispanic families: Social context and cultural influences. *Journal of Family Psychology, 18*(4), 651–657.

Vargas, E. D. & Ybarra, V. D. (2017). U.S. citizen children of undocumented parents: the link between state immigration policy and the health of Latino children. *Journal of Immigrant and Minority Health, 19*(4), 913–920.

Vega, W. A., Alderete, E., Kolody, B., & Aguilar-Gaxiola, S. (1998). Illicit drug use among Mexicans and Mexican Americans in California: The effects of gender and acculturation. *Addiction, 93*(12), 1839–1850.

Voisine, S., Parsai, M., Marsiglia, F. F., Kulis, S., & Nieri, T. (2008). Parental monitoring and adolescent substance use among Mexican/Mexican American adolescents in the Southwest United States. *Families in Society, 89,* 264–273.

Walsh, S. D., Djalovski, A., Boniel-Nissim, M., & HarelFisch, Y. (2014). Parental, peer and school experiences as predictors of alcohol drinking among first- and second-generation immigrant adolescents in Israel. *Drug and Alcohol Dependence, 138,* 39–47.

Warner, L. A., Canino, G., & Colón, H. M. (2001). Prevalence and correlates of substance use disorders among older adolescents in Puerto Rico and the United States: A cross-cultural comparison. *Drug and Alcohol Dependence, 63*(3), 229–243.

Washington State Institute for Public Policy. (2016). *keepin' it REAL*. Retrieved from: http://wsipp.wa.gov/BenefitCost/Program/379.

Williams, L. S., Alvarez, S. D., & Andrade Hauck, K. S. (2002). My name is not Maria: Young Latinas seeking home in the heartland. *Social Problems, 49*(4), 563–584.

Wright, A. J., Nichols, T. R., Graber, J. A., Brooks-Gunn, J., & Botvin, G. J. (2004). It's not what you say, it's how many different ways you can say it: Links between divergent peer resistance skills and delinquency a year later. *Journal of Adolescent Health, 35*(5), 380–391.

Yabiku, S., Kulis, S., Marsiglia, F. F., Lewin, B., Nieri, T., & Hussaini, S. (2007). Neighborhood effects on the efficacy of a program to prevent youth alcohol use. *Substance Use and Misuse, 42*(1), 65–87.

Zamboanga, B. L., Schwartz, S. J., Jarvis, L. H., & Van Tyne, K. (2009). Acculturation and substance use among Hispanic early adolescents: Investigating the mediating roles of acculturative stress and self-esteem. *Journal of Primary Prevention, 30*(3–4), 315–333.

Zapata-Roblyer, M. I., Grzywacz, J. G., Cervantes, R. C., & Merten, M. J. (2016). Stress and alcohol, cigarette, and marijuana use among Latino adolescents in families with undocumented immigrants. *Journal of Child and Family Studies, 25*(2), 475–487.

Zhang, X., Martinez-Donate, A. P., Nobles, J., Hovell, M. F., Rangel, M. G., & Rhoads, N. M. (2015). Substance use across different phases of the migration process: A survey of Mexican migrants flows. *Journal of Immigrant and Minority Health, 17*(6), 1746–1757.

Zong, J., & Batalova, J. (2016). *Frequently requested statistics on immigrants and immigration in the United States*. Washington, DC: Migration Policy Institute.

Chapter 6
Disability Among the Latinx Population: Epidemiology and Empowerment Interventions

Fabricio E. Balcazar, Sandra Magaña and Yolanda Suarez-Balcazar

Abstract The significant increase in the Latinx population in the USA has also resulted in an increase in Latinx persons with disabilities. This chapter provides an overview of the prevalence and the most common types of disability in the Latinx population and a review of the health care status and barriers to health care experienced by Latinx persons. Empowerment-based interventions to address some of the barriers are also discussed here. We close the chapter with a discussion of implications for future research.

Keywords Latinx · Disability · Health · Empowerment · Intervention

As the Latinx population in the USA has increased, so has the number of Latinx people with a disability. In 2013, 4,652,500 Latinx individuals of all ages reported one or more disabilities (Erickson, Lee, & von Schrader, 2014). According to the data from the U.S. Bureau of the Census, disability disproportionately affects members of racial and ethnic minority groups (Yee, 2011). For example, data from the 2013 American Community Survey show relatively high rates of disability for the black population (14.7%) and the American Indian/Alaskan Native population (18.4%) at all ages compared with the general population (12.6%); the rate is lower for the Latinx population (8.7%) than the general population (Erickson et al., 2014). However, evidence suggests that disability may be underreported by Latinx individuals because of sociocultural barriers; thus, these figures may not represent true prevalence. For example, Latinx people are underrepresented in autism surveillance efforts conducted by the Centers for Disease Control and Prevention (CDC) (2016), which reports a prevalence of autism of approximately 1.5% for non-Latinx white children and approximately 1% for Latinx children. Because these surveillance efforts are based

F. E. Balcazar (✉)
Department of Disability and Human Development, University of Illinois-Chicago, Chicago, IL, USA
e-mail: fabricio@uic.edu

S. Magaña
Steve Hicks School of Social Work, University of Texas-Austin, Austin, TX, USA

Y. Suarez-Balcazar
Department of Occupational Therapy, University of Illinois-Chicago, Chicago, IL, USA

on record reviews, the reported prevalence actually represents access to diagnosis and not the true prevalence of disability. Several researchers have argued that Latinx people face many barriers accessing diagnostic services, such as limited knowledge and information about disability, lack of resources and insurance for evaluations and medical consultations, language barriers, and varying immigration statuses among family members that often preclude them from seeking medical help (Magaña, Lopez, Aguinaga, & Morton, 2013; Zuckerman et al., 2014). Likewise, other disabilities may also be underreported within the Latinx population.

Despite the probable undercount of Latinx with disabilities, robust data suggest that the disability resulting from job-related injury is more likely for Latinx individuals than for individuals in other racial/ethnic populations (Grzywacz et al., 2012; Krause & Terza, 2006; Orrenius & Zavodny, 2009; Sears, Bowman, & Silverstein, 2012). Latinx people tend to work in the most hazardous environments in the USA—with little or no protection—such as construction, farming, and work with machinery or exposure to corrosive and/or dangerous chemicals. Furthermore, injuries on the job are likely to be underreported by Latinx individuals because of the fear of losing their job or recognition of their immigration status (Grzywacz et al., 2012).

Moreover, Latinx individuals with disabilities are more likely to live in poverty than white or Asian individuals with disabilities (Yee, 2011). In addition, health, rehabilitation, and independent living outcomes for people with disabilities are less favorable within the Latinx population than the non-Hispanic white population (Granados, Puwula, Berman, & Dowling, 2001; Lillie-Blanton & Hudman, 2001; Suarez-Balcazar, Balcazar, Taylor-Ritzler, Ali, & Hasnain, 2013). For example, Latinx individuals with disabilities are less likely to participate in their communities, be fully employed, and live independently (U.S. Department of Labor, Bureau of Labor Statistics, 2015).

The purpose of this chapter is threefold. First, we will provide an overview of the prevalence and the most common types of disability in the Latinx population. Second, we will review some of the health issues and barriers to community participation and independent living that Latinx people with disabilities face in the USA. Third, we will discuss empowerment-based interventions designed to address some of these challenges.

Prevalence of Disability in the United States

The Centers for Disease Control and Prevention (CDC) reports that the prevalence of disability in 2005 was 21.8%, which represents 47.5 million individuals (2015). The three most common causes of disability are arthritis or rheumatism (an estimated 8.6 million people), back or spine problems (7.6 million), and heart disease (3.0 million). The prevalence of disability is significantly higher for women (24.4%) than men (19.1%) at all ages and, for both men and women, the prevalence doubles with age (18–44 years: 11.0%; 45–64 years: 23.9%; and 65 years and older: 51.8%). The authors of the report conclude that by 2030, the number of adults aged 65 and older is expected to reach 71 million, which will greatly increase the demand for appropriate medical and public health services, as more persons (Baby Boomers) enter this age group at highest risk for disability.

Health Care Status of Latinx Individuals with Disabilities

The health profile of the Latinx population in the USA differs from that of the white population. For example, the death rate and smoking rate are lower, the prevalence of heart disease is 35% lower, and the prevalence of cancer is 49% lower among the Latinx population compared with the white population (Centers for Disease Control and Prevention [CDC], 2015). However, a variety of other health risks are higher within the Latinx population than within the white population, including a 23% increased likelihood of obesity; a 24% greater likelihood of poorly controlled blood pressure; and a 50% greater likelihood of dying from diabetes or liver disease (CDC, 2015). In addition, in 2015, 2.2 million Latinx individuals reported having asthma, and they were twice as likely than non-Hispanic white individuals with asthma to seek medical attention in an emergency department (Office of Minority Health, 2017).

Similarly, Latinx children are twice as likely to die from asthma compared with white children (Office of Minority Health, 2017). Many Latinx individuals experience disability as a consequence of a health disease (such as diabetes), are at higher risk to experience these diseases if they already have a disability, or are older (Markides et al., 1996). For Latinx individuals with a disability, a chronic health condition may become exacerbated. For example, compared with white adults with the intellectual or developmental disability, Latinx adults with intellectual or developmental disability are more likely to be obese, have diabetes, and have poor physical and mental health status (Magaña, Parish, Morales, Li, & Fujiura, 2016). Furthermore, the health outcomes for Latinx adults with the intellectual or development disability are worse than those for nondisabled Latinx adults (Magaña et al., 2016).

Access to Health Care

Among Latinx people with disabilities, in addition to disparities in health status and chronic health conditions, disparities also exist in access and utilization of health care and quality of care. For example, among children with disabilities, levels of health care access (e.g., insurance coverage, regular source of care, or a medical home) are lower for Latinx children than for white children (Parish, Magaña, Rose, Timberlake, & Swaine, 2012; Strickland, Jones, Ghandour, Kogan, & Newacheck, 2011). These findings mirror access issues in the nondisabled Latinx population. In the USA, about one in three Latinx individuals are uninsured, which is the highest proportion of any demographic group (Kaiser Foundation Commission on Medicaid and the Uninsured, 2013). In comparison, about one in five black and one in eight non-Latinx white individuals are uninsured. Half of the uninsured Latinx people report some type of temporary disability and 15–20% report a long-term disability (U.S. Census Bureau, Brief Disability Status, 2012). Research shows that the largest barrier in Latinx individuals' access to health care is cost (CDC, 2015). Unlike other demographic groups, the Latinx population in the USA is also far more likely to encounter challenges related to language, discrimination, economic status/finances, and immigration status, all of which contribute to poor access to health services.

Health Care Utilization and Quality of Life

With respect to health care utilization, Latinx individuals are underserved by health-related services and, as a result, they are less likely to receive preventive treatments and/or treatment for secondary conditions (Suarez-Balcazar et al., 2013). Disparities also exist in the quality of health care. Among parents of children with disabilities, Latinx parents reported that their health care provider was less likely to spend enough time with their child, makes the parent feel like a partner, and be culturally sensitive compared with white parents (Magaña, Parish, & Son, 2015).

Latinx people with disabilities also experience barriers to independent living and health services, such as the lack of culturally appropriate outreach and bilingual and culturally competent service providers (National Council on Disability, 2003). Because of these and other barriers, Latinx individuals with disabilities are often not well integrated into the society, and the workplace and negative health outcomes are more likely (Balcazar, Keys, & Suarez-Balcazar, 2001; Ludwig-Beymer, Blankemeier, Casas-Byots, & Suarez-Balcazar, 1996). As such, they are less likely to take advantage of both formal and informal resources/services and more likely to experience discrimination at multiple levels, primarily because of their disability, racial and ethnic background, lack of mastery of the English language, and/or socioeconomic status. Consequently, the disabling aspects of their impairment are significantly enhanced.

Cultural factors also influence the lack of access to health care for Latinx individuals with disabilities. Researchers assert that the lack of cultural competence among health care providers has had a negative impact on Latinx individuals, with greater likelihoods of discrimination, cultural mistrust, and poor communication with providers (Escarce & Kapur, 2006). In addition, many Latinx families lack knowledge about the availability of disability-related services in their community (Raymond-Flesch, Siemons, Pourat, Jacobs, & Brindis, 2014).

To conclude, Latinx individuals with disabilities, compared with individuals in other racial/ethnic groups, encounter unique barriers that contribute to negative health outcomes. These barriers are fundamentally tied to limited access to health insurance and therefore limited preventive care and high-quality health care and/or access to community services, a disparity that is even more pronounced among Latinx individuals with disabilities. Socioeconomic status and the types of jobs that Latinx individuals perform (most of which do not provide health insurance coverage for the worker and/or the family) become important contextual factors when the relationship between health and disability is examined in this population. Next, we discuss issues of community participation among Latinx individuals with disabilities.

Community Participation and Independent Living

Historically, individuals with disabilities have experienced marginalization in participation in community life, education, and employment, among other areas (Balcazar, Suarez-Balcazar, Keys, & Taylor-Ritzler, 2010). According to a report released by the U.S. Bureau of Labor Statistics for the year 2014, 17.1% of persons with a disability were employed in the USA compared with 64.6% of persons without a disability (U.S. Department of Labor, Bureau of Labor Statistics, 2015). In addition, relative to the overall population, individuals with disabilities who are employed typically hold jobs with lower wages than their peers without a disability (American Community Survey, 2013). Furthermore, poorer employment outcomes are associated with being a member of a minority race or ethnic group and being less well educated (Crisp, 2005). These disparities contribute to the pervasive poverty rate among individuals with disabilities (U.S. Census Bureau Newsroom, 2013), in particular among the Latinx population and other minority groups. Latinx individuals with disabilities experience stressors and expenses related to daily living with a disability that place them at risk for poverty (Suarez-Balcazar et al., 2013). These stressors include the need to purchase costly adaptive equipment, to modify the home for accessibility, and to pay for personal care services, as well as overall stressors associated with environmental, psychologic, and social barriers (Suarez-Balcazar & Cooper, 2005).

In addition, Latinx individuals with disabilities often experience challenges when applying for social services such as vocational rehabilitation, which provides support for pursuing employment and educational opportunities (Langi & Balcazar, 2017). Difficulties include obtaining all required documents needed to qualify for services (e.g., a valid Social Security number), meeting eligibility criteria, and receiving fewer services than some white consumers (Oberoi, Balcazar, Suarez-Balcazar, Langi, & Lukyanova, 2015; Taylor-Ritzler, Balcazar, Suarez-Balcazar, & Garcia-Iriarte, 2007). People with disabilities are also more likely than people without disabilities to experience disparity in community participation (Ouellette-Kuntz, 2005). Strong evidence indicates that, in general, active participation in making decisions about one's life and community has an impact on an individual's health and well-being (Krahn, Hammond, & Turner, 2006). The concept of full participation in society for all individuals with disabilities often represents a key goal for advocates, researchers, and rehabilitation specialists (Hammel, Magasi et al., 2008). Full participation includes active engagement in everyday situations at the societal and personal levels as well as the meaningfulness and satisfaction that results from those engagements (Hammel, Jones et al., 2008). Successful community participation for people with disabilities generally involves social relationships, employment, leisure activities, and family and community life (Cardol, De Jong, & Ward, 2002; Heinemann, Kurenbach, &

Quist, 2011). True community participation depends on a culture of inclusion as well as opportunities for meaningful contact and activities that range across the life span (Magasi, Hammel, Heinemann, Whiteneck, & Bogner, 2009).

In summary, Latinx individuals with disabilities are less likely to participate in their communities and use disability-related services than the general population of individuals with disabilities (Raymond-Flesch et al., 2014). As mentioned, barriers to the use of disability services include perceived discrimination, a lack of culturally responsive providers and outreach personnel, cultural mistrust, language and communication difficulties, distrust of government policies, and a lack of knowledge about policies and programs. The combination of these barriers results in less community living and independent living outcomes compared with white individuals with disabilities (Cardoso, Romero, Chan, Dutta, & Rahimi, 2007; Sander, Pappadis, Clark, & Struchen, 2011; Suarez-Balcazar, Balcazar, & Willis, 2012).

Despite these challenges, Latinx people with disabilities often rely on protective factors that enhance their satisfaction with and quality of life. For example, they often view disability not as an individual matter, but as the responsibility of the entire family—including extended family members such as grandparents and other relatives; in addition, Latinx adults with disabilities are more likely to be living at home and may rely on support and assistance, if needed, from their kinship and family networks (Tejero-Hughes, Martinez Valle-Riestra, & Arguelles, 2008); Latinx individuals are also protected by values such as familism and collective well-being and receive ongoing tangible and social support from family members (Marin, Organista, & Chun, 2003). These protective factors, however, place a significant amount of pressure on women in the family, who are more likely to care for the person with a disability (Magaña & Smith, 2006). A side effect for mothers of children with disabilities is that these mothers often lack the respite and support they need, which places their own well-being and health at risk (Magaña & Smith, 2008). In the next section, we discuss the social model of disability and the empowerment model as frameworks underpinning the interventions described. The interventions are designed to address some of the challenges and barriers mentioned in the introduction. We now review several approaches based on a conceptual framework of empowerment to address some of the unmet needs of Latinx people with disabilities.

The Empowerment Model and Related Interventions

Rappaport (1987) defined empowerment as the process of enhancing people's active control over their lives. He suggested that empowerment is the process by which individuals, communities, or organizations gain mastery over their interactions in such a way that they discover their own ability to look for solutions rather than helplessly living with their concerns. Empowerment is a multilevel construct emerging at the individual, group, organizational, and/or community levels. It is affected by a person's previous experiences, is contextual, and is limited by spatial and temporal boundaries (Rappaport, 1987). In the context of disability, empowerment strategies are developed with consideration of the interactions between individual and/or group strengths and challenges in relation to the contextual supports and/or barriers that determine the degree of control that one can attain in his or her life (Fawcett et al., 1994). This definition is consistent with the social model of disability (Oliver, 2013), which emphasizes disability as a function of the limitations in the environment that determine the individual's degree of participation and community engagement. According to this framework, the disabling experience (impairment) is related to an individual's degree of functioning in his or her particular environment (Hahn, 1993). In this case, the physical, cognitive, or psychologic impairment of the individual becomes secondary to the capacity of the environment to allow and support full participation and integration into working, independent living, and community activities. For that reason, disability-related challenges are viewed primarily as a product of limiting environments and negative societal attitudes (Gill & Cross, 2010). From this perspective, individuals with disabilities need enabling and accessible environments that provide them with the resources and opportunities for full participation in everyday life activities and the achievement of personal goals (Albrecht, 2007).

Several scholars in the disability field, such as Fine and Asch (1988) and Charlton (1998, 2006), argue that the conditions that keep people with disabilities marginalized can be eliminated only through changing unequal power relations and the redistribution of wealth. Power can be defined as the ability to access material and psychosocial resources; it is also a social regulation system that provides people the opportunity and capacity to achieve a state of well-being (Montero, 2009). However, some groups often use power to accumulate privileges over the groups they oppress. This oppression happens through deprivation, exclusion, violence, discrimination, and control of the oppressed group (Nelson & Prilleltensky, 2005). These conditions contribute to the psychosocial profile of an oppressed group, which often perceives itself as a victim of uncontrollable superior forces (e.g., political, military, cultural, ethnic, religious, and/or social) that lacks competence and the ability to pursue a successful life. These perceptions are common among people with disabilities. According to Paulo Freire (1970), the unfortunate dilemma is that most people who experience oppression do not necessarily act to transform their social reality because they have internalized their oppression. Freire also argues that marginalized individuals do not have a *critical awareness* that allows them to see the injustices or the oppressions in their lives. A marginalized individual often accepts his or her existence based on perceptions of destiny, bad luck, and/or supernatural forces that are beyond his or her control. Challenging these perceptions becomes a central part of the empowerment process. Therefore, the capacity of the individual with a disability to fully participate in the community and become integrated into the fabric of society is a function of the environment's accessibility, the supports and services available for him or her to function and perform effectively, and the individual's ability to advocate for himself or herself. Empowerment interventions to address the challenges people with disabilities face are well framed under the social model of disability.

Empowering Interventions

Several approaches to addressing the marginalization of Latinx people with disabilities are consistent with an empowerment framework (Fawcett et al., 1994; Fetterman, 2015; Suarez-Balcazar et al., 2013; Zimmerman & Eisman, 2016). For example, Fawcett et al. (1994) proposed a contextual-behavioral model of empowerment and illustrated their model with several case studies in which individuals with disabilities engaged in the process of empowerment at the individual, group, and organizational level to remove barriers to or enhance facilitators of independence. Within the contextual model of empowerment of Fawcett et al. (1994), the interaction between the efforts to strengthen individual characteristics such as knowledge and advocacy skills and the removal of contextual barriers that hinder community integration and independent living can contribute to enhancing empowerment outcomes among individuals with disabilities.

Many people with disabilities have organized and united to advocate for their rights. They have followed the tradition of so-called identity politics to find common ground on which to organize their national disability rights movements. Identity politics originally grew out of collective movements for equality on the basis of gender, race, and sexuality. In the USA, white middle-class individuals with physical disabilities have primarily led the movement; Latinx people with disabilities have remained at the sidelines of this movement. Overall, Latinx people with disabilities have had little involvement in disability rights and advocacy movements. However, Latinx individuals with disabilities and their parents have created service programs and support groups to address the needs that were unmet by the disability service system. For example, in Chicago, Illinois, El Valor—a nationally recognized nonprofit organization that serves people with disabilities and their families—was founded in 1973 by the late Guadalupe Reyes, who was a mother and visionary leader. According to El Valor's website (www.elvalor.org), she dreamed of a community that would be inclusive of her son and others with disabilities. Similarly, Fiesta Educativa (www.fiestaeducativa.org), a nonprofit organization founded in 1978 in California, was formed by family members and professionals who recognized the need to empower and educate parents of children with disabilities. More recently, Latinx parents of children with autism have formed support groups in different communities to provide information and assistance; these groups include Grupo Salto in Chicago and Grupo de Autismo in Milwaukee, Wisconsin. A recent effort to build a movement of Latinx people with disabilities was launched by an organization called Cambiando Vidas, housed at Access Living, the Chicago-based center for independent living. This organization held its first national conference, "Building a National Network: Empowering Latinos with Disabilities," in the spring of 2016 and brought Latinx individuals with disabilities from several states. This group plans to hold annual conferences and expands its network (www.latinxdisabilitycoalition.com).

Balcazar and Suarez-Balcazar (2016) adapted the model of power redistribution of Bennett-Cattaneo and Chapman (2010) as a framework of analysis for efforts in the redistribution of resources in a historically asymmetric context, such as the one experienced by Latinx individuals with disabilities. The model is a dialectical and contextual model that can provide an explanation for some of the factors that lead people to seek power redistribution. The process starts when the group or individual with a disability identifies and articulates an injustice that he or she has experienced in a particular context, such as the workplace. This articulation is often the result of awareness or the realization of historical inequalities or grievances that have not been addressed. Once the individual, or group of persons with disabilities, decides to pursue power redistribution, the goals may be articulated in terms of what is desired in a particular situation or context. For example, a person with a spinal cord injury and two other employees with disabilities in a small company may be notified that the next year their insurance premiums will go up more than the ones for other employees because they use more services. Depending on the degree of motivation and critical awareness, the affected employees may decide to act on the situation once they realize they are being discriminated against. Different degrees of motivation are associated with the group's goal, depending on the circumstances or sense of urgency experienced. Also, several factors determine the degree of competence and effectiveness of the group in seeking power redistribution. These factors include knowledge of rights and responsibilities (including the policies or laws that may be associated with the particular situation); level of competence and skills (often associated with previous experience in pursuing redress of injustices or addressing power imbalances); and the degree of self-efficacy (which is related to previous experiences and successes) in attaining personal and/or group goals. Actions and counteractions are taken depending on the way in which the organization reacts to the group's empowerment efforts.

In this example, the employer may decide that the insurance policy is too expensive and the employees should pay more for it. At this point, conflict or compromise (depending on the situation) takes place, and the direct result is power redistribution (which may vary, depending on the effectiveness of the advocacy efforts and related actions and counteractions). For example, the employees may file a lawsuit under the American with Disabilities Act of 1990 (ADA) against the employer, which may result in fines for the employer. Sometimes, the individuals with a disability run out of options exhaust their resources, are repressed or fired, or become demoralized and concede defeat. Therefore, there is no guarantee that the process will result in greater power to the aspiring individual or group. The resulting changes in power redistribution may stop the process if the parties are satisfied or may restart the process again in order to pursue better results. Individuals or groups may seek more knowledge or advocacy training or they may need to increase their own levels of awareness and organization in order to succeed. The sense of efficacy of those involved in the process is affected by their degree of success in conducting advocacy activities over time.

In general, advocacy tactics can create opportunities for capacity building and empowerment, allowing participants to pursue changes in policies, programs, or services, and providing opportunities to engage in self-efficacy efforts as well. (See https://ccbmdr.ahslabs.uic.edu/products/ for several guides for consumer involvement in advocacy organizations.) To promote empowerment at the community and societal level, it is important to examine national, state, and local policies, programs, and/or services that unexpectedly or intentionally raise barriers for people with disabilities, eliminate or reduce services, and/or exclude them from opportunities. National advocacy groups such as the American Association of People with Disabilities (www.aapd.com) or the National Disability Rights Network (www.ndrn.org) are vigilant about promoting the empowerment of people with disabilities.

The Promotoras de Salud Model

The *promotora* (promoter) model has been widely used in the field of public health as a way to educate Latinx people about chronic health conditions and health promotion (Rhodes, Foley, Zometa, & Bloom, 2007). *Promotoras* are typically lay people from the Latinx community who serve as a bridge between the community and health professionals (Otiniano, Carroll-Scott, Toy, & Wallace, 2012). *Promotoras* may be employed by health care providers and trained in general health issues or may work on projects related to specific chronic conditions. They typically receive training on the health issues related to their project and may receive training to help patients navigate complex health care systems.

Magaña, Lopez, and Machalicek (2017) adapted the model to educate mothers of children with autism spectrum disorder (ASD) about better ways to help their children develop and learn. The researchers believed it was important to include peer leaders as *promotoras* as a way to empower the community of Latinx individuals with the disability. The intervention, *Parents Taking Action* (PTA), follows a psychoeducational approach to educate parents who have children with ASD (Magaña et al., 2017). The peer leaders approach ensures that the *promotoras* have shared experiences that go beyond the ethnic community because they also share the challenges for parents raising a child with ASD. This shared experience, or in Spanish, *convivencia*, is powerful in promoting self-efficacy among participants in the intervention, a key element of the empowerment framework presented here. One *promotora* summed it up in a focus group after her experience with delivering the intervention: *"It's the shared experience (convivencia), also the support between families. Because in whatever form, we are the same...We share at the same time that we learn from each other."*

This method of intervention delivery works particularly well in Latinx immigrant communities in which community members rely on persons they can trust to provide information and education and help them navigate the sometimes daunting service system.

Although parents who participate in PTA become empowered on an individual and family level to take action in helping their children learn, the program can also lead to change at the community level, which relates to the empowerment model and the social model of disability. *Promotoras* work with other parents on how to advocate for services in schools and in the community. The collective impact of parents using their advocacy skills can change the approach that providers and school staff take with parents, as the providers see parents more as change agents rather than passive recipients of services. These changes may lead to conflict, which as outlined earlier, is a driver for change. For example, PTA is currently being piloted in Bogota, Colombia. Children in this project attend one school, the only school that includes children with disabilities in the city. One of the challenges at the school is that, although the school is inclusive, the administration does not provide resources to the teachers about how to work with children with disabilities. At the same time, parents from the PTA program began to make demands to the teachers about the treatment of their children in the school. Because this is an ongoing project, the conflict may lead teachers to advocate for resources from the school administration so that they can gain the training needed to work better with children with disabilities.

Another example of an intervention that follows the *promotora* model is *By Caring for Myself, I Can Better Care for My Family* (Magaña, Li, Miranda, & Paradiso, 2015). This intervention focuses on the idea of family to orient mothers of children and adults with intellectual and developmental disabilities (IDD) toward their own health promotion. As mentioned earlier, research shows that many Latinx mothers of children with IDD are very focused on their main role in life being to care for their child with a disability, as well as caring for other family members (Magaña & Smith, 2006). By engaging peer-based *promotoras* who are mothers of children with IDD, the program emphasizes the importance for mothers to see a doctor for checkups and screenings and to practice healthy habits related to diet, exercise, and stress reduction. These habits are discussed in the context of the child with the disability and the whole family based on the premise that mothers are engaging in healthy habits will lead to family healthy habits (Magaña, Li, et al., 2015).

Healthy Families: Promoting Healthy Lifestyles

Building further on the idea of incorporating the family into interventions for people with IDD, another intervention example under the empowerment framework is a healthy lifestyles program called *Familias Saludables* (Suarez-Balcazar et al., 2016). The program, implemented in collaboration with a local community agency, is based on an adaptation of *Health Matters* (Marks, Sisirak, & Heller, 2010) and includes three main components: dance as physical activity, health education, and goal setting/self-management. The program targets the whole family, including siblings, parents, and other relatives of youth and young adults with developmental disabilities. The program focuses on culturally relevant healthy lifestyles activities. The program empowers family members who are trained on how to lead dance sessions and/or assist in implementing the intervention. It also focuses on creating capacity at the community level so that the program can be sustained at the community level. Preliminary data show that the program has an impact on family routines and family goal setting (Suarez-Balcazar et al., 2016).

Conclusion

The Latinx community in general and Latinx individuals with disabilities, in particular, often encounter many challenges in accessing health services and receiving many needed social and community supports. As mentioned, the actual and projected growth of the Latinx population is only going to exacerbate these problems. Poverty, lack of health insurance, immigration status, and lack of bilingual and culturally competent providers limit the access to health and social services for Latinx individuals with disabilities. Despite these challenges, many Latinx families rely on their own strengths and culture to cope with the challenges.

Empowerment is a valuable framework for the development of interventions designed to address some of these challenges. Several researchers have alluded to the impact of participatory research strategies on one's perceived sense of empowerment (Balcazar, Keys, Kaplan, & Suarez-Balcazar, 1998) and on building the capacity of participants to address their unmet needs through advocacy. Because many Latinx women are likely to be involved in providing support to their family members with disabilities throughout the life course, it is important that interventions such as *promotoras de salud* and *Familias Saludables* seek to empower families and the persons with disabilities they care for as a way to benefit the family as a whole. The other important benefit of these types of interventions is that they address the cultural and linguistic barriers that are likely to appear if other types of individuals are involved in the service delivery. Cultural competency is a critical dimension that allows for the trust and *confianza* that is central to effective engagements, teaching, and learning.

Directions for Future Research

To date, little information is available on community-based strategies that can facilitate the empowerment of Latinx individuals with disabilities. New research methods and strategies within an empowerment approach are needed to enhance the capacity of Latinx people with disabilities and their families to improve their own health, community participation, and independent living outcomes. Interventions designed to empower consumers, such as the ones described here, are yielding promising results, but these interventions are not widely disseminated and reach only small segments of the population. In effect, more research is needed to evaluate ways in which Latinx families of individuals with disabilities are coping and addressing their needs or not and how promising interventions can be made available to them (outreach). Ways to improve the cultural and linguistic competence of the health care, educational, and social services systems are needed. A much wider use of peers as mentors, guides, or sources of support and information is required. Service systems could benefit from engaging peers who are already culturally and linguistically competent to deliver needed guidance and support. Such a model is being shown as effective with the *promotoras* intervention but was also successful in an intervention with individuals with spinal cord injuries resulting from gun violence (Balcazar, Hayes-Kelly, Keys, & Balfanz-Vertiz, 2011). Using local resources and the strength of the community itself should continue to be evaluated as a way to address key unmet needs and promote the health of Latinx individuals with disabilities.

References

Albrecht, T. J. (2007). *Challenges and service needs of undocumented Mexican undergraduate students: Students' voices and administrators' perspectives.* The University of Texas at Austin, Austin, TX. Retrieved from http://repositories.lib.utexas.edu/handle/2152/3542.

American Community Survey. (2013). *2013 American community survey 1-year estimates* [Data file]. Retrieved from https://factfinder.census.gov/faces/tableservices/jsf/pages/productview.xhtml?src=bkmk.

Balcazar, F. B., Hayes-Kelly, E., Keys, C. B., & Balfanz-Vertiz, K. (2011). Using peer mentoring to support the rehabilitation of individuals with violently acquired spinal cord injuries. *Journal of Applied Rehabilitation Counseling, 42,* 3–11.

Balcazar, F. E., Keys, C. B., Kaplan, D. L., & Suarez-Balcazar, Y. (1998). Participatory action research with disabilities: Principles and challenges. *Canadian Journal of Rehabilitation, 12,* 105–112.

Balcazar, F. E., Keys, C., & Suarez-Balcazar, Y. (2001). Empowering Latinos with disabilities to address issues of independent living and disability rights: A capacity building approach. *Journal of Prevention and Intervention in the Community, 21*(2), 53–70.

Balcazar, F.E., & Suarez-Balcazar, Y. (2016). Promoting empowerment among individuals with disabilities. In M. A. Bond, C. B. Keys, & I. Serrano-García (Eds.), *APA handbook of community psychology* (Vol. 2). Washington, DC: American Psychological Association. Retrieved from: http://www.apa.org/pubs/books/4311524.aspx?tab=2.

Balcazar, F. E., Suarez-Balcazar, Y., Keys, C., & Taylor-Ritzler, T. (2010). *Race, culture, and disability: Rehabilitation science and practice.* Sudbury, MA: Jones and Bartlett Publishers.

Bennett-Cattaneo, L., & Chapman, A. R. (2010). The process of empowerment: A model for use in research and practice. *American Psychologist, 65*(7), 646–659.

Cardol, M., De Jong, B. A., & Ward, C. D. (2002). On autonomy and participation in rehabilitation. *Disability and Rehabilitation, 24,* 970–974.

Cardoso, R., Romero, M., Chan, F., Dutta, A., & Rahimi, M. (2007). Disparities in vocational services for Latino clients with traumatic brain injury. *Journal of Head Trauma Rehabilitation, 22,* 85–94.

Centers for Disease Control and Prevention. (2015). *CDC vital signs—Hispanic health.* Retrieved from https://www.cdc.gov/vitalsigns/pdf/2015-05-vitalsigns.pdf.

Centers for Disease Control and Prevention. (2016). *Prevalence and characteristics of autism spectrum disorder among children aged 8 years—Autism and developmental disability monitoring network, 11 sites, United States, 2012.* Retrieved from http://www.cdc.gov/mmwr/volumes/65/ss/ss6503a1.htm.

Charlton, J. (1998). *Nothing about us without us: Disability oppression and empowerment.* Berkeley, CA: University of California Press.

Charlton, J. (2006). The dimensions of disability oppression: An overview. In L. J. Davis (Ed.), *The disability studies reader* (pp. 147–159). New York: Routledge.

Crisp, R. (2005). Key factors related to vocational outcome: Trends for six disability groups. *Journal of Rehabilitation, 71*(4), 30–37.

Erickson, W., Lee, C., & von Schrader, S. (2014). *2013 Disability status report: United States.* Ithaca, NY: Cornell University Employment and Disability Institute.

Escarce, J. J., & Kapur, K. (2006). Access to and quality of health care. In M. Tienda & F. Mitchell (Eds.), *Hispanics and the future of America* (pp. 410–446). Washington, DC: National Academies Press.

Fawcett, S. B., White, G. W., Balcazar, F., Suarez-Balcazar, Y., Mathews, M. R., & Paine, A. (1994). A contextual-behavioral model of empowerment: Case studies involving people with disabilities. *American Journal of Community Psychology, 22*, 471–496.

Fetterman, D. M. (2015). *Empowerment evaluation: Knowledge and tools for self-assessment, evaluation capacity building, and accountability*. Thousand Oaks, CA: Sage.

Fine, M., & Asch, A. (1988). *Women with disabilities: Essays in psychology, culture and politics*. Philadelphia: Temple University Press.

Freire, P. (1970). *Pedagogy of the oppressed*. New York, NY: Continuum International.

Gill, C. J., & Cross, W. E. (2010). Disability identity and racial-cultural identity development: Points of convergence, divergence, and interplay. In F. E. Balcazar, Y. Suarez-Balcazar, T. Taylor-Ritzler, & C. B. Keys (Eds.), *Race, culture, & disability* (pp. 33–52). Sudbury, MA: Jones and Bartlett.

Granados, G., Puwula, J., Berman, N., & Dowling, P. (2001). Health care for Latino children: Impact of child and parental birthplace on insurance status and access to health services. *American Journal of Public Health, 91*, 1806–1820.

Grzywacz, J., Quandt, S., Marin, A., Summers, P., Lang, W., Mills, T., Arcury, T. (2012). Occupational injury and work organization among immigrant Latino residential construction workers. *American Journal of Industrial Medicine, 55*, 698–706. https://doi.org/10.1002/ajim.22014.

Hahn, H. (1993). The potential impact of disability studies on political science (as well as vice versa). *Policy Studies Journal, 21*, 740–751.

Hammel, J., Jones, R., Smith, J., Sanford, J., Bodine, C., & Johnson, M. (2008). Environmental barriers and supports to the health, function, and participation of people with developmental and intellectual disabilities: Report from the state of the science in aging with developmental disabilities conference. *Disability & Health, 1*(3), 143–149.

Hammel, J., Magasi, S., Heinemann, A., Whiteneck, G., Bogner, J., & Rodriguez, E. (2008). What does participation mean? An insider perspective from people with disabilities. *Disability and Rehabilitation, 30*(19), 1445–1460. https://doi.org/10.1080/09638280701625534.

Heinemann, J. A., Kurenbach, B., & Quist, D. (2011). Molecular profiling—A tool for addressing emerging gaps in the comparative risk assessment of GMOs. *Environment International, 37*, 1285–1293.

Kaiser Foundation Commission on Medicaid and the Uninsured. (2013). Health coverage by race and ethnicity: The potential impact on the affordable care act. Retrieved from http://kff.org/disparities-policy/issue-brief/health-coverage-by-race-and-ethnicity-the-potential-impact-of-the-affordable-care-act/.

Krahn, G. L., Hammond, L., & Turner, A. (2006). A cascade of disparities: Health and health care access for people with intellectual disabilities. *Mental Retardation and Developmental Disabilities Research Review, 12*(1), 70–82.

Krause, J. S., & Terza, J. V. (2006). Injury and demographic factors predictive of disparities in earnings after spinal cord injury. *Archives of Physical Medicine and Rehabilitation, 87*(10), 1318–1326. https://doi.org/10.1016/j.apmr.2006.07.254.

Langi, F. L., & Balcazar, F. E. (2017). Risk factors for failure to enter vocational rehabilitation services among individuals with disabilities. *Disability and Rehabilitation, 39*(26), 2640–2647.

Lillie-Blanton, M., & Hudman, J. (2001). Untangling the web: Race/ethnicity, immigration, and the nation's health. *American Journal of Public Health, 91*, 1736–1739.

Ludwig-Beymer, P., Blankemeier, J., Casas-Byots, C., & Suarez-Balcazar, Y. (1996). Community assessment in a suburban Hispanic community: A description of method. *Journal of Transcultural Nursing, 8*, 19–27.

Magaña, S., Li, H., Miranda, E., & Paradiso, R. (2015). Improving health behaviors of Latina mothers of youths and adults with intellectual and developmental disabilities. *Journal of Intellectual Disability Research, 59*, 397–410. https://doi.org/10.1111/jir.12139.

Magaña, S., Lopez, K., Aguinaga, A., & Morton, H. (2013). Access to diagnosis and treatment services among Latino children with autism spectrum disorders. *Intellectual and Developmental Disabilities, 51,* 141–153. https://doi.org/10.1352/1934-9556-51.3.141.

Magaña, S., Lopez, K., & Machalicek, W. (2017). Parents taking action: A psycho-educational intervention for Latino parents of children with autism spectrum disorders. *Family Process, 56*(1), 59–74. https://doi.org/10.1111/famp.12169.

Magaña, S., Parish, S., Morales, M., Li, H., & Fujiura, G. (2016). Racial and ethnic health disparities among people with intellectual and developmental disabilities. *Intellectual and Developmental Disabilities, 54,* 161–172. https://doi.org/10.1352/1934-9556-54.3.161.

Magaña, S., Parish, S., & Son, E. (2015). Have racial and ethnic disparities in the quality of health care relationships changed for children with developmental disabilities and ASD? *American Journal of Intellectual and Developmental Disabilities, 120,* 504–513. https://doi.org/10.1352/1944-7558-120.6.504.

Magaña, S., & Smith, M. J. (2006). Psychological distress and well-being of Latina and non-Latina white mothers of youth and adults with an autism spectrum disorder: Cultural attitudes towards co-residence status. *American Journal of Orthopsychiatry, 76,* 346–357. https://doi.org/10.1037/0002-9432.76.3.346.

Magaña, S., & Smith, M. (2008). Health behaviors, service utilization, and access to care among older mothers of color who have children with developmental disabilities. *Intellectual and Developmental Disabilities, 46,* 267–280. https://doi.org/10.1352/1934-9556(2008)46%5b267:HBSUAA%5d2.0.CO;2.

Magasi, S., Hammel, J., Heinemann, A., Whiteneck, G., & Bogner, J. (2009). Participation: A comparative analysis of multiple rehabilitation stakeholders' perspectives. *Journal of Rehabilitation Medicine, 41*(11), 936–944. https://doi.org/10.2340/16501977-0450.

Marin, G., Organista, P. B., & Chun, K. M. (2003). *Handbook of racial and ethnic minority psychology.* Thousand Oaks, CA: Sage.

Markides, K. S., Stroup-Benham, C. A., Goodwin, J. S., Perkowski, L. C., Lichtenstein, M., & Ray, L. A. (1996). The effect of medical conditions on the functional limitations of Mexican-American elderly. *Annals of Epidemiology, 6*(5), 386–392.

Marks, B., Sisirak, J., & Heller, T. (2010). *Health matters: The exercise and nutrition health education curriculum for people with developmental disabilities.* Baltimore, MD: Brookes.

Montero, M. (2009). Methods for liberation: critical consciousness in action. In M. Montero & C. C. Sonn (Eds.), *Psychology of liberation* (pp. 73–92). New York, NY: Springer.

National Council on Disability (2003). Outreach and people with disabilities from diverse cultures: A review of the literature. Retrieved from http://www.ncd.gov/newsroom/advisory/cultural/cdi_litreview.html.

Nelson, G., & Prilleltensky, I. (Eds.). (2005). *Community psychology: In pursuit of liberation and wellbeing.* New York, NY: Palgrave MacMillan.

Oberoi, A. K., Balcazar, F., Suarez-Balcazar, Y., Langi, F., & Lukyanova, V. (2015). Employment outcomes among African American and White women with disabilities: Examining the inequalities. *Women, Gender and Families of Color, 3,* 144–164. https://doi.org/10.5406/womgenfamcol.3.2.0144.

Office of Minority Health. (2017). *Asthma and Hispanic Americans.* Retrieved from http://minorityhealth.hhs.gov/omh/browse.aspx?lvl=4&lvlid=60.

Oliver, M. (2013). The social model of disability: thirty years on. *Disability & Society, 28*(7), 1024–1026. http://dx.doi.org/10/1080/09687599.2013.818773.

Orrenius, P. M., & Zavodny, M. (2009). Do immigrants work in riskier jobs? *Demography, 46*(3), 535–551.

Otiniano, A. D., Carroll-Scott, A., Toy, P., & Wallace, S. P. (2012). Supporting Latino communities' natural helpers: A case study of promotoras in a research capacity building course. *Journal of Immigrant and Minority Health/Center for Minority Public Health, 14,* 657–663. https://doi.org/10.1007/s10903-011-9519-9.

Ouellette-Kuntz, H. (2005). Understanding health disparities and inequities faced by individuals with intellectual disabilities. *Journal of Applied Research in Intellectual Disabilities, 18*(2), 113–121.

Parish, S., Magaña, S., Rose, R., Timberlake, M., & Swaine, J. (2012). Health care of Latino children with autism and other developmental disabilities: Quality of provider interaction mediates utilization. *American Journal on Intellectual and Developmental Disabilities, 117,* 304–315. https://doi.org/10.1352/1944-7558-117.4.304.

Rappaport, J. (1987). Terms of empowerment/exemplars of prevention: Toward a theory for community psychology. *American Journal of Community Psychology, 15*(2), 121–148.

Raymond-Flesch, M., Siemons, R., Pourat, N., Jacobs, K., & Brindis, C. D. (2014). There is no help out there and if there is, it's really hard to find": A qualitative study of the health concerns and healthcare access of Latino "DREAMers". *Journal of Adolescent Health, 55*(3), 323–328. https://doi.org/10.1016/j.jadohealth.2014.05.012.

Rhodes, S. D., Foley, K. L., Zometa, C. S., & Bloom, F. R. (2007). Lay health advisor interventions among Hispanics/Latinos: A qualitative systematic review. *American Journal of Preventive Medicine, 33,* 418–427. https://doi.org/10.1016/j.amepre.2007.07.023.

Sander, A. M., Pappadis, M. R., Clark, A. N., & Struchen, M. A. (2011). Perceptions of community integration in an ethnically diverse sample. *Journal of Head Trauma Rehabilitation, 26*(2), 158–169.

Sears, J., Bowman, S., & Silverstein, B. (2012). Trends in the disproportionate burden of work-related traumatic injuries sustained by Latinos. *Journal of Occupational and Environmental Medicine, 54,* 1239–1245. https://doi.org/10.1097/JOM.0b013e31825a34ed.

Strickland, B. B., Jones, J. R., Ghandour, R. M., Kogan, M. D., & Newacheck, P. W. (2011). The medical home: Health care access and impact for children and youth in the United States. *Pediatrics, 127,* 604–611. https://doi.org/10.1542/peds.2009-3555.

Suarez-Balcazar, Y., Balcazar, F. B., Taylor-Ritzler, T., Ali, A., & Hasnain, R. (2013). Race, poverty, and disability: A social justice dilemma. In B. J. Betancur & C. Herring (Eds.), *Reinventing race, reinventing racism* (pp. 351–367). Boston, MA: Brill.

Suarez-Balcazar, Y., Balcazar, F., & Willis, C. (2012). Cultural considerations for MS rehabilitation. In M. Finlayson (Ed.), *Multiple sclerosis rehabilitation: From impairment to participation.* Boca Raton, FL: CRC Press, Taylor & Francis Group.

Suarez-Balcazar, Y., & Cooper, M. B. (2005). Poverty. In G. Albrecht (Ed.), *Encyclopedia of disability* (Vol. 2, pp. 1281–1284). Thousand Oaks, CA: Sage.

Suarez-Balcazar, Y., Hoisington, M., Orozco, A. A., Garcia, C., Smith, K., Arias, D., Bonner, B. (2016). Benefits of a culturally tailored health promotion program for Latino youth with disabilities and their families. *American Journal of Occupational Therapy, 70*(5), 1–8. https://doi.org/10.5014/ajot.2016.021949.

Taylor-Ritzler, T., Balcazar, F. E., Suarez-Balcazar, Y., & Garcia-Iriarte, E. (2007). Conducting disability research with people from diverse ethnic groups: Challenges and opportunities. *Journal of Rehabilitation, 74*(1), 4–11.

Tejero-Hughes, M., Martinez Valle-Riestra, D., & Arguelles, M. E. (2008). The voices of Latino families raising children with special needs. *Journal of Latinos and Education, 7*(3), 241–257.

U.S. Census Bureau, Brief Disability Status. (2012). *Americans with disabilities: 2010.* Retrieved from http://www.census.gov/prod/2012pubs/p70-131.pdf.

U.S. Census Bureau, Newsroom. (2013). *Workers with a disability Less Likely to be employed, more likely to hold jobs with lower earnings.* Census Bureau Reports, 14 March 2013. Retrieved from: https://www.census.gov/newsroom/press-releases/2013/cb13-47.html.

U.S. Department of Labor, Bureau of Labor Statistics. (2015). *Employment and unemployment among youth summary.* Retrieved from: www.bls.gov/news.release/youth.nr0.htm.

Yee, S. (2011). Health and health care disparities among people with disabilities. *Disability Rights Education & Defense Fund,* 1–6.

Zimmerman, M., & Eisman, A. (2016). Empowerment theory. In M. A. Bond, C. B. Keys, & I. Serrano-García (Eds.), *APA handbook of community psychology* (Vol. 1). Washington, DC:

American Psychological Association. Retrieved from: http://www.apa.org/pubs/books/4311524.aspx?tab=2.

Zuckerman, K. E., Sinche, B., Mejia, A., Cobian, M., Becker, T., & Nicolaidis, C. (2014). Latino parents' perspectives on barriers to autism diagnosis. *Academic Pediatrics, 14,* 301–308. https://doi.org/10.1016/j.acap.2013.12.004.

Chapter 7
Aging and Health in the Latinx Population in the USA: Changing Demographics, Social Vulnerabilities, and the Aim of Quality of Life

Iveris L. Martinez and Adriana Baron

Abstract In this chapter, we outline the health status and experiences of aging among Latinx persons. Aging among Latinx persons is heterogeneous, based on country of origin, place of residence, generation, socioeconomic status, social support networks, and life experiences. Despite having higher life expectancies than White non-Hispanics, this population suffers from a greater burden of disability, their utilization of existing health services is lower, and the proportion of Latinx older adults living at the poverty level is greater compared to other racial/ethnic groups. With fewer economic resources, Latinx older adults may be highly dependent on family and social services for long-term care. We conclude by providing alternative frameworks for examining aging in the Latinx population.

Keywords Latinx aging · Caregivers · Care recipients · Disability · Social vulnerability

The number of Latinx older adults in the USA is projected to increase rapidly from the current 8% (or 3.5 million in 2014) of all persons 65 years and older to 22% (or 21.5 million) by 2060 (Federal Interagency Forum on Aging-Related Statistics, 2016). Life expectancy is also increasing for Latinx persons. In 2014, life expectancy at birth was estimated to be 81.8 years; by 2050, Latinx persons are expected to live, on average, 87 years (Federal Interagency Forum on Aging-Related Statistics, 2016). Although "old age" cannot be universally defined, in most of the developed world, the chronological age of 65 years and older is usually used. In some contexts, however, because of health conditions, retirement age, or living conditions, 55 or 60 may be used as the threshold. As the Latinx population continues to grow and age, it is particularly important to understand the overall structure of the population, its health status, and available resources. The experience

---

I. L. Martinez (✉)
Center for Successful Aging, California State University, Long Beach, CA, USA
e-mail: Iveris.Martinez@csulb.edu

A. Baron
Benjamin Leon Center for Geriatric Education and Research, Florida International University, Miami, FL, USA

of aging among Latinx persons is heterogeneous, based on country of origin, place of residence, generation, socioeconomic status, social support networks, and diverse life experiences. However, for Latinx older adults as a group, the burden of disability is higher, the utilization of existing health services is lower, and the proportion of Latinx older adults living at the poverty level are greater than Whites (Guendelman & Wagner, 2000). With fewer economic resources, Latinx older adults may be highly dependent on family and social services for long-term care. Because most families have older adults residing with them as caregivers and/or care recipients, the well-being of Latinx older adults should be of importance to anyone studying or otherwise interested in the Latinx population in the USA.

When we describe Latinx older adults, we cast a wide net that includes older Mexican American persons living on the US–Mexico border; Cuban American, Puerto Rican, and Dominican-origin persons residing predominantly in Florida and the northeastern region of the country; and persons of Central American and South American origin living throughout the country, in both rural areas and urban centers. Latinx persons, therefore, do not make up a homogenous group, as is too often assumed. In fact, the percentage of Latinx older adults varies greatly by country of origin and region of the USA. Nonetheless, Latinx older adults are tied together with some commonalities, including both social vulnerabilities and potential cultural strengths that have an impact on the quality of life during aging.

Using 2008 census data, Mendes de Leon and colleagues found that the Latinx population is growing in areas not traditionally thought of as strongholds for Latinx communities, such as the Midwest, Central Florida, and the Southeast, and declining in other areas, such as the Northeast and Southwest (Mendes de Leon, Eschbach, & Markides, 2011). The Latinx population in the Midwest has tripled since 1980 and now constitutes 6.6% of the entire Midwest population. Latinx older adults in the Midwest are predominantly male, somewhat younger overall, and are more likely to be foreign-born than Latinx adults living in the Southwest (Mendes de Leon et al., 2011). In comparison, the Latinx population in Florida has grown fivefold since 1980, from 858,158 persons to 4.2 million in 2010 (Martinez & Varella, 2017). Between 2000 and 2010, the state saw a nearly 60% growth of the Latinx population, which is currently 22.5% of the total population. Meanwhile, the growth of the Latinx population in the Northeast has remained consistent with the growth of the overall population growth of 3% in the last decade. As of 2010, 14% of all Latinx persons in the USA lived in the Northeast, down from 18% 30 years ago. The Latinx population in Florida is slightly older, has a higher percentage of women, and is more likely to be foreign-born (76.9%) than Latinx individuals in the Northeast (52.8%) and the country overall (54.2%); in addition, poverty rates are higher for Latinx, despite higher educational attainment (Martinez & Varella, 2017).

Comparative Demography of Aging in the Latinx Population

Age Structure

The size of the Latinx population 65 years and older in the USA was estimated to be nearly 3.8 million persons in 2015 (U.S. Census Bureau: American Community Survey [ACS], 2015). Mexican American older adults make up more than half of this population, with nearly two million persons 65 and older. Puerto Rican and Cuban American persons make up the other two largest groups of older adults, followed by persons of South American origin (Table 7.1). These figures reflect the total population size for these subgroups and the percent of older adults within each group.

Compared with the overall population of the USA, as of 2015, the Latinx population as a whole is relatively young, with a median age of 28.7 years, indicating that half of the population is younger than that age. For the entire US population, the median age is 37.8 years. However, a different picture emerges when Latinx subgroups are evaluated according to the place of origin. The median age varies greatly by subgroup, ranging from 26.9 years for Mexican American persons to 40.8 years for Cuban American persons. Similarly, 6.6% of the Latinx population is 65 years or older compared with 14.9% of the US population. The percentage of Latinx older adults is lowest for those of Central American and Mexican origin and much higher for those of Cuban origin (Table 7.1) (U.S. Census Bureau: ACS, 2015).

Poverty

The proportion of the population 65 years or older is not the only factor to consider when looking at Latinx aging. One must also factor in the conditions of aging, such as poverty, that may affect the quality of life of people as they grow older. Latinx older adults are more likely to live in poverty than the overall population of older adults in the USA. In 2015, 18.5% of Latinx older adults lived in poverty compared with 9% of all older adults in the USA. Among Latinx subgroups, the percentage of older adults living in poverty is highest for the Dominican and Cuban American populations and lower for populations of South American and Mexican descent (Table 7.1). Compared with the overall US population, the Latinx population has a slightly higher percentage of older women, for whom the poverty rate is higher (Cubanski, Casillas, & Damico, 2015). Therefore, attention to gender in the study of aging in the Latinx population is important. Financial strain is a key element in the social vulnerability and health of Latinx older adults, as we later describe.

Table 7.1 Comparative demography of Latino[a] subgroups

	USA	All Latinos	Latino Origin					
			Mexican	Puerto Rican	Central American	South American	Cuban	Dominican
Total population	321,418,821	56,496,122	35,797,080	5,372,759	5,210,908	3,403,619	2,106,501	1,873,097
Median age (years)	37.8	28.7	26.9	29.5	30.1	35.6	40.8	30.1
No. (%) of persons $\geq$65 years	47,732,480 (14.9)	3,755,328 (6.6)	1,966,230 (5.5)	432,091 (8.0)	245,260 (4.7)	318,550 (9.4)	354,740 (16.8)	137,341 (7.3)
Percentage of persons $\geq$75 years	6.3	2.6	2.1	3.1	1.6	3.5	8.7	2.8
Percentage of women among adults $\geq$65 years	55.9	57.1	55.2	57.1	64.0	60.2	57.3	60.1
Rate of disability for adults $\geq$65 years (per 100,0000)	35.4	39.0	40.2	42.8	33.2	28.7	37.8	40.3
Percentage of adults $\geq$65 years living in poverty	9.0	18.5	16.9	21.3	18.2	16.9	23.6	31.4
Age-dependency ratio[b]	60.66	58.70	66.90	64.05	51.68	49.16	58.69	55.99
Old age-dependency ratio[b]	23.85	10.84	9.16	13.19	7.13	13.96	26.72	11.43

[a]Hispanic/Latino is the ethnic category used in the American Community Survey
[b]Calculated using an age of 18 years as the cut-off for youth and 65 and older to define older adults
Source 2015 American Community Survey 1-Year Estimates, S0201 Selected Population Profile in the United States

Dependency Ratios

Dependency ratios offer a glimpse of the proportion of a population that requires care and financial support compared with the proportion that is economically active or in the labor force. Dependency ratios are calculated here as the number of persons economically dependent or not of working age (defined as younger than 18 years and 65 years or older) divided by the total number of persons of expected working age (18–64 years). The ratio indicates the number of individuals outside the workforce who depend on 100 people of working age. The lower the ratio, the larger the proportion of individuals 18–64 years old, with relatively fewer children and/or older adults. The dependency ratio is approximately 61 for the entire country and 59 for the overall Latinx population (Table 7.1). The ratio ranges among Latinx subgroups, from 49 for persons of South American origin, to 67 for the Mexican American subgroup. However, when only the proportion of the population 65 years or older is considered, the results differ. The so-called old-age dependency ratio is calculated as the number of persons 65 and older per the number of persons of working age. A high ratio indicates that the number of older adults is proportionately higher than the number of adults of working age. This ratio is highest for the Cuban American population (approximately 27) (Table 7.1). Notably, the number of children in the Cuban American population is only slightly higher than the number of older adults. The old-age dependency ratio is much lower among populations of Mexican and Central American descent (Table 7.1). However, this ratio is likely to change as the percentage of older adults grows, with important implications for work, family, and the economy (He, Goodkind, & Kowal, 2016).

Life Expectancy, Morbidity, and Mortality

Despite higher rates of poverty, the life expectancy in the Latinx population was higher than that in the white and black (non-Hispanic) populations (81.8 years, 79.0 years, and 75.6 years, respectively), based on 2014 data (Kochanek, Murphy, Xu, & Tejada-Vera, 2016). Life expectancy at birth is highest for Latinx women (84.0 years), followed by white (81.4 years), and black (78.4) women (Kochanek et al., 2016). The longer life expectancy at birth for the Latinx population compared with the white population is associated with lower death rates from cancer, heart disease, chronic lower respiratory diseases, unintentional injuries, suicides, Alzheimer disease, and Parkinson disease (Heron, 2016). The top five leading causes of death for Latinx older adults are heart disease, cancer, stroke, Alzheimer disease, and diabetes. Latinx individuals are living longer, but increasing longevity may lead to a greater number of them with disability and dependence.

Health Concerns of Latinx Older Adults

Burden of Select Chronic Diseases

Among older adults, the prevalence of certain chronic conditions, such as arthritis, chronic obstructive pulmonary disease, and heart disease is lower in the Latinx population than in the white population (Federal Interagency Forum on Aging-Related Statistics, 2016). However, the prevalence of asthma, hypertension, stroke, and diabetes is higher among Latinx older adults compared with white older adults. Moreover, the prevalence of chronic conditions differs among Latinx subgroups. For example, the prevalence of stroke is highest in Dominican-origin men and Puerto Rican women (Daviglus et al., 2012). Obesity, a risk factor for diabetes, is also more common among Latinx older adults (33.4%) than among white older adults (28.6%) (Daviglus et al., 2012).

Diabetes is a major health issue for Latinx persons. One in three Latinx older adults has diabetes (32.3%); this rate is similar to that for black older adults (32.1%) and much higher than that for white older adults (18.3%) (Federal Interagency Forum on Aging-Related Statistics, 2016). The Hispanic Community Health Study/Study of Latinos (HCHS/SOL) found that the prevalence of type 2 diabetes was lower for persons of Central American (17.7%), South American (10.2%), and Cuban origin (13.4%) but higher for persons of Mexican (18.3%) and Puerto Rican (18.1%) origin. The prevalence of diabetes within the Latinx population increases with age; the prevalence is 38.7% for individuals 60–69 years old and 48.6% for individuals 70–74 years old (Schneiderman et al., 2014). Risk of diabetes increases with age because of increasing insulin resistance associated with sarcopenia and physical inactivity, as well as impaired pancreatic function. Diabetes in older adults has been associated with a high prevalence of cardiovascular disease, depression, falls, Alzheimer disease, multi-infarct dementia, persistent pain, and polypharmacy with more risk of side effects and drug-to-drug interaction. Furthermore, diabetes has been linked to functional decline in older adults, perhaps because of the interaction between peripheral neuropathy, vision and hearing impairment, gait and balance problems, and other medical conditions (Kirkman et al., 2012). According to data from the National Health and Nutrition Examination Surveys (NHANES) 2007–2010, the percentage of individuals with controlled diabetes (hemoglobin A1C of less than 7%) was lower for Latinx individuals (47.3%) than for black (52.6%) or white (52.9%) individuals (Casagrande, Fradkin, Saydah, Rust, & Cowie, 2013).

Cancer

The overall prevalence of cancer is lower among Latinx older adults (12.5%), than among either black (16.7%) or white (26.0%) older adults. However, the prevalence of cancers associated with infectious diseases is higher in the Latinx population compared with the general population (National Cancer Institute, 2016).

- Stomach cancer associated with chronic infection with *Helicobacter pylori* (50.24 per 100,000 population)
- Liver cancer associated with hepatitis B and C infection (59.68 vs. 27.85 per 100,000 population)
- Cervical cancer associated with human papillomavirus infection (16.22 vs. 7.09 per 100,000 population)
- Gallbladder cancer associated with chronic *Salmonella typhi* infection (11.8 vs. 5.49 per 100.000 population) (Randi, Franceschi, & La Vecchia, 2006).

Cancer of the prostate, breast, colon, and lung and bronchus are the most prevalent invasive cancers reported among Latinx older adults (Siegel et al., 2015). The following disparities have been reported for these cancers.

- The incidence and mortality rate for colon cancer are 10–20% lower in the Latinx population compared with the white population.
- The incidence and mortality rate for lung cancer are approximately 50% lower among Latinx persons than among white persons and may be due to a lower rate of smoking in the Latinx population.
- The mortality rate for lung cancer for Cuban American men is almost double that for Mexican American men because of a higher prevalence of smoking and greater cigarette consumption (Kaplan et al., 2014).
- The incidence of breast cancer is 40% lower for Mexican American women than for Cuban American and Puerto Rican women.
- The incidence of colon cancer is lower for Mexican American men than among Cuban American and Puerto Rican men.

The rate of late-stage cancer at the time of diagnosis is higher among Latinx individuals than the general population; however, despite less access to high-quality health care in the Latinx population, the overall cancer-related death rate in that population is 30% lower than that in the white population (Quesnel-Vallée, Farrah, & Jenkins, 2011).

Mental Health and Aging

Depression is one of the most common and treatable mental health problems in aging. However, the burden of depressive symptoms is a major clinical and public health problem in older populations because of its common occurrence, adverse impact on the quality of life of older adults and their families, and increased demand for formal and informal healthcare services (Noël et al., 2004). The prevalence of clinically significant depressive symptoms may range from 8 to 16% in community-dwelling older adults (Blazer, 2003). Substantial heterogeneity in the prevalence of depression has been documented within older populations. Researchers have consistently found a prevalence of depressive symptoms among Latinx older adults that was substantially higher than the population average. For Latinx adults 50 years and older, the rate of current depression is higher than that for white and black adults of the same age (Centers for Disease Control and Prevention [CDC], 2008). Several studies among community-dwelling Mexican American older adults have shown a prevalence of depression of about 25.5% (González, Haan, & Hinton, 2001). Differences have been reported by subgroup or heritage. For example, in a study of Latinx adults 59 years and older in the USA, the prevalence of depression was higher in the Puerto Rican subgroup than in the Cuban American, Mexican, or other Latinx subgroups (Yang, Cazorla-Lancaster, & Jones, 2008). In a study of Latinx older adults in Miami-Dade County, Florida, researchers found a high prevalence of depressive symptomatology (33%) and noted that such symptoms may go unrecognized (Martinez, Baron, Largaespada, Ceruto, & Chaves, 2017). This rate is more than double the overall rate of 14.7% for older Floridians (CDC, 2015).

Social factors associated with depression in Latinx older adults include female sex, being widowed or divorced, living alone, providing care for a parent, presence of chronic diseases, functional limitations, poor health behaviors, lower educational attainment, and unemployment or underemployment, lower income, and lack of health insurance coverage (Jang, Chiriboga, Kim, & Phillips, 2008; Rodriguez-Galan & Falcón, 2009). Furthermore, with the Latinx population, depressive symptoms have been associated with increased dependency as measured by instrumental activities of daily living (complex skills needed to live independently, such as shopping, money management, and taking medications), and activities of daily living (ADL) (basic self-care tasks required to live independently, such as bathing, self-feeding, and dressing) (Bowen & Ruch, 2015). Higher levels of depressive symptoms have been associated with adverse health outcomes, including cardiovascular diseases; geriatric syndromes, including frailty, physical disability, and cognitive impairment; and mortality, independently from the impact of comorbidities and other health indicators. Additionally, healthcare utilization and costs have been shown to be substantially higher for older adults with higher levels of depressive symptomatology (Bock et al., 2014).

In older adults, symptoms of depression may include depressed mood; loss of interest in activities or hobbies; changes in appetite, with weight gain or loss; changes in sleep patterns; memory and concentration difficulties; feelings of worthlessness or guilt; psychomotor agitation or retardation; fatigue; somatic symptoms; and recurrent suicidal ideation (American Psychiatric Association, 2013). Cognitive symptoms may be particularly prominent, and less affective symptoms have been reported as "depression without sadness" among older adults (Gallo & Rabins, 1999). However, symptoms of depression may be slightly different for Latinx older adults, particularly, with heightened somatization. Fatigue, weakness, multiple aches, pain, dizziness, palpitations, and sleep disturbance are the most common symptoms of depression among Latinx older adults (Lewis-Fernández, Das, Alfonso, Weissman, & Olfson, 2005).

The role of social support, including loneliness, in depression among Latinx older adults has gone relatively unexplored (Gerst-Emerson, Shovali, & Markides, 2014; Russell & Taylor, 2009). In a study of community-dwelling Latinx older adults in Miami-Dade County, poor health was independently associated with depressive symptomatology (Martinez et al., 2017). Social isolation, loneliness, and lack of social support were associated with a higher level of depressive symptoms, even after adjusting for prevalent chronic diseases and physical function; these findings highlight the importance of the social world in the mental health of older adults. Depressive symptoms were not explained by age or physical health, and social support is an important factor that is often overlooked in studies of depression.

Disability

Disability, as defined by the Americans with Disabilities Act (ADA), is a physical or mental impairment that substantially limits one or more of an individual's major life activities. Major life activities include, but are not limited to, caring for oneself, performing manual tasks, seeing, hearing, eating, sleeping, walking, standing, lifting, bending, speaking, breathing, learning, reading, concentrating, thinking, communicating, and working (United States Department of Justice, 2009). The American Community Survey (ACS) defines a person to have disability if any one of the following areas is impaired: hearing, vision, cognition, ambulation, self-care, and independent living. Cognitive disability is defined as having difficulty remembering, concentrating, or making decisions because of a physical, mental, or emotional problem (United States Census Bureau, 2010).

The so-called Hispanic paradox refers to the fact that health outcomes appear to be better and the mortality rate is lower in the Hispanic population, despite its poorer socioeconomic status compared with other racial/ethnic groups (Abraído-Lanza, Dohrenwend, Ng-Mak, & Turner, 1999). The Hispanic paradox in mortality does not appear to extend to disability (Hayward, Hummer, Chiu, González-González, & Wong, 2014). Although Latinx older adults are living longer, they experience greater disability as they age (Angel, Angel, & Hill, 2014), which means that these adults live longer with a disability and have a longer period of time being dependent on others compared with white older adults (Markides & Rote, 2014/2015).

According to the 2015 American Community Survey, the proportion of the older population reporting one or more disabilities is slightly higher for Latinx older adults (39%) than for non-Hispanic older adults (35.4%). The proportion is considerably higher among persons of Puerto Rican, Dominican, and Mexican origin than among other Hispanic subgroups (Table 7.1). Disability rates among individuals of Cuban and Central American descent are closer to the overall rates in the USA, and the rate is lowest for individuals of South American origin (Table 7.1). The relatively high disability rates among Latinx older adults raises several questions: Who will care for Latinx older adults as they become older? How will the family be able to provide care, given the competing demands of work and children? How does immigration to the

USA and movements within the country affect family structure and the availability of kin to provide care?

The disability rate within the Latinx population also varies by region, place of birth, and gender. In one study, the disability rates for women of Puerto Rican and Dominican origin were higher than the rate for white women (Tucker, Falcon, Bianchi, Cacho, & Bermudez, 2000). Other factors also appear to play a role, such as language spoken, with non-English-speaking Latinx persons reporting higher levels of some types of disability (Dunlop, Song, Manheim, Daviglus, & Chang, 2007; Haan & Weldon, 1996; Tirodkar, Song, Chang, Dunlop, & Chang, 2008). When Latinx subgroups are compared at a national level, the overall prevalence of disability and the rates of mobility and cognitive disability are highest in the Puerto Rican population. The disability rate is second-highest in the Mexican American population, and the lowest rate is found in the Cuban American subgroup. Differences also exist among US-born and foreign-born populations, with higher rates of disability for foreign-born individuals (Sheftel, 2017). Some researchers have hypothesized that the higher rate is associated with early-life exposures to malnutrition, poverty, and infectious diseases (Palloni, McEniry, Wong, & Pelaez, 2006) and lower levels of education (Crimmins, Hayward, & Seeman, 2004; Hummer, Benjamins, & Rogers, 2004).

Comparison of disability rates across regions point to heterogeneity among Latinx persons according to region, place of birth, and gender (Martinez & Varella, 2017; Mendes de Leon et al., 2011). As examples, the following differences have been found in Florida and the northeastern region of the USA (Martinez & Varella, 2017).

- The rate of overall disability is higher for Latinx older adults than for white older adults.
- The rate of cognitive disability is almost twice as high among Latinx persons than among white persons; the rate is highest among Cuban American and Puerto Rican women and similar to the rate among black women.
- The rates of mobility and self-care disability for the Latinx population are higher than the rates for the white population, but lower than the rates for the black population.

Trajectories of cognitive functioning vary by gender (Bryant, Shetterly, Baxter, & Hamman, 2002), nativity (foreign born vs. U.S. born), and time in the USA (Hill, Angel, Balistreri, & Herrera, 2012; Martinez & Varella, 2017; Mendes de Leon et al., 2011). Cognitive impairment appears to be associated with an increased risk of ADL-related disability over time (Raji, Snih, Ray, Patel, & Markides, 2004). The findings of several studies indicate that the prevalence of dementia may be higher in the Latinx and black populations compared with the white population (Gurland et al., 1999; Tang et al., 2001). Higher rates of vascular disease, diabetes, high blood pressure, and high cholesterol are all factors that place Latinx persons at greater risk for the development of Alzheimer disease and related dementias.

Bryant and colleagues (2002) note that "Greater prevalent disability in the Hispanic cohort, especially in women, may reflect a reservoir accumulated during younger years and related to culture and socioeconomic status as well as to older age" (p. 361). Although women live longer, they have the highest rates of disability (Hayward et al., 2014; Sheftel, 2017). Gender differences as Latinx persons age may reflect a history of cumulative disadvantages and stressors, both biological and social. These differences are often driven by the "constrained choices" that women face throughout their life course (Rieker & Bird, 2005).

When the rate of disability is compared across income levels, the rate is highest for people living below 100% of the poverty line. There appears to be a modest dose response across the type of disability for most origin groups; the lower the income-to-poverty ratio, the higher the frequency of disability. A gradient between socioeconomic status and health has been previously described in several populations (Marmot, 1996) and is usually clearly seen when health outcomes for Latinx populations are evaluated according to socioeconomic groups (Crimmins et al., 2007).

The differences in disability rates may reflect different migration and occupational histories. The histories of migration, economic, employment, and occupational characteristics; health insurance status; and life course health status of a population can affect the health status of older adults. Better understanding of the disability status among different Latinx subgroups might better guide programs to foster social support networks and to address needs for health and social services, leading ultimately to optimal aging across populations.

Alternative Frameworks for Examining Aging in the Latinx Population

From Cultural Values to Cultural Humility

The literature on Latinx aging, particularly in relation to aging and long-term care, often refers to the cultural values of *familismo, personalismo, respeto, confianza,* and *dignidad* (familism, personalism, respect, trust, and dignity), which can influence caregiver perceptions of appropriate care and therefore decision-making (Gelman, 2014). For example, low levels of formal service utilization in the Latinx population have been associated with *personalismo,* or the tendency to trust people rather than institutions. Latinx persons may not feel connected to a home health agency; rather, they want home health services from someone they already know (Herrera, George, Angel, Markides, & Torres-Gil, 2013). However, the focus on *familismo* or a cultural tendency toward strong emphasis on the family, can lead to the assumption that the family should be the natural support network for older adults, and therefore, health and social systems of care may ignore the specific needs of the Latinx population. The structural, cultural, and psychosocial impact of immigration on the family can also be problematic (Bastida, 1988), and thus needs to be considered when developing systems of care. Research shows that although familial values may be upheld in principle, these values may also be changing and contradicted by actual behavior (Martinez, 2002; Ruiz, 2012; Sabogal, Marín, Otero-Sabogal, Marín, & Perez-Stable,

1987). For example, Ruiz (2012) noted the following about a sample of self-identified Latinx elders in the Los Angeles area.

> The general consensus was that sons and daughters were busy with work and families, and so the elders withheld making any demands on them. These elders encouraged their sons and daughters to focus on their own nuclear families although they appeared saddened by the limited contact. Still, these elders stressed that younger family members would come around, if and when the elders "needed them." Despite these significant health limitations, the majority of Latinx elders (80%) reported very infrequent contact with their significant younger family members. These findings clarify and add depth to the Latinx elders' melancholy tone uncovered in the focus group discussions and their need for expanded exchanges of support outside of the traditional family sphere (p. 54).

Similarly, in her study of Cuban-origin older adults in Miami, Martinez (2002) found an increasing tendency toward older adults living alone and a resignation to the lack of contact with children and grandchildren. The elders expressed not wanting to be perceived as a nuisance and therefore accepted the changing situation. The focus on familism and the perspective that Latinx persons do not need or want formal services may prevent providers from developing appropriate resources for this population and inadvertently increasing inequalities (Ruiz, 2012). Evidence suggests instead that "minority seniors and caregivers may require a larger menu of services and better coordination of care posing potential challenges to aging services providers" (Herrera et al., 2013).

We must move beyond familism in thinking of the needs of Latinx older adults and their families, recognizing that cultural values are dynamic and change over time and space. Culture, broadly defined, consists of patterns of behaviors and values, implicit or explicit, acquired and transmitted, independent of genes. Some of the reasons caregivers use or decline formal support services are known, but the role of culture is relatively unexplored. The majority of literature on caregivers focuses on individual caregivers, the role of stress and coping model, with the subjective well-being of the caregiver as the outcome (Pearlin et al., 1990). Studies of formal services have been based largely on Andersen's healthcare utilization model (1995) and expanded to take into account the characteristics of not only the caregiver but also the care recipient; e.g., the level of need and dependency, length of time of care (Mullan, 1993; Stephens, 1993). However, decisions regarding care are not made by individuals in isolation nor in the absence of the influence of familial ties, cultural values, and other social influences. Cultural values may influence not only the use of support services but also its availability. Caregivers have life experiences that may influence their perceived burden or judgment of psychologic distress. In this respect, the National Institutes of Health "The Cultural Framework for Health" may provide helpful guidance in operationalizing culture as a dynamic entity in relation to health research (Kagawa-Singer, Dressler, George, & Elwood, 2014).

In current theoretical models and frameworks of caregiving and culturally competent care, caregivers' needs, stressors, and decision-making are considered separately from organizational and structural barriers. Missing from many theoretical models of caregiving is the acknowledgment that the cultural values are also represented in the service system. These values may not be congruent with those of caregivers and their families or reflected in current assessment and offering of services. Cultural congruence is "a process of effective interaction between the provider and client levels" (Schim & Doorenbos, 2010). Culturally congruent care is a care that is customized to fit with the client or patient's own values, beliefs, traditions, practices, and lifestyle. From a practice perspective, the concept of cultural humility also offers an alternative, one that is slowly replacing cultural competence as a goal in health profession education. Cultural humility is an ongoing process of self-reflection and lifelong learning about one's own biases and lack of absolute knowledge about a patient's experience. It encourages one to ask questions about and learn from patients' experiences. It also recognizes power imbalances in the patient/provider relation (Tervalon & Murray-Garcia, 1998). As the Latinx population ages and becomes increasingly diverse, cultural humility in both research and provision of health and social services will be crucial.

Social Vulnerability, Social Support, and Engagement Theory

Social vulnerability in aging includes but is not limited to social isolation, stress, limited life space (i.e., physical and psychologic environment), and limited financial resources that may have an impact on the quality of life as well as clinical vulnerability. Life space is a measure of spatial mobility area and the frequency with which an individual travels in his or her daily life, in a specific time frame (Baker, Bodner & Allman, 2003). Sensitization to the social vulnerability associated with aging is central to the development of cultural humility. In the concept of social vulnerability, how social factors holistically influence health outcomes is considered. Social vulnerability in aging stems from an accumulation of social problems throughout the life course and has been shown to be a significant predictor of mortality and disability (Wallace, Theou, Pena, Rockwood, & Andrew, 2015), cognitive function (Andrew, Fisk, & Rockwood, 2011), and frailty (Andrew, 2015). Social factors that contribute to social vulnerability are multilevel, ranging from family and broader social networks to institutions and environmental and societal factors and can be linked to the current understanding of frailty from a medical and basic science perspective (see Andrew, 2015). An approach of cultural humility allows recognition of not only potential cultural differences but also the social vulnerabilities in persons with realities very different from ours.

In older adults, both socioeconomic status and social integration have been related to a range of important health outcomes, including mortality and cognitive and physical functioning (see Cohen, 2004; House, Kessler, & Herzog, 1990, for two seminal articles). An extensive discussion of social integration and health is beyond the scope of this chapter; however, evidence suggests that participation in social activities may increase social networks and opportunities for social support and interaction. Feeling productive and engaged in regular structured activities as one ages is important to psychologic health; promotes life satisfaction; and protects against mortality, disability, and cognitive decline. Social engagement through participation in formal activities and the potential health benefits derived may vary by gender, socioeconomic gradient, and ethnicity. Recognizing the limits of behavioral interventions aimed at improving health outcomes, social scientists, and gerontologists are starting to combine efforts to better understand psychologic motivations and environmental contexts of health-promotion efforts (Glass, 2000). Factors that motivate or prohibit persons from being socially active are not always obvious and may be culturally specific. For example, research conducted in Baltimore on civic engagement and participation in activities among black and white women and men of lower and middle income showed differences in preferences, motivators, and barriers (Martinez, Crooks, Kim, & Tanner, 2011; Martinez, Kim, Tanner, Fried, & Seeman, 2009). Mobility limitations at younger ages, health concerns, limited economic resources, lack of transportation, and the lack of appeal of structured hours and tasks, as well as of activities were some of the barriers mentioned. However, research also demonstrates that it is possible to target specific audiences with health-promotion messages and motivate older adults and engage them in activities that benefit their health (Fried et al., 2013; Martinez et al., 2006).

Unfortunately, relatively little is known about health-promoting opportunities, such as volunteering and social engagement, among Latinx populations. In addition to the barriers to social and civic engagement imposed by poverty, Latinx older adults may also face language barriers to participating in activities. Cultural preferences for different types of activities may also play a role in participation. Research has shown that preferences in types of activities, as well as level of participation in activities, are influenced by ethnic preferences or values and marginalization as a result of age, class, ethnicity, race, or gender, which limits access to activities (Floyd, 1998). Although there appears to be little consensus on the impact of race and ethnicity in participation in leisure activity in general, and among older adults in particular, a comprehensive review of the literature of race and ethnicity conducted by Floyd (2007) indicated a shift toward ethnic and cultural differences and a move away from racial differences. Patterns established in earlier life may continue into later life. Barriers to participation in social activities may include the perceived capability for participating, normative social roles, and available opportunities in post-retirement years. In other words, what older adults can and cannot do is driven not only by physical and cognitive capacities but also by sociocultural expectations and opportunities that may vary by gender norms, as well as ethnicity and class status. Images of aging may, therefore, have important long-term implications for health promotion throughout the life course.

A life course perspective may be helpful as a theoretical framework for understanding social engagement among Latinx older adults. The life course or life cycle perspective stems from a conceptualization of the life course as a "changing constellation of roles and perspectives governed by a cognitive map for ordering major life events and expectations appropriate to age" (Spencer, 1990). However, these so-called maps are culturally specific and change with time, and expectations for later years in life are not universal. For example, the concept of successful aging (Rowe and Kahn 1997) promoted in the 1990s centered on individual factors of physical and cognitive health and social participation. This concept has since come under attack for its Western, individualistic focus. A life course perspective on aging can help one understand the experiences that shape an individual's life experiences, exposures, and their resulting health outcomes, as well as expectations for old age.

Furthermore, Carstensen (1991) put forth the socioemotional selectivity theory, which posits that people "proactively manage their social worlds" engaging in social contact motivated by two goals: information (or obtaining useful knowledge) and emotional regulation (or engaging in satisfying social relations). The theory suggests that participation in certain activities or social goals depends on the conditions the individual perceives, especially perceived time. With limited perceived time, as people age, they are more likely to seek social partners in terms of emotional gratification rather than informational value. Baltes and Carstensen (1999) later proposed the theory of selective optimization and compensation (SOC) to describe how individuals successfully adapt to aging.

The basic assumption of the SOC model is that the three processes form a system of behavioral action or regulate development and aging. Whereas selection processes address the choice of goals, life domains, and life tasks, both compensation and optimization are concerned with the means to maintain or enhance chosen goals. (p. 218). Therefore, engagement in activities may be modulated by life course experience and cultural constructions of proper roles in old age. Thus, it is important to consider life trajectories and goals of older adults in understanding aging.

The research on social vulnerability, social engagement, and aging in the Latinx population is not yet fully developed, and it should be, as intervening on social factors may be the most effective way of improving quality of life for older adults. From the Hispanic Established Population for the Epidemiological Study of the Elderly (H-EPESE), we know, for example, that social support and financial stressors play a nuanced role on frailty depending on the trajectories of decline (Peek, Howrey, Ternent, Ray, & Ottenbacher, 2012). The experience of aging is influenced by gender, which appears to play a role in the relation between social support and mortality, with a stronger association for men (Hill, Uchino, Eckhardt, & Angel, 2016). Given that women tend to live longer, experience higher disability levels in aging, and are also more likely to serve as caregivers, future research needs to more closely evaluate aging in women.

Research and Intervention Needs and Priorities

Data Needs

First and foremost, data across regions and subgroups of older Latinx older adults are needed. Several good datasets exist on Latinx aging, such as the H-EPESE and the Sacramento Area Latino Study on Aging (SALSA Study). However, these are limited to Mexican American persons and to the Southwestern region of the USA.

A more recent study, the HCHS/SOL, includes sites throughout the USA (Miami, San Diego, Chicago, and the Bronx [NY]) and with subgroups beyond the Mexican American population, including persons of Cuban, Puerto Rican, Dominican, and Central and South American origin; however, the upper limit of the study is 74 years of age. The sites also include Latinx persons living in urban areas and do not reflect newer growth areas of the Latinx population. Therefore, the HCHS/SOL study may prove of limited utility for understanding aging among Latinx adults. In addition to quantitative data that shed light on the experience of aging among diverse groups of Latinx persons, qualitative studies are needed to better understand the dynamics of population aging and the cultural nuances that may have an impact on the quality of life for Latinx older adults.

In addition, more information is needed about the conditions that are relatively new to the Latinx aging population. Alzheimer disease is a prime example. The rates of Alzheimer disease and related dementias are higher among Latinx persons than among white and black persons, particularly in older age groups (Alzheimer's Association, 2014). Higher rates of vascular disease, diabetes, high blood pressure, and high cholesterol are all factors that place Latinx persons at greater risk for the development of Alzheimer disease or related dementias (Gurland et al., 1999). We would expect variability among Latinx subgroups. The prevalence and care of dementia are areas that are relatively understudied in certain regions and subgroups. Of particular importance is a better understanding of appropriate caregiving models for Latinx older adults and their families; that is, models that are in line with the cultural values for this population, as well as the reality of their economic and work situations.

Health Promotion

Existing models of prevention and health promotion interventions need to be tested in Latinx subgroups in order to translate the models successfully to diverse populations. For example, *Tomando Control de su Salud* (Taking Control of Your Health), developed by a team of Stanford University researchers, is a self-management education intervention for Spanish-speaking Latinx persons with a variety of chronic health conditions, such as arthritis, diabetes, heart disease, and lung disease. Participants learn problem-solving, decision-making, and other techniques for managing problems common to Latinx persons with chronic disease. Topics covered in the program include appropriate use of the healthcare system; how to evaluate new treatments; communicating effectively with family, friends, and health professionals; healthy eating; appropriate use of medications; techniques to deal with problems; and appropriate exercises for maintaining and improving strength, flexibility, and endurance. The education is available through the CDC website (https://www.cdc.gov/arthritis/interventions/self_manage.htm).

Some of the most exciting and promising interventions in aging address not only the physical and mental health of older adults but also the social engagement needs of older adults, who are often isolated. For example, *Bailamos* is a dance intervention program for community-dwelling inactive Latinx adults 55 years and older who self-identified as having mobility limitation. The dance program includes 12 weeks of one-hour dance sessions. The developers noted self-reports of higher levels of physical activity, greater cognitive function, and improved physical quality of life (Marquez, Bustamante, Aguiñaga, & Hernandez, 2015).

Furthermore, several interventions have been shown to be efficacious in managing depression among older adults and include social connectedness as a strategy. Healthy IDEAS (Identifying Depression, Empowering Activities for Seniors) provides depression care in the participant's home. Participants and their caregivers receive education about depression treatment, self-care, and assistance in obtaining further treatment from primary care and mental health providers. They encourage participants to manage their depression through a behavioral activation approach that includes involvement in meaningful social activities (CDC, 2009). The Program to Encourage Active, Rewarding Lives for Seniors, or PEARLS, is a home-based program that teaches depression management techniques that include (1) problem-solving treatment, in which participants are taught to recognize depressive symptoms, define problems that may contribute to depression, and devise steps to solve these problems; (2) social and physical activity planning; and (3) pleasant event planning and scheduling (CDC, 2009). Many of these interventions have yet to be systematically tested in Latinx populations and may be an important investment of resources, particularly given the relatively high rates of depression among Latinx older adults.

Caregiving

Caregiving is poised to be one of the biggest challenges for the aging Latinx population. A growing population of Latinx older adults, who are living longer and experiencing more chronic illness and dementia, is likely to increase the use of costly but preventable emergency room visits, as well as increase the need for long-term care and social support systems. Home and community-based services (HCBS) refers to assistance with ADLs and are intended to offer cost savings for the patient and healthcare system by meeting an older disabled person's needs in the home. However, the rate of unmet hours of care is the highest for Latinx persons in comparison with African American and whites (Herrera et al., 2013). For example, only one-third of Latinx caregivers used HCBS and less than 17% used meal delivery, transportation, and respite (Casado, van Vulpen, & Davis, 2011). Latinx caregivers tend to be in higher burden situations, provide more hours of care, and provide care with more ADLs. At the same time, they report less stress and more fulfillment with their caregiving role (Herrera et al., 2013). Among Latinx caregivers, 40% report that they have to stop working, cut back work hours, or change jobs in order to fulfill their roles as caregivers (Evercare Study and National Alliance for Caregiving, 2008). These changes can have profound economic ramifications for caregiving families. Furthermore, caregiving is associated with declines in physical health and psychologic well-being of caregivers, an increase in the use of healthcare services, and even higher mortality. Caregiver burden is associated with dementia of higher severity and lower satisfaction with social networks; whereas increased symptoms of depression among caregivers is associated with comorbidities and lower satisfaction with social networks (Luchsinger et al., 2015).

Potential reasons for underuse of HCBS include lack of awareness of available services, language barriers, health beliefs that promote informal care, financial limitations, perceived insensitivity to cultural factors, stigma, and the belief that what HCBS provides is not needed (Casado et al., 2011). The disparity in the utilization of services may be partially due to the cultural incongruence between what service providers offer and the needs of Latinx caregivers of older adults. For example, support groups, based largely on a mental health model, are one of the primary formal supports offered to caregivers of persons with Alzheimer disease. Support groups are used primarily by white middle-class caregivers and have been met with varying success among Latinx caregivers because of the stigma associated with mental illness, notions of privacy, and familial obligations (Henderson, 1984). The availability of effective supports for Latinx caregivers, including respite care, training in caregiving activities, care coordination, and financial support, has implications not only for older adults and their family caregivers but also for state and local area agencies on aging, local long-term care and aging services providers, and insurance companies.

Health and Social Policy

Approximately 5% of Latinx older adults are uninsured, which is significant given that older adults at this age qualify for Medicare. Adults in this age-group without insurance are likely those with legal permanent residency for less than five years or undocumented immigrants. The rate of uninsured Latinx persons younger than 65 is much higher; the rate decreased by half between 2010 and 2016 (from 43.2 to 24.8%) with the implementation of the Affordable Care Act (Zammitti, Cohen, & Martinez, 2016). Uninsured rates vary by states. Many Latinx persons work in occupations that do not offer access to employee-based health insurance or offer such insurance at an unaffordable rate. Access to health insurance at younger ages can affect the quality of life of Latinx adults as they age. Therefore, government policies that expand access to affordable health insurance continue to be needed to facilitate access to high-quality care and contribute to the financial security of individuals and families.

Social services such as HCBS for low-income older adults in the USA are offered mainly through the Older Americans Act (OAA) of 1965. This act has been continuously threatened with elimination and/or budget cuts in recent years. Services provided by OAA include home-delivered meals, congregate meals, caregiver support, home assistance, job training, volunteer opportunities, and protection from elder abuse. Home and community-based services are more cost-effective than nursing homes and other skilled-care facilities. At-home health services allow people to save their personal and government income, making HCBS a more practical monetary approach. Government-funded HCBS through the network of Area Agencies on Aging (AAA), on estimate, provide services at one-third the amount of costly institutional care, which is normally covered by Medicaid exclusively. Many AAAs are creating partnerships with other healthcare agencies, so they will not depend solely on funding sources such as the OAA. These partnerships increase the likelihood of better health outcomes and quality of health care while keeping costs contained (National Survey of Area Agencies on Aging, 2017a, 2017b).

Furthermore, from a longer term perspective, policy makers should consider the impact of education on health and aging. The high school dropout rate for Latinx youth is more than twice that for white youth (12% vs. 5%) (Krogstad, 2016). Only 15% of Latinx persons have a Bachelor's degree or higher (compared with 22% of black persons and 41% of white persons) (Krogstad, 2016). Access to education has been shown to have an impact on lifelong earning potential. Wage policies that prohibit discrimination can also have a lifelong effect on the health and opportunities of Latinx older adults. Currently, Latinx women working full-time make 54 cents for every dollar that a white non-Hispanic man makes (National Partnership for Women & Families, 2018). Access and opportunities to higher education, which have historically been lower for the Latinx population, also have important implications for health promotion and disease prevention throughout the life course, as persons with lower educational attainment engage in higher risk behavior and have lower health literacy.

We also need to consider the influence of policies more broadly beyond health policies, such as social policies and immigration policies, particularly in terms of family structure, economic resources, and availability of social support to secure the quality of life of Latinx individuals as they continue to age. For example, the increasing number of deportations of undocumented immigrants may weaken family ties, deprive older adults of caregivers, and leave families without breadwinners. Undocumented status can limit access to healthcare and social services and subject persons to harsh working conditions. Hummer and Hayward (2015) have noted that the current situation of a large number of undocumented residents in the USA is the result of government policies. These authors also argue that the future social and economic health of the Latinx population in the USA depends on a normalization of their immigration status and a path to citizenship. In conclusion, we need to think beyond traditional issues in health and aging, and to promote the quality of life for Latinx older adults, we need an understanding of Latinx aging and the social vulnerabilities this population faces, including the impact of immigration policy and status on risk factors for health.

References

Abraído-Lanza, A. F., Dohrenwend, B. P., Ng-Mak, D. S., & Turner, J. B. (1999). The Latino mortality paradox: A test of the "salmon bias" and healthy migrant hypotheses. *American Journal of Public Health, 89,* 1543–1548. https://doi.org/10.2105/AJPH.89.10.1543.

Alzheimer's Association. (2014). Alzheimer's disease facts and figures. *Alzheimer's and Dementia, 10,* 47–92.

American Psychiatric Association. (2013). *Diagnostic and statistical manual of mental disorders (DSM-5).* Washington, DC: American Psychiatric Publishing.

Andersen, R. M. (1995). Revisiting the behavioral model and access to medical care: Does it matter? *Journal of Health and Social Behavior, 36,* 1–10.

Andrew, M. K. (2015). Frailty and social vulnerability. In O. Theou & K. Rockwood (Eds.), *Frailty in aging. Biological, clinical and social implications* (pp. 186–195). Basel, Switzerland: Karger Publishers.

Andrew, M. K., Fisk, J. D., & Rockwood, K. (2011). Social vulnerability and prefrontal cortical function in elderly people: A report from the Canadian Study of Health and Aging. *International Psychogeriatrics, 23,* 450–458.

Angel, R. J., Angel, J. L., & Hill, T. D. (2014). Longer lives, sicker lives? Increased longevity and extended disability among Mexican-origin elders. *Journals of Gerontology Series B: Psychological Sciences and Social Sciences, 70*(4), 639–649.

Baker, P. S., Bodner, E. V., & Allman, R. M. (2003). Measuring life-space mobility in community-dwelling older adults. *Journal of the American Geriatrics Society, 51,* 1610–1614.

Baltes, M. M., & Carstensen, L. L. (1999). Social-psychological theories and their applications to aging: From individual to collective. In V. L. Bengtson & K. W. Schaie (Eds.), *Handbook of theories of aging* (pp. 209–226). New York, NY: Springer Publishing.

Bastida, E. (1988). Reexamining assumptions about extended familism: Older Puerto Ricans in a comparative perspective. In M. Sotomayor & H. Curiel (Eds.), *Hispanic elderly: A cultural signature* (pp. 163–181). Edinburg, TX: Pan American University Press.

Blazer, D. G. (2003). Depression in late life: Review and commentary. *Journals of Gerontology. Series A, Biological Sciences and Medical Sciences, 58,* M249–M265.

Bock, J. O., Luppa, M., Brettschneider, C., Riedel-Heller, S., Bickel, H., Fuchs, A., et al. (2014). Impact of depression on health care utilization and costs among multimorbid patients–results from the multicare cohort study. *PLoS ONE, 9,* e91973.

Bowen, M. E., & Ruch, A. (2015). Depressive symptoms and disability risk among older white and Latino adults by nativity status. *Journal of Aging and Health, 27,* 1286–1305.

Bryant, L. L., Shetterly, S. M., Baxter, J., & Hamman, R. F. (2002). Changing functional status in a biethnic rural population: The San Luis Valley health and aging study. *American Journal of Epidemiology, 155,* 361–367.

Carstensen, L. L. (1991). Selectivity theory: Social activity in life-span context. *Annual Review of Gerontology and Geriatrics, 11,* 195–217.

Casado, B. L., van Vulpen, K. S., & Davis, S. L. (2011). Unmet needs for home and community-based services among frail older Americans and their caregivers. *Journal of Aging and Health, 23,* 529–553.

Casagrande, S. S., Fradkin, J. E., Saydah, S. H., Rust, K. F., & Cowie, C. C. (2013). The prevalence of meeting A1C, blood pressure, and LDL goals among people with diabetes, 1988–2010. *Diabetes Care, 36,* 2271–2279.

Centers for Disease Control and Prevention. (2015). Behavioral Risk Factor Surveillance Survey (BRFSS) prevalence & trends data. https://www.cdc.gov/brfss/brfssprevalence/.

Centers for Disease Control and Prevention and National Association of Chronic Disease Directors. (2008). *The state of mental health and aging in America. Issue Brief #1: What do the data tell us?* Atlanta, GA: National Association of Chronic Disease Directors. https://www.cdc.gov/aging/pdf/mental_health.pdf.

Centers for Disease Control and Prevention and National Association of Chronic Disease Directors. (2009). *The state of mental health and aging in America. Issue Brief #2: Addressing depression in older adults: Selected evidence-based programs*. Atlanta, GA: National Association of Chronic Disease Directors. https://www.cdc.gov/aging/pdf/mental_health_brief_2.pdf.

Cohen, S. (2004). Social relationships and health. *American Psychologist, 59,* 676.

Crimmins, E. M., Hayward, M. D., & Seeman, T. E. (2004). Race/ethnicity, socioeconomic status, and health. *Critical Perspectives on Racial and Ethnic Differences in Health in Late Life,* 310–352.

Crimmins, E. M., Kim, J. K., Alley, D. E., Karlamangla, A., & Seeman, T. (2007). Hispanic paradox in biological risk profiles. *American Journal of Public Health, 97,* 1305–1310.

Cubanski, J., Casillas, G., & Damico, A. (2015). Poverty among seniors: An updated analysis of national and state level poverty rates under the official and supplemental poverty measures. http://files.kff.org/attachment/issue-brief-poverty-among-seniorsan-updated-analysis-of-national-and-state-level-poverty-ratesunder-the-official-and-supplemental-poverty-measures.

Daviglus, M. L., Talavera, G. A., Avilés-Santa, M. L., Allison, M., Cai, J., Criqui, M. H., et al. (2012). Prevalence of major cardiovascular risk factors and cardiovascular diseases among Hispanic/Latino individuals of diverse backgrounds in the United States. *Journal of the American Medical Association, 308,* 1775–1784.

Dunlop, D. D., Song, J., Manheim, L. M., Daviglus, M. L., & Chang, R. W. (2007). Racial/ethnic differences in the development of disability among older adults. *American Journal of Public Health, 97,* 2209–2215. https://doi.org/10.2105/AJPH.2006.106047. [pii].

Evercare Study and National Alliance for Caregiving. (2008). *Evercare study of Hispanic family caregiving in the U.S.: Findings from a national study*. http://www.caregiving.org/data/Hispanic_Caregiver_Study_web_ENG_FINAL_11_04_08.pdf.

Federal Interagency Forum on Aging-Related Statistics. (2016). *Older Americans 2016: Key indicators of well-being*. Washington, DC: U.S. Government Printing Office. https://agingstats.gov/docs/LatestReport/Older-Americans-2016-Key-Indicators-of-WellBeing.pdf.

Floyd, M. F. (1998). Getting beyond marginality and ethnicity: The challenge for race and ethnic studies in leisure research. *Journal of Leisure Research, 30,* 3.

Floyd, M. F. (2007). Research on race and ethnicity in leisure: Anticipating the fourth wave. *Leisure/loisir, 31,* 245–254.

Fried, L. P., Carlson, M. C., McGill, S., Seeman, T., Xue, Q. L., Frick, K., et al. (2013). Experience Corps: A dual trial to promote the health of older adults and children's academic success. *Contemporary Clinical Trials, 36,* 1–13.

Gallo, J. J., & Rabins, P. V. (1999). Depression without sadness: Alternative presentations of depression in late life. *American Family Physician, 60,* 820–826.

Gelman, C. R. (2014). Familismo and its impact on the family caregiving of Latinos with Alzheimer's disease: A complex narrative. *Research on Aging, 36,* 40–71.

Gerst-Emerson, K., Shovali, T. E., & Markides, K. S. (2014). Loneliness among very old Mexican Americans: Findings from the Hispanic established populations epidemiologic studies of the elderly. *Archives of Gerontology and Geriatrics, 59,* 145–149.

Glass, T. A. (2000). Psychosocial interventions. In L. F. Berkman & I. Kawachi (Eds.), *Social epidemiology* (pp. 267–305). New York, NY: Oxford University Press.

González, H. M., Haan, M. N., & Hinton, L. (2001). Acculturation and the prevalence of depression in older Mexican Americans: Baseline results of the Sacramento Area Latino Study on Aging. *Journal of the American Geriatrics Society, 49,* 948–953.

Guendelman, S., & Wagner, T. H. (2000). Health services utilization among Latinos and white non-Latinos: Results from a national survey. *Journal of Health Care for the Poor and Underserved, 11,* 179–194.

Gurland, B. J., Wilder, D. E., Lantigua, R., Stern, Y., Chen, J., Killeffer, E. H., et al. (1999). Rates of dementia in three ethno-racial groups. *International Journal of Geriatric Psychiatry, 14,* 481–493.

Haan, M. N., & Weldon, M. (1996). The influence of diabetes, hypertension, and stroke on ethnic differences in physical and cognitive functioning in an ethnically diverse older population. *Annals of Epidemiology, 6,* 392–398.

Hayward, M. D., Hummer, R. A., Chiu, C. T., González-González, C., & Wong, R. (2014). Does the Hispanic paradox in US adult mortality extend to disability? *Population Research and Policy Review, 33*, 81–96.

He, W., Goodkind, D., & Kowal, P. U. S. (2016). *Census Bureau, international population reports.* P95/16-1, An Aging World: 2015, Washington, DC: US Government Publishing Office.

Henderson, J. N. (1984). Creating culturally relevant Alzheimer's support groups for racial and ethnic minorities.

Heron, M. (2016). Deaths: leading causes for 2014. *National Vital Statistics Reports, 65*, 1–95. https://www.cdc.gov/nchs/data/nvsr/nvsr65/nvsr65_05.pdf.

Herrera, A. P., George, R., Angel, J. L., Markides, K., & Torres-Gil, F. (2013). Variation in Older Americans Act caregiver service use, unmet hours of care, and independence among Hispanics, African Americans, and Whites. *Home Health Care Services Quarterly, 32*, 35–56.

Hill, T. D., Angel, J. L., Balistreri, K. S., & Herrera, A. P. (2012). Immigrant status and cognitive functioning in late-life: An examination of gender variations in the healthy immigrant effect. *Social Science and Medicine, 75*, 2076–2084.

Hill, T. D., Uchino, B. N., Eckhardt, J. L., & Angel, J. L. (2016). Perceived social support trajectories and the all-cause mortality risk of older Mexican American women and men. *Research on Aging, 38*, 374–398.

House, J. S., Kessler, R. C., & Herzog, A. R. (1990). Age, socioeconomic status, and health. *Milbank Quarterly, 68*, 383–411.

Hummer, R. A., Benjamins, M. R., & Rogers, R. G. (2004). Racial and ethnic disparities in health and mortality among the US elderly population. *Critical Perspectives on Racial and ethnic differences in health in late life*, 53–94.

Hummer, R. A., & Hayward, M. D. (2015). Hispanic older adult health & longevity in the United States: Current patterns & concerns for the future. *Daedalus, 144*(2), 20–30.

Jang, Y., Chiriboga, D. A., Kim, G., & Phillips, K. (2008). Depressive symptoms in four racial and ethnic groups: The Survey of Older Floridians (SOF). *Research on Aging*.

Kagawa-Singer, M., Dressler, W. W., George, S. M., & Elwood, W. N. (2014). *The cultural framework for health: An integrative approach for research and program design and evaluation.*

Kaplan, R. C., Bangdiwala, S. I., Barnhart, J. M., Castañeda, S. F., Gellman, M. D., Lee, D. J., et al. (2014). Smoking among US Hispanic/Latino adults: The Hispanic Community Health Study/Study of Latinos. *American Journal of Preventive Medicine, 46*, 496–506.

Kirkman, M. S., Briscoe, V. J., Clark, N., Florez, H., Haas, L. B., Halter, J. B., et al. (2012). Diabetes in older adults. *Diabetes Care, 35*, 2650–2664.

Kochanek, K. D., Murphy, S. L., Xu, J. Q., Tejada-Vera, B. (2016). Deaths: Final data for 2014. *National Vital Statistics Reports, 65*, 1–121. https://www.cdc.gov/nchs/data/nvsr/nvsr65/nvsr65_04.pdf.

Krogstad, J. M. (2016). 5 Facts about Latinos and education. http://www.pewresearch.org/fact-tank/2016/07/28/5-facts-about-latinos-and-education/.

Lewis-Fernández, R., Das, A. K., Alfonso, C., Weissman, M. M., & Olfson, M. (2005). Depression in US Hispanics: Diagnostic and management considerations in family practice. *Journal of the American Board of Family Practice, 18*, 282–296.

Luchsinger, J. A., Tipiani, D., Torres-Patiño, G., Silver, S., Eimicke, J. P., Ramirez, M., et al. (2015). Characteristics and mental health of Hispanic dementia caregivers in New York City. *American Journal of Alzheimer's Disease and Other Dementias, 30*, 584–590.

Markides, K. S., & Rote, S. (2014/2015). Aging, minority status, and disability. *Generations, 38*, 19–24.

Marmot, M. (1996). The social pattern of health and disease. In D. Blane, E. Brunner, & R. Wilkinson (Eds.), *Health and social organization: Towards a health policy for the twenty-first century* (pp. 42–67). London, UK: Routledge.

Marquez, D. X., Bustamante, E. E., Aguiñaga, S., & Hernandez, R. (2015). BAILAMOS: Development, pilot testing, and future directions of a Latin dance program for older Latinos. *Health Education & Behavior, 42*, 604–610.

Martinez, I. L. (2002). The elder in the Cuban American family: Making sense of the real and ideal. *Journal of Comparative Family Studies*, 359–375.

Martinez, I. L., Baron, A., Largaespada, V., Ceruto, J., & Chaves, P. H. (2017). Prevalence of depression and its related social factors among Hispanic older adults. *Gerontologist, 56*, 90–100.

Martinez, I. L., Crooks, D., Kim, K. S., & Tanner, E. (2011). Invisible civic engagement among older adults: Valuing the contributions of informal volunteering. *Journal of Cross-Cultural Gerontology, 26*, 23–37.

Martinez, I. L., Frick, K., Glass, T. A., Carlson, M., Tanner, E., Ricks, M., & Fried, L. P. (2006). Engaging older adults in high impact volunteering that enhances health: Recruitment and retention in the Experience Corps® Baltimore. *Journal of Urban Health, 83'*, 941–953.

Martinez, I. L., Kim, K., Tanner, E., Fried, L. P., & Seeman, T. (2009). Ethnic and class variations in promoting social activities among older adults. *Activities, Adaptation & Aging, 33*, 96–119.

Martinez, I. L., & Varella, M. (2017). Latino population trends and late-life disability in Florida and the Northeast. Unpublished manuscript.

Mendes de Leon, C. F., Eschbach, K., & Markides, K. S. (2011). Population trends and late-life disability in Hispanics from the Midwest. *Journal of Aging and Health, 23*, 1166–1188.

Mullan, J. T. (1993). *Barriers to the use of formal services among Alzheimer's caregivers* (pp. 241–259). Caregiving systems: Informal and formal helpers.

National Association of Area Agencies on Aging. (2017a). *Local leaders in aging and community living*. Washington, DC: National Association of Area Agencies on Aging. https://www.n4a.org/content.asp?contentid=287.

National Association of Area Agencies on Aging. (2017b). National Survey of Area Agencies on Aging: 2017 (Report and Toolkit). https://www.n4a.org/2017aaasurvey.

National Cancer Institute. (2016). Surveillance, Epidemiology, and End Results Program (SEER) cancer statistics. https://seer.cancer.gov/explorer/application.php.

National Partnership for Women and Families. (2018). Fact sheet. Latinas and the wage gap. http://www.nationalpartnership.org/research-library/workplace-fairness/fair-pay/latinas-wage-gap.pdf.

Noël, P. H., Williams, J. W., Unützer, J., Worchel, J., Lee, S., Cornell, J., et al. (2004). Depression and comorbid illness in elderly primary care patients: Impact on multiple domains of health status and well-being. *Annals of Family Medicine, 2*, 555–562.

Palloni, A., McEniry, M., Wong, R., & Pelaez, M. (2006). The tide to come: Elderly health in Latin America and the Caribbean. *Journal of Aging and Health, 18*, 180–206.

Pearlin, L. I., Mullan, J. T., Semple, S. J., & Skaff, M. M. (1990). Caregiving and the stress process: An overview of concepts and their measures. *The gerontologist, 30*(5), 583–594.

Peek, M. K., Howrey, B. T., Ternent, R. S., Ray, L. A., & Ottenbacher, K. J. (2012). Social support, stressors, and frailty among older Mexican American adults. *Journals of Gerontology. Series B, Psychological Sciences and Social Sciences, 67*, 755–764.

Quesnel-Vallée, A., Farrah, J. S., & Jenkins, T. (2011). Population aging, health systems, and equity: Shared challenges for the United States and Canada. *Handbook of sociology of aging* (pp. 563–581). New York, NY: Springer.

Raji, M. A., Snih, S. A., Ray, L. A., Patel, K. V., & Markides, K. S. (2004). Cognitive status and incident disability in older Mexican Americans: Findings from the Hispanic established population for the epidemiological study of the elderly. *Ethnicity and Disease, 14*, 26–31.

Randi, G., Franceschi, S., & La Vecchia, C. (2006). Gallbladder cancer worldwide: Geographical distribution and risk factors. *International Journal of Cancer, 118*, 1591–1602.

Rieker, P. P., & Bird, C. E. (2005). Rethinking gender differences in health: Why we need to integrate social and biological perspectives. *Journals of Gerontology Series B: Psychological Sciences and Social Sciences, 60*(Special Issue 2), S40–S47.

Rodriguez-Galan, M. B., & Falcón, L. M. (2009). Perceived problems with access to medical care and depression among older Puerto Ricans, Dominicans, other Hispanics, and a comparison group of non-Hispanic Whites. *Journal of Aging and Health, 21*, 501–518.

Rowe, J. W., & Kahn, R. L. (1997). *Successful aging*. The gerontologist, 37(4), 433–440.

Ruiz, M. E. (2012). Latino elders reframing familismo: Implications for health and caregiving support. *Journal of Cultural Diversity, 19,* 50.

Russell, D., & Taylor, J. (2009). Living alone and depressive symptoms: The influence of gender, physical disability, and social support among Hispanic and non-Hispanic older adults. *Journals of Gerontology. Series B, Psychological Sciences and Social Sciences, 64,* 95–104.

Sabogal, F., Marín, G., Otero-Sabogal, R., Marín, B. V., & Perez-Stable, E. J. (1987). Hispanic familism and acculturation: What changes and what doesn't? *Hispanic Journal of Behavioral Sciences, 9,* 397–412.

Schim, S. M., & Doorenbos, A. Z. (2010). A three-dimensional model of cultural congruence: Framework for intervention. *Journal of Social Work in End-of-Life & Palliative Care, 6,* 256–270.

Schneiderman, N., Llabre, M., Cowie, C. C., Barnhart, J., Carnethon, M., Gallo, L. C., et al. (2014). Prevalence of diabetes among Hispanics/Latinos from diverse backgrounds: The Hispanic Community Health Study/Study of Latinos (HCHS/SOL). *Diabetes Care, 37,* 2233–2239.

Sheftel, M. G. (2017). Prevalence of disability among Hispanic immigrant populations: New evidence from the American community survey. *Population Review, 56*(1).

Siegel, R. L., Fedewa, S. A., Miller, K. D., Goding-Sauer, A., Pinheiro, P. S., Martinez-Tyson, D., & Jemal, A. (2015). Cancer statistics for Hispanics/Latinos, 2015. *CA: Cancer Journal for Clinicians, 65,* 457–480.

Spencer, P. (1990). The riddled course: Theories of age and its transformations.

Stephens, M. A. P. (1993). Understanding barriers to caregivers' use of formal services: The caregiver's perspective. *Caregiving systems: Informal and formal helpers* (pp 261–272).

Tang, M. X., Cross, P., Andrews, H., Jacobs, D. M., Small, S., Bell, K., et al. (2001). Incidence of AD in African-Americans, Caribbean Hispanics, and Caucasians in northern Manhattan. *Neurology, 56,* 49–56.

Tervalon, M., & Murray-Garcia, J. (1998). Cultural humility vs. cultural competence: A critical distinction in defining physician training outcomes in multicultural education. *Journal of Health Care for the Poor and Underserved, 9,* 117–125.

Tirodkar, M. A., Song, J., Chang, R. W., Dunlop, D. D., & Chang, H. J. (2008). Racial and ethnic differences in activities of daily living disability among the elderly: The case of Spanish speakers. *Archives of Physical Medicine and Rehabilitation, 89,* 1262–1266. https://doi.org/10.1016/j.apmr.2007.11.042.

Tucker, K. L., Falcon, L. M., Bianchi, L. A., Cacho, E., & Bermudez, O. I. (2000). Self-reported prevalence and health correlates of functional limitation among Massachusetts elderly. *Journals of Gerontology. Series A, Biological Sciences and Medical Sciences, 55,* M90–M97.

United States Department of Justice. (2009). American With Disabilities Act of 1990, As Amended. United States Department of Justice, Civil Rights Division. https://www.ada.gov/pubs/adastatute08.htm#12102.

United States Census Bureau (2010). American Community Survey (ACS), 2010. https://www.census.gov/people/disability/%20methodology/acs.html.

United States Census Bureau (2015). American Community Survey (ACS), 2015.

Wallace, L. M., Theou, O., Pena, F., Rockwood, K., & Andrew, M. K. (2015). Social vulnerability as a predictor of mortality and disability: Cross-country differences in the survey of health, aging, and retirement in Europe (SHARE). *Aging Clinical and Experimental Research, 27,* 365–372.

Yang, F. M., Cazorla-Lancaster, Y., & Jones, R. N. (2008). Within-group differences in depression among older Hispanics living in the United States. *The Journals of Gerontology Series B: Psychological Sciences and Social Sciences, 63,* P27–P32.

Zammitti, E. P., Cohen, R. A., & Martinez, M. E. (2016). *Health insurance coverage: Early release of estimates from the National Health Interview Survey, January–June 2016.* Washington, DC: National Center for Health Statistics. https://www.cdc.gov/nchs/data/nhis/earlyrelease/insur201611.pdf.

Chapter 8
Health Threats that Can Affect Hispanic/Latino Migrants and Immigrants

Thomas M. Painter

Abstract Various health threats can affect Hispanic/Latino migrants and immigrants en route to and from, and following their arrival in the United States (US). In this chapter, I describe several of these health threats and examples of approaches that have been used to address some of them, and describe social-structural and circumstantial factors that can affect migrant and immigrant health. I then briefly describe factors that than can affect two Hispanic/Latino immigrant subpopulations that may be particularly vulnerable to health threats: women and children/minors. I also suggest that the concept of structural vulnerability is useful for characterizing and understanding the varied circumstances of Hispanic/Latino migrants and immigrants in their countries of origin and the US. I conclude the chapter with a brief reprise of several topics that merit further study.

Keywords Hispanic · Latinx · Latino · Health threats · Immigrants · Migrants · Women · Children · Structural · Vulnerability

In this chapter, I describe various health threats that can affect Hispanic/Latino migrants and immigrants en route to and from, and following their arrival in the US as they seek opportunities to secure resources they and their families need for their livelihoods. These threats include multiple dangers in their countries of origin and during their travels to the US and, once arrived, hazardous working conditions, exposure to chronic and infectious diseases, and substance abuse. In several instances, I describe examples of approaches that have been used to address these health threats. I also describe social–structural and circumstantial factors that can affect their health and access to and participation in healthcare services in the US. These include factors related to what is termed the Hispanic paradox, i.e., the deterioration of pre-immigration health patterns among Hispanic/Latino immigrants over time after they

---

Disclaimer The findings and conclusions in this report are those of the author and do not necessarily represent the official position of the Centers for Disease Control and Prevention (CDC).

T. M. Painter (✉)
Division of HIV/AIDS Prevention, U.S. Centers for Disease Control and Prevention, 1600 Clifton Rd, NE MS US8-5, Atlanta, GA 30329, USA
e-mail: tcp2@cdc.gov

© Springer Nature Switzerland AG 2020
A. D. Martínez and S. D. Rhodes (eds.), *New and Emerging Issues in Latinx Health*, https://doi.org/10.1007/978-3-030-24043-1_8

arrive in the US; racial and ethnic bias; language barriers and linguistic, cultural appropriateness of healthcare promotion and services; and policy-related factors. I then briefly discuss issues among two Hispanic/Latino immigrant subpopulations that may be particularly vulnerable to health threats: women and children/minors. The examples are intended to illustrate the kinds of health threats and conditions that can affect the well-being of Hispanic/Latino migrants and immigrants and do not pretend to exhaust the possibilities. Toward the end of the chapter, I suggest that the concept of structural vulnerability is useful for characterizing and understanding the varied circumstances of Hispanic/Latino migrants and immigrants in their countries of origin and the US. Structural vulnerability, which is created and sustained over time by multiple factors, can increase the liability of migrants and immigrants to the negative effects of various health risks as they engage in transnational mobility. I conclude the chapter with a brief reprise of several topics identified while describing health threats that can affect Hispanic/Latino migrants and immigrants and that merit further study.

Hispanic/Latino Migrants and Immigrants in the US

The Hispanic/Latino population is the largest, fastest growing ethnic minority group in the US, numbering nearly 57 million and representing 17.6% of the total US population in 2015 (U.S. Census Bureau, 2016); the number is projected to reach 119 million in 2060 (U.S. Census Bureau, 2014). Most Hispanics/Latinos are US-born (Zong & Batalova, 2017). In 2015, the number of foreign-born Hispanics/Latinos in the US was estimated to be 19.4 million: 11.5 million from Mexico, 5.3 million from Central and South America, and 2.6 million from Caribbean countries (Flores, López, & Radford, 2017).

Hispanic/Latino migrants travel to the US with the intention of eventually returning to their countries of origin to reside and may make several return trips to their home countries during their time in the US (Massey, Durand, & Malone, 2002; Rodríguez, Sáenz, & Menjívar, 2008). These cyclical migration patterns have declined because of (a) the effects of the Great Recession, dating from 2007, resulting in a major contraction of employment opportunities for Hispanic/Latino migrants in the US, and (b) stricter enforcement of US immigration policies, which have made movement across the US–Mexican border more difficult, contributing to a de facto settling out by some migrants in the US (Stepler & Lopez, 2016).

Hispanic/Latino immigrants travel to the US with the intention of staying permanently in this country (Organista, Carillo, & Ayala, 2004; Valverde et al., 2015). Both Hispanic/Latino migrants and immigrants participate in the migration process in search of resources needed for their and their families' livelihoods within transnational social fields or spaces that include their communities and countries of origin, cross-border areas, and their destination countries (Lopez, 2007; Massey, 2008; Newland, 2009; Painter, 1996, 1999). The migration process entails mobility of individuals and groups (e.g., families, co-residents from the same neighborhoods or communities) between their countries of origin and their destination countries. The process also includes factors associated with the mobility of these individuals and groups, e.g., their physical itineraries, transit areas, places where they live and work, duration of residence at their destinations, and movement within destination countries.

Once in the US, Hispanic/Latino migrants and immigrants may be actively engaged in the labor force. Their labor force participation rate (the percentage of a given population that is of working age and are members of the workforce) in 2016 was 67.9%, compared with 64% for US-born Hispanics/Latinos, 62.4% for US-born Whites, and 60.1% for US-born Blacks (U.S. Department of Labor, 2017). Hispanic/Latino migrants and immigrants find a wide variety jobs in the US, many of which pay low wages; these jobs include day labor or work in urban- and suburban-based service or agro-processing industries areas, or farmwork. Other Hispanic/Latino migrants and immigrant may accumulate sufficient capital to begin small businesses such as shops or restaurants. Despite their frequently low earning levels, their active engagement in the US economy is important both for their livelihoods and those of their families in the US and their countries of origin, and for the economies of their countries of origin. Mexican immigrants, for example, remitted $28.5 billion to Mexico in 2016, accounting for 2.3% of the country's gross domestic product (GDP). The absolute size of immigrant remittances to the Central American countries of El Salvador, Guatemala, and Honduras was smaller, but accounted for 10% to more than 18% of the countries' GDPs (World Bank, 2017).

Hispanic/Latino migrant and immigrant mobility may also be fueled by extra-economic factors, such as political instability and violence in their countries of origin. Hispanic/Latino immigration to the US as a means of escaping extreme circumstances such as political or drug gang-related violence in their countries of origin has increased since the 1990s and with it, requests from these persons for asylum. Asylum requests from Mexican immigrants numbered nearly 18,000 in 2015. Asylum requests from El Salvadoran, Guatemalan, and Honduran immigrants during 2013–2015 exceeded those recorded during all of the previous 15 years. An estimated 26,600 children from these three countries sought asylum in the US in 2015 (Zong & Batalova, 2017). Unauthorized Hispanic/Latino immigrants (those who enter the country without legal permission and those who overstay their legal visas) were estimated to number nearly 8.4 million in 2015 (Passel & Cohn, 2017), with the number of those who overstayed their visas being greater than those who illegally entered the US (Warren & Kerwin, 2017).

For purposes of this chapter, I use the term "Hispanic/Latino immigrants" to refer to foreign-born Hispanic/Latino individuals in the US who are migrants or immigrants as characterized above, whose movement may be driven by economic or extra-economic factors, or some combination of both.

Opportunities and Risks in the US

Participation in the migration process as a means of locating income-earning opportunities or escaping dangerous situations in their countries of origin can potentially expose Hispanic/Latino immigrants to health threats en route to and from, and within the US. Examples of in-transit dangers to which undocumented individuals may be particularly susceptible include gang assaults, rapes, robberies, falls from freight cars while riding long-haul trains through Mexico toward the US–Mexican border, and mistreatment by smugglers (Fernandez, Pérez-Peña, & Montgomery, 2017; Medecins sans Frontieres, 2017; Tuckman, 2014). Other transit-related dangers that can affect these individuals after they cross the US–Mexican border include accidents and deaths due to excess heat exposure, thirst, and starvation that can occur during their long treks over desert areas in the US border states of California, Arizona, New Mexico, and Texas (Taylor et al., 2018). In a study that covered the period 2002–2003, for example, exposure to excessive heat accounted for more than 70% of deaths among immigrants who attempted unauthorized border crossings into these four states (Sapkota et al., 2006). Lastly, some immigrants are apprehended by border patrol agents or local authorities (International Organization for Migration, 2014).

Health Vulnerabilities of Hispanic/Latino Immigrants in the US

Hazardous Work Conditions

Disparities in economic opportunities can lead to disproportionate exposure by members of racial/ethnic minority groups in the US to risks of workplace injury. In the construction industry, for example, Hispanics/Latinos accounted for one-fifth of the US workforce in 2013; of these, 75% were foreign-born immigrants who frequently worked in jobs with high levels of injury risks (Flynn, Cunningham, et al., 2015; Seabury, Terp, & Boden, 2017). Among urban construction workers, Hispanic/Latino immigrant workers have been affected disproportionately by both traumatic (nonfatal) and fatal occupational injuries. Rates for the latter were nearly twice that for US-born Hispanic/Latino workers during the mid-2000s. Particularly, dangerous lines of construction work are roofing and ironworking (Forst, Avila, Anozie, & Rubin, 2010).

Hispanic/Latino immigrant workers who are engaged in agriculture and food processing industries, including poultry, pork, and beef processing (Kandel & Parrado, 2005), can also face exposure to a range of work-related health threats. Multiple factors can contribute to their vulnerability and create barriers to their accessing and participating in healthcare services. Work-related hazards include long-term exposure to herbicides and pesticides, dermatitis, excessive heat exposure, repetitive motion-related injuries, dental diseases, inadequate preventive care, and social and mental health problems (Gibson, 2016; Hall, Lee, Clark, & Perilla, 2016; Hansen & Donohoe, 2003; Taylor et al., 2018; Walton et al., 2017). Their working conditions can be harsh (e.g., long summer days spent harvesting row crops) and potentially dangerous (harvesting tree crops; processing poultry and livestock) (Arcury & Quandt, 2007; Gibson, 2016; U.S. Government Accountability Office, 2016). Children of immigrant farmworkers can also be negatively affected by work-related factors. They are exempted from federal child labor laws that limit the amount of time that children under 16 years of age may work in agriculture (Marlenga, Berg, Linneman, Brison, & Pickett, 2007; Quandt, 2009). Factors that can negatively affect access by these Hispanic/Latino immigrants to health care include their unstable employment, lack of access to transportation, and residence in isolated rural areas with limited health services. Other factors that can negatively affect access to health care include low incomes, lack of health insurance, limited education and English language skills, a lack of access to health-related information, and being in the US without proper documentation (Arcury & Quandt, 2007; Guevara & Sangaramoorthy, 2017; Martinez-Donate et al., 2017; Summers, Quandt, Talton, Galván, Arcury, 2015). Detailed data on health and utilization of formal health services by workers in agriculture and related industries are limited; in particular, little is known about how and the extent to which these immigrants self-treat and self-manage their health (Arcury & Quandt, 2007).

Data from a nationally representative US Department of Labor survey in 2012–2014 of the estimated one million-plus migrant and immigrant agricultural workers in the US provides a snapshot of this labor force (U.S. Department of Labor, 2016). Most (80%) were Hispanic/Latino, more than two-thirds of whom were born in Mexico. Most were men (72%), although the proportion of women has increased. Most are married (63%), have children (57%), have settled in US locations (84%), and speak no or limited English (70%). More than one-third (39%) are unaccompanied by nuclear family members. Men are nearly three times as likely to be unaccompanied as women (47% vs. 16%). They work in fruit and nut crops (41%), vegetable crops (21%), field or mixed crops (16%), and horticulture (22%); 49% earned less than $20,000 from agricultural work the previous year, and two-thirds do not have health insurance (U.S. Department of Labor, 2016).

Vulnerability of Hispanic/Latino immigrants to work-related hazards, particularly immigrants who are newly arrived and without documentation, can result from multiple factors in addition to exposure to the work hazards per se. These factors were described in a study of Hispanic/Latino immigrants in Santa Fe, New Mexico, and Cincinnati, Ohio (Flynn, Eggerth, & Jacobson, 2015). The factors include concerns about being able to stay in the US by avoiding detention and deportation and feeling pressure to find a job to maintain themselves, supporting family members in their countries of origin, and possibly paying off debts to smugglers. As a result of being in these precarious circumstances, Hispanic/Latino immigrants may accept unsatisfactory and unsafe working conditions, even work-related injuries, without complaining for fear of losing their jobs, or having employers report them to authorities. Fear of job loss can also lead to overperforming on the job, leading to an unsustainable work pace, fatigue, and injury. The circumstances of undocumented

Hispanic/Latino immigrants can also be affected by laws and levels of enforcement that vary from one jurisdiction to another and may create barriers to their knowing about and accessing resources to which they are legally entitled. These resources may include workers' compensation, emergency medical care, or protections facilitated by the Occupational Safety and Health Administration. Some undocumented immigrants may avoid or disengage from potentially helpful occupational safety and health-related institutions for fear that seeking assistance may "create more problems than solutions" (Flynn, Eggerth, & Jacobson, 2015).

A collaboration between the US National Institute for Occupational Safety and Health (NIOSH) and the Mexican Ministries of Health and Foreign Affairs illustrates an initiative to address work-related hazards that can affect immigrant workers. The program aims to promote occupational safety and reduce occupational health disparities that affect Mexican workers in the construction and hospitality industries (Flynn, Check, Eggerth, & Tonda, 2013) and has resulted in a continuing focus on occupational safety and health in the *Ventanillas de Salud* (Health Windows) programs of the Mexican Consular Network in the US (Rangel Gomez et al., 2017).

Chronic Diseases

A review of multiple datasets for the years 2009–2013 found that Hispanics/Latinos overall in the US (both US- and foreign-born) had better health outcomes than Whites for most analyzed health factors, despite facing worse socioeconomic barriers that included a greater likelihood of living below the poverty line, not having completed high school, not having health insurance, and delaying or not receiving needed health care because of cost considerations. These outcomes included lower death rates for seven of the 10 leading causes of death, including cancer and heart disease. The prevalence of cancer and heart disease is also lower for Hispanics/Latinos than for white persons (Dominguez et al., 2015). However, compared with the White population, the Hispanic/Latino population overall had higher death rates from diabetes (51% higher), and chronic liver disease and cirrhosis (48% higher), and a higher prevalence of diabetes (133% higher) and obesity (23% higher). Among Hispanics/Latinos, the prevalence of obesity, hypertension, smoking, heart disease, and cancer is lower for foreign-born individuals than for US-born individuals. In a separate study of eight major federal health data systems, foreign-born Hispanics/Latinos were found to have a longer life expectancy than US-born Hispanics/Latinos (Singh, Rodriguez-Lainz, & Kogan, 2013). In both of the aforementioned studies, no distinction was made between migrants and immigrants among foreign-born individuals and changes in health outcomes over time were not evaluated. I will discuss changes in health status over time among Hispanic/Latino immigrants in the US when examining acculturation and related factors later in the chapter.

The observed differences between foreign- and US-born individuals point to a need for improved strategies to collect public health data and data on health promotion programs that more effectively capture and respond to the diversity of Hispanic/Latino individuals in the US based on differences such as birth status (foreign- or US-born), countries of origin, sex at birth, age, spoken languages and language proficiency, education, health literacy, types of work, and income levels (Dominguez et al., 2015; Fenelon, Chinn, & Anderson, 2017). A study of efforts by undocumented Mexican immigrants with end-stage renal disease to obtain dialysis care in South Texas illustrates the difficulties that can occur when seeking needed care for a chronic disease. Because of their undocumented status and their inability to pay for outpatient care, some individuals in the study were obliged to seek care in emergency rooms. Due to limited medical staff serving large numbers of patients in these settings, often involving long wait times, these individuals faced an increased likelihood of missed or delayed access to treatment (Melo, 2017).

Community Health Workers The use of community health workers (*promotoras/es de salud*) is an approach that can be useful for efforts to increase access to and participation by underserved Hispanic/Latino immigrant populations in initiatives that address a range of health conditions, including chronic diseases (Dominguez et al., 2015). This approach may lend itself to culturally appropriate health promotion and prevention efforts that include education, outreach, enrollment, screening, and service delivery for Hispanic/Latino immigrants. Findings from a randomized community trial study in El Paso, Texas is illustrative. A group of primarily foreign-born, female Hispanic/Latino participants in a *promotoras de salud* intervention reported higher levels of awareness about cardiovascular disease risk factors, consumed less salt, engaged in better weight control practices, and had slightly lower cholesterol levels at follow-up, compared with women who did not participate in the intervention (Balcázar et al., 2010). A *promotora* intervention delivered to uninsured Hispanic/Latino immigrant women living in a rural US–Mexican border area of Arizona resulted in significant increases in participants' compliance with annual examinations for prevention of chronic diseases compared with nonparticipants (Hunter et al., 2004). Finally, a *promotores de salud* intervention produced promising results for reducing progression to type 2 diabetes and managing diabetes after disease onset among Hispanic/Latino populations that included both foreign-born and US-born individuals (Community Guide, 2016, 2017). The potential contribution of approaches that use community health workers for health promotion may be based in part on the degree to which they can focus on a range of health-related conditions and support client efforts to overcome social–structural as well as behavioral factors, rather than focusing on a single disease or condition (Kangovi et al., 2017).

Infectious Diseases

HIV and Other Sexually Transmitted Diseases Studies have repeatedly described the vulnerability of Hispanic/Latino immigrants in the US to HIV and other sexually transmitted diseases (STDs) (Kissinger et al., 2012; Organista et al., 2012; Painter, 2008; Quesada, Hart, & Bourgois, 2011; Valverde et al., 2015). In addition, research has shown that HIV infection among foreign-born Hispanics/Latinos is more likely to have occurred in the US than in their countries of origin (Espinoza, Hall, & Hu, 2012; Katz, 2012; Wiewel, Torian, Hanna, Bocour, & Shepard, 2015). Once infected, these individuals may contribute to HIV infection in their home communities when they return temporarily or permanently. Changing patterns of HIV infection in Mexico, the source of most Hispanic/Latino immigrants in the US, illustrates the potential role of return migrants as a bridge population. Researchers in the mid- to late 2000s described how the return of HIV-infected men from the US contributed to HIV in Mexico becoming increasingly rural and heterosexual in nature (Bastos, Cáceres, Galvão, Veras, & Castilho, 2008; Rodríguez, Garcia et al., 2008; Salgado de Snyder et al., 2010; Sowell, Holtz, & Velasquez, 2008).

Involvement in risk behaviors by individual Hispanic/Latino immigrants can increase their vulnerability to HIV/STD infection or transmission; however, social–structural and circumstantial factors can also influence their likelihood of engaging in actions that can increase their HIV/STD risks. These factors include social and geographic isolation (Sanchez et al., 2012), loneliness (Hirsch, Muñoz-Laboy, Nyhus, Yount, & Bauermeister, 2009; Muñoz-Laboy, Hirsch, & Quipse-Lazaro, 2009; Rhodes et al., 2011), disrupted family relationships (Hirsch, Higgins, Bentley, & Nathanson, 2002; Hirsch et al., 2007, 2009; Organista, 2007), and attenuated or missing family-based or community-based social controls (norms and sanctions) that may moderate risk behaviors in their US destinations (Parrado & Flippen, 2010). The effects of social–cultural displacement, and associated desperation (*desesperación*) or depression that can occur, on Hispanic/Latino immigrants' potential HIV/STD risk behaviors (Aranda-Naranjo, Gaskins, Bustamante, Lopez, & Rodriguiz, 2000; Organista, 2007; Shedlin, Decena, & Oliver-Velez, 2005) may be amplified among those who travel to destinations in the South and Midwestern US, where Hispanic/Latino communities are more recent, often dating from the early 1990s. Newer Hispanic/Latino immigrant destinations may not afford the same levels of social support and social integration that can be found in more established communities, such as those in the southwestern US (Frasca, 2009; Hirsch et al., 2009; Kochhar, Suro, & Tafoya, 2005; Massey, 2008; Painter, 2008; Parrado & Flippen, 2010). Limited education, English language proficiency, and health literacy among some immigrants, and little or no Spanish proficiency among immigrants from indigenous Mixtec, Zapotec, or Triqui-speaking populations in southern Mexico and Central America (Cornelius, Fitzgerald, & Fisher, 2007; Holmes, 2013) can contribute to inadequate knowledge and erroneous beliefs about HIV/STD transmission and prevention, low levels of perceived infection risks, and a lack of information about care and treatment options (Organista, Alvarado, Balbutin-Burnham, Worby, & Martinez, 2006; Parrado, Flippen, & McQuiston, 2004). For Hispanic/Latino immigrant men, particularly those who travel to the US unaccompanied by spouses or partners, vulnerability to HIV/STD risks can be increased by residence and socializing in areas such as urban apartment complexes and rural agricultural camps where men may outnumber women (Grzywacz et al. 2004; Hirsch et al., 2002; Parrado et al. 2004). These settings may be associated with an increased likelihood of alcohol consumption, binge drinking (Loury, Jesse, & Wu, 2011; Organista, 2007; Organista & Kubo, 2005; Worby et al., 2014), and noninjection drug use (Apostolopoulos et al., 2006). These circumstances may also be conducive to sexual risk behaviors, including condomless sex with heterosexual, same-sex, and transgender partners who may or may not be sex workers (Kissinger et al., 2008, 2012; Parrado & Flippen, 2010; Sanchez et al., 2012; Valverde, DiNenno, Schulden, Oster, & Painter, 2016). For Hispanic/Latina immigrant women, the greatest source of HIV/STD infection risk may be condomless sex with a regular partner, including their husbands, the result of limited sexual decision-making power within couple relationships and deference to partners (Hirsch et al., 2002, 2007, 2009; Montealegre, Risser, Selwyn, McCurdy, & Sabin, 2012; Valverde et al., 2015). Gay, bisexual, and transgender Hispanic/Latino immigrants may be disproportionately affected by discrimination because of their status as immigrants, as members of an ethnic/racial minority, their gender identification, and actions that can increase their risks of transmitting or being infected by HIV/STDs (Rhodes et al., 2017; Rhodes, 2018).

HIV testing and knowledge of one's HIV serostatus are gateways to effective HIV prevention and potential access to HIV care and related services. A 2017 Centers for Disease Control and Prevention (CDC) study demonstrated the efficacy of pre-exposure prophylaxis (PrEP) for preventing HIV infection among individuals who are known to be HIV-negative through HIV testing, but whose actions may increase their risks of HIV infection (CDC, 2017). The use of PrEP, together with consistent condom use, offers HIV prevention options for potential use by some Hispanic/Latino immigrants. For individuals who are infected with HIV and not aware of their HIV serostatus, HIV testing is a key step toward accessing treatment with antiretroviral therapy (ART) and referrals to supportive services (CDC, 2011). The outcome of ART for persons living with HIV may be longer, healthier lives. In addition, ART substantially reduces the risk of sexual transmission of HIV. Persons living with HIV who receive ART as prescribed, and achieve and maintain an undetectable viral load have effectively no risk of transmitting HIV to their HIV-negative sexual partners (CDC, 2018). However, conditions associated with being undocumented in the US can create barriers to uptake of HIV care. This fact is illustrated by a study of mostly Hispanic/Latino immigrants in the Bronx, NY, in which undocumented individuals were more likely than those with documentation to enter HIV care with advanced disease. Contributing factors included a lack of access to health insurance and prescription medications (Ross, Felsen, Cunningham, Patel, & Hanna, 2017). More research and culturally competent public health outreach are needed to better understand the varied circumstances of Hispanic/Latino immigrant populations in the US and increase their awareness of and participation, as appropriate, in these approaches to HIV prevention and care. Outreach efforts may be particularly challenging when reaching immigrants who are mobile and, in some cases, in the US without documentation and potentially wary of engaging with formal healthcare services. Initiatives are also needed to support efforts by Hispanic/Latino immigrants to overcome the negative effects of social-structural factors on their access to and participation in HIV-related services, and the potential contribution of forms of social support to their coping with these factors and to HIV protective actions (Althoff et al., 2013, 2017; Kissinger et al., 2012, 2013; Painter, 2018).

A limited number of behavioral HIV/STD prevention interventions have been developed specifically for and have demonstrated efficacy for use with Hispanic/Latino immigrants. These interventions may promote condom use and HIV testing and have been developed for use with Hispanic/Latino immigrant heterosexual men (Rhodes, Hergenrather, Bloom, Leichliter, & Montaño, 2009; Rhodes et al., 2011; Sánchez, De La Rosa, & Serna, 2013); gay, bisexual, and other men who have sex with men (O'Donnell, Stueve, Joseph, & Flores, 2014; Rhodes et al., 2010, 2012, 2017); and women (Wingood et al., 2011). There is some evidence, however, that the use of these interventions by service providers who work with Hispanic/Latino immigrant populations may be limited (Painter et al., 2012; Painter, 2018).

Tuberculosis The tuberculosis (TB) case rate per 100,000 population among Hispanics/Latinos in the US in 2015 (4.8) was eight times higher than that among Whites (0.6) (CDC, 2016b). The number of TB cases among foreign-born Hispanics/Latinos that year was three times greater than that among US-born Hispanics/Latinos (2,030 vs. 658). Among all foreign-born populations in the US, the second largest number of TB cases in 2014 was in the Hispanic/Latino population, representing nearly one-third of all cases. During the period 2011–2015, Mexico had the largest number of TB cases among 30 countries listed by CDC (2016a). Factors that can create challenges to TB prevention and that may be particularly pertinent to Hispanic/Latino immigrants include delayed detection and diagnosis, inadequate treatment, nonprioritization of treatment among those with asymptomatic latent infection, socioeconomic factors that limit access to health care and housing, limited health literacy, language and cultural barriers, and TB-related stigma that may deter people from seeking medical care (CDC, 2016a).

Substance Abuse

Loneliness, separation from family members, difficult living and working conditions, and chronic stress and fear associated with being in the US without documentation can contribute to substance abuse, particularly problem drinking, among Hispanic/Latino immigrants (Loury et al., 2011; Worby et al., 2014). Binge drinking by male Hispanic/Latino immigrants has been associated with unprotected sex with heterosexual partners (Organista, 2007; Worby et al., 2014) and, among gay, bisexual, and other men who have sex with men, with unprotected anal sex with partners whose HIV serostatus is serodiscordant or unknown (Mizuno, Borkowf, Ayala, Carballo-Diéguez, & Millett, 2015). In some studies of Hispanic/Latino immigrants, the length of time they have been in the US has been associated with increased alcohol consumption (Lara, Gamboa, Kahramanian, Morales, & Hayes Bautista, 2005). However, this association has not been described consistently, suggesting a need for fine-grained analyses that examine differences in drinking patterns among Hispanics/Latinos by country of origin and in the US (Sanchez et al., 2014). Researchers have reported variable rates of drug use, principally noninjection drug use, by male Hispanic/Latino immigrants (Kissinger et al., 2013). Apostolopoulos et al. (2006) reported that Hispanic/Latino migrant men in South Carolina used alcohol and noninjection drugs (principally marijuana and crack cocaine) as a means of coping with the social isolation that can result from living in farmworker camps. These authors noted that although many of the men had used alcohol in Mexico, drug use often started after they arrived in the US. The lifetime prevalence of drug use may be lower for immigrants than for US-born Hispanics/Latinos; however, drug-using immigrants may be less likely than US-born individuals to participate in treatment programs and more likely to use family or social services as sources of support (Mancini, Salas-Wright, & Vaughn, 2015).

Effects of Social-Structural and Circumstantial Factors

Factors Related to the Hispanic Paradox

The deterioration of pre-immigration health status among Hispanic/Latino immigrants over time in the US has been referred to variously as the Hispanic paradox, the Latino mortality paradox, and the healthy immigrant paradox (Abraído-Lanza, Chao, & Flórez, 2005; Castro, 2013; Markides & Coreil, 1986). Greater degrees of acculturation—the adoption by Hispanic/Latino immigrants of mainstream American cultural (or subcultural) values, norms, and behaviors—or longer residence in the US (sometimes used as a proxy for acculturation) have been associated with increased vulnerability to a range of health threats (Brown, Wilson, & Angel, 2015; Goldman et al., 2014; Singh et al., 2013; Thomson & Hoffman-Goetz, 2009). Examples include increased alcohol use and smoking, obesity (Abraído-Lanza et al., 2005; Guendelman, Ritterman-Weintraub, Fernald, & Kaufer-Horwitz, 2013), increased risks of HIV/STD infection (Galvan, Ortiz, Martinez, & Bing, 2008; Haderxhanaj, Rhodes, Romaguera, Bloom, & Leichliter, 2015; McCoy, Shehadeh, Rubens, & Navarro, 2014; Mizuno et al., 2015; Sanchez et al., 2012), and anxiety and depression (Orozco, Borges, Medina-Mora, Aguilar-Gaxiola, & Breslau, 2013). However, research findings concerning the association between acculturation and health outcomes among Hispanic/Latino immigrants are not consistent. In contrast to the patterns just described, some researchers have found that acculturation can be associated with positive health outcomes, including less frequent problematic food consumption patterns (Arandia, Nalty, Sharkey, & Dean, 2012), reduced rates of hypertension (Hall et al., 2016), and less frequent HIV/STD infection risk behaviors (Parrado et al., 2004; Viadro & Earp, 2000). The relationship between time in the US, acculturation processes, and the likelihood of negative health outcomes or health-protective actions requires further study. The relationship between predeparture conditions in immigrants' countries of origin and their health outcomes in the US also needs to be better understood (Torres & Wallace, 2013).

Lastly, patterns of declining health over time among Hispanic/Latino immigrants in the US have also been evaluated in terms of contributing factors other than the effects of acculturation (Viruell-Fuentes, Miranda, & Abdulrahim, 2012). (Also see Chapter 15.) This perspective is illustrated by Creighton et al. (2012), who evaluated the increasing prevalence of obesity over time among Hispanic/Latino immigrants in the US. They propose that obesity and associated negative health outcomes may result more from the cumulative effects of economic factors having a broader and disproportionate impact on Hispanic/Latino immigrant communities than from their incorporation of US host culture values and behaviors. Federal government agricultural subsidies favoring the production of inexpensive high-calorie foods, and the aggressive marketing and widespread ease of access to these foods and beverages in Hispanic/Latino immigrant and other predominantly racial/ethnic minority communities in the US, may also contribute to the deterioration of their health status over time (Creighton, Goldman, Pebley, & Chung, 2012). Relatively low-income levels and limited access to retailers that carry healthier foods in some Hispanic/Latino immigrant communities may constrain their access to health-protective choices and better quality foods. The mass marketing of inexpensive ultraprocessed foods is a transnational phenomenon, and has been associated with the development of negative dietary practices and the widespread prevalence of obesity in developing countries, including those from which some Hispanic/Latino immigrants originate (Jacobs & Richtel, 2017; Martínez, 2013). Lastly, involvement in the disruptive, stressful migration process itself, and the experiences of Hispanic/Latino immigrants as they cope with challenges they face during the immediate postmigration period may also detrimentally affect their health status (Goldman et al., 2014). These processes and their effects on health outcomes among Hispanic/Latino immigrants require further study.

Racial/Ethnic Bias

Hispanic/Latino immigrants in the US may be subject to stigmatization, social marginalization, racism, and discrimination because of their appearance, language use, the kinds of work they do, and their known or perceived status as immigrants, whether documented or undocumented. These processes may also make it difficult for them to gain access to any number of resources they and their families need for their well-being, including health-related services. Implicit and explicit biases among healthcare providers as manifested in, for example, perceptions, values, and verbal behavior during patient-provider interactions, can also negatively affect their contacts with Hispanic/Latino immigrants, creating barriers to health care delivery at the provider-patient interface and contributing to negative health outcomes for immigrants. Research has been limited concerning the effects of implicit provider bias and actions on Hispanic/Latino immigrants' health care outcomes over time (Hall et al., 2015; Martinez et al., 2017).

Language Barriers and Linguistic, Cultural Appropriateness of Healthcare Promotion and Services

Spanish-speaking persons accounted for nearly two-thirds of the nearly 26 million individuals with limited English proficiency living in the US in 2013 (Zong & Batalova, 2017). Access to healthcare-related information by Hispanic/Latino immigrants can be negatively affected by the limited availability of culturally appropriate information in Spanish or the indigenous languages they use in everyday life. These barriers can also occur at the point of healthcare delivery, when providers may not have the language proficiency required to understand and address the needs of patients who are immigrants when trained interpreters are not available, or when immigrants' family members are enlisted on the spot to serve as translators. These family members may not understand medical terminology and filter out responses that are perceived as unsatisfactory because of deference to medical staff (Nápoles et al., 2015). The lack of information collected by public health organizations concerning linguistic and national origin-related diversity among Hispanic/Latino immigrants and the health issues that can affect them may result in unsatisfactory understandings of these issues and inadequate programmatic activities to address them (Beltran, Harrison, Hall, & Dean, 2011; CDC, 2014; Rodriguez-Lainz, McDonald, Penman-Aguilar, & Barrett, et al., 2016).

Policy-Related Factors

National, state, and local-level policies and procedures, including those that address immigration, can affect healthcare access and outcomes among documented and undocumented Hispanic/Latino immigrants (Galeucia & Hirsch, 2016). The findings of a systematic review indicate that immigration policies can negatively affect healthcare access by undocumented immigrants and contribute to negative mental health outcomes, including depression, anxiety, and post-traumatic stress disorder (Martinez et al., 2015). Many Hispanic/Latino immigrants in the US do not have health insurance. The Patient Protection and Affordable Care Act aimed to expand health coverage; however, the estimated 11 million undocumented immigrants in the country are not covered by the legislation (Brown et al., 2015). Nearly, 80% of these undocumented immigrants are from Mexico or Central or South American countries (Rosenblum & Ruiz Soto, 2015). Findings from studies in California (Vargas Bustamante et al., 2012) and North Carolina (Rhodes et al., 2015) illustrate the potential effects of immigration policies. In California, undocumented Mexican immigrants were found to be less likely than documented immigrants to report having a usual source of medical care and having visited a physician during the previous year (Vargas Bustamante et al., 2012). The North Carolina study was designed to examine the effects of the local implementation of section 287(g) of the Immigration and Nationality Act. It authorizes Immigration and Customs Enforcement to develop agreements with state and local law enforcement agencies to enforce federal immigration law during their routine law enforcement activities. A total of 83 Hispanic/Latino immigrants, mostly women (64%), in six North Carolina counties participated in focus groups and individual interviews, and qualitative analysis of their responses demonstrated recurring themes relative to section 287(g) enforcement. The policy was perceived as exacerbating distrust of formal services, including health services; creating barriers to accessing and using health services; contributing to the use of non-standard and potentially risky sources of care; reducing physical and mental health; and compromising the health of the immigrants' children (Rhodes et al., 2015). In a separate analysis by the same authors of vital records data, Hispanic/Latina women were more likely than non-Hispanic/Latina women to seek prenatal care later during their pregnancies and to receive inadequate care; however, the database did not contain information on country of origin; thus, the authors were unable to distinguish foreign-born (immigrant) from US-born Hispanic/Latina women. The findings of two other studies further illustrate the role of health insurance access to healthcare-related outcomes among immigrants. In a study of HIV-infected adults in the Bronx, mostly Hispanic/Latino undocumented immigrants, having access to health insurance was associated with positive outcomes of HIV care. In this instance, healthcare access was facilitated by the New York State AIDS Drug Assistance Program (Ross et al., 2017). By contrast, in a study of Mexican migrants in Tijuana, Mexico, a lack of access to health insurance, as well as the presence of transportation barriers were associated with a reduced likelihood of receiving health care, having a usual source of care, and higher rates of foregone health care (Martinez-Donate et al., 2017).

Hispanic/Latino Subpopulations with Particular Vulnerabilities

Women Hispanic/Latina immigrant women play a crucial role in their communities and families. Women in agricultural families may be actively engaged in farm work and, like their male partners, be exposed to some of the same health hazards, including pesticides and other agricultural chemicals. Despite the greater susceptibility of women of reproductive age to these hazards, they may not benefit from special protections.

Women's status in Hispanic/Latino immigrant family structures, and the occasional lack of authorization to be in the US, may increase their dependence on spouses or partners, create barriers to seeking and accessing health care, and possibly to reporting and seeking assistance when intimate partner violence occurs (Quandt, 2009). Hispanic/Latina immigrant women's vulnerability to intimate partner violence may also be the result of additional factors that can create barriers to their efforts to seek assistance or leave abusive partners. These factors include values and associated social norms that positively sanction deference to male partners and remaining in a marriage, particularly where there are children (Alvarez, Davidson, Fleming, & Glass, 2016). Women's access to and participation in support services may be limited, occurring only after a prolonged abusive relationship (Alvarez & Fedock, 2018). Research on intimate partner violence among Hispanic/Latina immigrant women has focused principally on barriers to seeking help. There is limited research on factors that facilitate women's actions to seek help and issues related to access and acceptability of health and support services for survivors of intimate partner violence. Greater attention to these topics may facilitate the development of supportive interventions for Hispanic/Latina immigrant women who confront intimate partner violence. Currently, these interventions are few in number (Alvarez et al., 2016; Alvarez & Fedock, 2018).

Children and Minors Earlier in the chapter, while describing health threats to Hispanic/Latino immigrant agricultural workers, I briefly described factors that can increase the vulnerability of their children to work-related hazards in the US. A very different set of factors has contributed to large numbers of Hispanic/Latino children traveling to the US alone or with family members. Increasing numbers of unaccompanied children and minors traveled to the US from the Central American countries of El Salvador, Guatemala, and Honduras and from Mexico during the mid-2000s. There is a paucity of information on the estimated numbers of unaccompanied Hispanic/Latino immigrant children who travel to the US; however, data on apprehensions at the US–Mexican border provide a sense of the magnitude of these movements. Since October 1, 2013, more than 47,000 unaccompanied children have been apprehended at the southwest US border, part of a surge that can also include children accompanied by their parents (Robles, 2014).

Multiple social and structural factors have contributed to this large scale mobility-as-escape. Among these factors are faltering economies: poverty, limited employment opportunities, food insecurity, rising crime, gang, and drug trafficking activity, including the forceful recruitment of children and minors under the threat of death to them or their families. The results are high death rates; domestic abuse; political turmoil; and limited capacity of local authorities (who may be allied with criminal and gang elements) to protect families from violence. The desire for family reunification has also contributed to the increased numbers. Adult Hispanic/Latino immigrants who have settled in the US send for the children they left behind to join them. Other factors may have contributed to the increasing numbers. One has been the perception among Central Americans that, until recently, the US government's treatment of minors, as well as minors traveling in family units had softened (Chishti & Hipsman,

2014). Another factor is the limited capacity of Mexican organizations (e.g., the *Sistema para el Desarrollo Integral de la Familia* [Mexican System for Integral Family Development]) to house and provide services to children who are apprehended by Mexican authorities as they travel to the US (Dominguez-Villegas, 2017).

Concluding Thoughts

Structural Vulnerability and Hispanic/Latino Immigrant Health

As noted earlier, Hispanic/Latino immigrants travel to and may remain in the US because they are seeking opportunities to improve their livelihoods and those of their families. Their livelihoods—and their very lives—in their countries of origin may also be negatively affected by social and political instability. Hispanic/Latino immigrants engage in the migration process as a strategy for dealing with one or both of these circumstances. These conditions and the processes that drive the migration process from their countries of origin can contribute to what Organista et al. (2012, 2013) and Quesada et al. (2011) refer to as structural vulnerability, which can broadly and negatively affect the lives and livelihoods of Hispanic/Latino immigrants. Structural vulnerability results initially from the immigrants' location in a hierarchical social order in their countries of origin that can be affected by both economic and noneconomic factors. It increases the likelihood that these immigrants will be negatively affected by any number of threats to their health and well-being and face barriers to accessing needed health care and other supportive services (Organista et al., 2012, 2013; Quesada et al., 2011).

As illustrated repeatedly in the examples considered above concerning health threats to Hispanic/Latino immigrants and the factors that can affect their access to health-related services, their structural vulnerability continues after they arrive in the US. The social order (or orders) in the US within which Hispanic/Latino immigrants can find themselves, their everyday lives, and those of their families and communities may be shaped by their social class position, harsh living and working conditions, severely restricted access to work authorization, lack of stable employment paying a living wage, and poverty. Other contributing factors to structural vulnerability among Hispanic/Latino immigrants in the US include a lack of or limited access to healthcare providers or health insurance, racism, and social stigma that may be associated with being perceived and treated negatively by others as an immigrant and a person having limited education and English language proficiency (Quesada et al., 2011). For Hispanic/Latino immigrants who are in the US without authorization, the structural vulnerability of their lives and livelihoods may be further increased by their liability of being apprehended, detained, and deported.

Research to Promote Hispanic/Latino Immigrant Health

While illustrating the kinds of health threats that can affect Hispanic/Latino immigrants, I have described several areas where further research is needed to clarify the circumstances, causes, and consequences of these threats to immigrants' health, the factors that can contribute to their structural vulnerability, and the implications for health promotion among these populations. These areas of needed research include the following.

- Ensuring a clearer picture of the diversity of Hispanic/Latino immigrant populations in the US, how they are affected by health threats, and what they do to address these threats in order to develop effective disease prevention and health promotion policies, programs, and interventions for and with them
- Causes of disparities in workplace injury risk that affect Hispanic/Latino immigrants, and developing and evaluating interventions to reduce them
- Interactions of immigration-related processes and outcomes with other social determinants of health that can affect Hispanic/Latino immigrants on and off the job
- Improving understandings concerning the varied circumstances that can affect HIV risks and HIV-protective actions among Hispanic/Latino populations in the US, and increasing their awareness of and participation, as appropriate, in HIV prevention and care
- Extent to which evidence-based behavioral HIV prevention interventions designed for specific Hispanic/Latino immigrant subpopulations (gay, bisexual, and other men who have sex with men, and heterosexual men and women) are actually being delivered to them by healthcare service providers
- Factors that facilitate efforts by Hispanic/Latino immigrant women to obtain support when dealing with intimate partner violence
- Extent to which implicit bias and associated actions by healthcare providers can affect Hispanic/Latino immigrants' health-related actions and outcomes
- Degree to which Hispanic/Latino agricultural and nonagricultural workers use health services or self-manage their health and resulting health outcomes
- Structural and behavioral factors that contribute to patterns of diet and alcohol use in Hispanic/Latino immigrants' countries of origin and in the US. A clearer picture of these factors may improve current understandings of the relationship between premigration and postmigration use patterns and options for supporting health-promoting actions in these settings
- Effectiveness of using *promotora/es de salud* to reach underserved Hispanic/Latino immigrants to address a range of disease prevention and health promotion issues in diverse settings.

Readers who share a particular interest in Hispanic/Latino immigrant health will quickly conclude that this list of research topics is brief. They are invited to expand and improve it, set priorities for the topics in terms of salience, and evaluate these topics and others. More generally, however, research is needed to better understand the production and persistence of structural vulnerability that can affect Hispanic/Latino immigrants and how it influences their likelihood of being affected by risks to their health and having access to and participating in health and supportive services. The improved understandings that result may provide the basis for developing policies, programs, and interventions to address these threats and support efforts by Hispanic/Latino immigrants to overcome them. Success in these areas will require, among other things, that studies and programs develop a sharper focus on subgroups within Hispanic/Latino immigrant populations, based on, for example, their country of origin, foreign-born or US-born status, and ethnicity, as manifested by language, values, and traditions of indigenous or dominant groups. Studies and programs also need to take into account factors that characterize immigrants' participation in the migration process and its effects on their health outcomes.

Lastly, studies and programs that aim to promote Hispanic/Latino immigrant health may benefit from a better understanding of factors such as social support and circumstances that can contribute to social support and lead to resilience among Hispanic/Latino immigrant communities in the face of multiple health threats, and to their ability to engage in health-promoting actions (Althoff et al., 2017; Ross et al., 2017). In several studies of heterosexual Hispanic/Latino immigrants that were cited earlier, social support was associated with various HIV-protective actions by study participants (Althoff et al., 2013, 2017; Hirsch et al., 2009; Kissinger et al., 2012, 2013; Painter, 2018). More recent, focused analysis points to the contributing role that social support and related factors may play in HIV testing by Hispanic/Latino immigrants who have sex with other men (Painter et al., 2019). Studies that focus on these factors may be useful more generally for health promotion efforts among Hispanic/Latino immigrants. More research may also clarify what can be done to draw from and potentially strengthen these social support relationships and processes to promote health-protective actions by Hispanic/Latino populations.

Acknowledgments I am grateful to Ken Dominguez, Michael Flynn, Airin Martinez, and Scott D. Rhodes for their comments on sections in earlier versions of this chapter; however, I am solely responsible for any interpretations contained herein.

References

Abraído-Lanza, A. F., Chao, M. T., & Flórez, K. R. (2005). Do healthy behaviors decline with greater acculturation? Implications for the Latino mortality paradox. *Social Science and Medicine, 61*(6), 1243–1255.

Althoff, M. D., Anderson-Smits, C., Kovacs, S., Salinas, O., Hembling, J., Schmidt, N., et al. (2013). Patterns and predictors of multiple sexual partnerships among newly arrived Latino migrant men. *AIDS and Behavior, 17*(7), 2416–2425. https://doi.org/10.1007/s10461-012-0315-x.

Althoff, M. D., Theall, K., Schmidt, N., Hembling, J., Gebrekristos, H. T., Thompson, M. M., et al. (2017). Social support networks and HIV/STI risk behaviors among Latino immigrants in a new receiving environment. *AIDS and Behavior, 21*(12), 3607–3617. https://doi.org/10.1007/s10461-017-1849-8.

Alvarez, C., & Fedock, G. (2018). Addressing intimate partner violence with Latina women: A call for research. *Trauma, Violence, & Abuse, 19*(4), 488–493.

Alvarez, C. P., Davidson, P. M., Fleming, C., & Glass, N. E. (2016). Elements of effective interventions for addressing intimate partner violence in Latina women: A systematic review. *PLoS ONE, 11*(8), e0160518. https://doi.org/10.1371/journal.pone.0160518.uj.

Apostolopoulos, Y., Somnez, S., Kronenfeld, J., Castillo, E., McLendon, L., & Smith, D. (2006). STI/HIV risks for Mexican migrant laborers: Exploratory ethnographies. *Journal of Immigrant and Minority Health, 8,* 291–302.

Aranda-Naranjo, B., Gaskins, S., Bustamante, L., Lopez, L. C., & Rodriguiz, J. (2000). La desesperación: Migrant and seasonal farm workers living with HIV/AIDS. *Journal of the Association of Nurses of AIDS Care, 11*(2), 22–28.

Arandia, G., Nalty, C., Sharkey, J. R., & Dean, W. R. (2012). Diet and acculturation among Hispanic/Latino older adults in the United States: A review of literature and recommendations. *Journal of Nutrition in Gerontology and Geriatrics, 31*(1), 16–37. https://doi.org/10.1080/21551197.2012.647553.

Arcury, T. A., & Quandt, S. A. (2007). Delivery of health services to migrant and seasonal farmworkers. *Annual Review of Public Health, 28,* 345–363.

Balcázar, H. G., de Heer, H., Rosenthal, L., Aguirre, M., Flores, L., Puentes, F. A., et al. (2010). A promotores de salud intervention to reduce cardiovascular disease risk in a high-risk Hispanic border population, 2005–2008. *Preventing Chronic Disease, 7*(2), A28.

Bastos, F. I., Cáceres, C., Galvão, J., Veras, M. A., & Castilho, E. A. (2008). AIDS in Latin America: Assessing the current status of the epidemic and the ongoing response. *International Journal of Epidemiology, 37,* 729–737.

Beltran, V. M., Harrison, K. M., Hall, H. I., & Dean, H. D. (2011). Collection of social determinant of health measures in U.S. national surveillance systems for HIV, viral hepatitis, STDs, and TB. *Public Health Reports, 126*(Suppl 3), 41–53.

Brown, H. S., III, Wilson, K. J., & Angel, J. L. (2015). Mexican immigrant health: Health insurance coverage implications. *Journal of Health Care for the Poor and Underserved, 26,* 990–1004.

Castro, F. G. (2013). Emerging Hispanic health paradoxes. *American Journal of Public Health, 103*(9), 1541. https://doi.org/10.2105/AJPH.2013.301529.

Centers for Disease Control and Prevention (CDC). (2011). *High-impact HIV prevention: CDC's approach to reducing HIV infections in the United States.* Atlanta, GA: Centers for Disease Control and Prevention, National Center for HIV/AIDS, Viral Hepatitis, STD, and TB Prevention, Division of HIV/AIDS Prevention. http://www.cdc.gov/hiv/pdf/policies_NHPC_Booklet.pdf.

CDC. (2014). *Immigrant/migrant/foreign-born health: Addressing health disparities. Seminar Proceedings.* Seminar Planning Committee. Unpublished report. Atlanta, GA: Centers for Disease Control and Prevention.

CDC. (2016a). *Tuberculosis in Hispanics/Latinos.* https://www.cdc.gov/tb/publications/pdf/tbhispanics_rev.pdf.

CDC. (2016b). *Reported tuberculosis in the United States, 2015.* Atlanta, GA: CDC, Division of Tuberculosis Elimination. https://www.cdc.gov/tb/statistics/reports/2015/pdfs/2015_surveillance_report_fullreport.pdf.

CDC. (2017). *Pre-exposure prophylaxis (PrEP).* https://www.cdc.gov/hiv/risk/prep/index.html.

CDC. (2018). Evidence of HIV treatment and viral suppression in preventing the sexual transmission of HIV. https://www.cdc.gov/hiv/pdf/risk/art/cdc-hiv-art-viral-suppression.pdf.

Chishti, M., & Hipsman, F. (2014). *Dramatic surge in the arrival of unaccompanied children has deep roots and no simple solutions.* http://www.migrationpolicy.org/article/dramatic-surge-arrival-unaccompanied-children-has-deep-roots-and-no-simple-solutions.

Community Guide. (2016). *Diabetes prevention: Interventions engaging community health workers improve risk factors and health outcomes.* https://www.thecommunityguide.org/content/community-health-worker-interventions-help-prevent-diabetes.

Community Guide. (2017). *Diabetes management: Interventions engaging community health workers*. https://www.thecommunityguide.org/sites/default/files/assets/OnePager-Diabetes-Management-CommunityHealthWorkers.pdf.

Cornelius, W. A., Fitzgerald, D. S., & Fisher, P. W. (Eds.). (2007). *Mayan journeys: The new migration from Yucatán to the United States*. La Jolla, CA: Center for Comparative Immigration Studies, University of California, San Diego.

Creighton, M. J., Goldman, N., Pebley, A. R., & Chung, C. Y. (2012). Durational and generational differences in Mexican immigrant obesity: Is acculturation the explanation? *Social Science and Medicine, 75*(2), 300–310. https://doi.org/10.1016/j.socscimed.2012.03.013.

Dominguez, K., Penman-Aguilar, A., Chang, M. H., Moonesinghe, R., Castellanos, T., Rodriguez-Lainz, A., et al. (2015). Vital signs: Leading causes of death, prevalence of diseases and risk factors, and use of health services among Hispanics in the United States—2009–2013. *Morbidity and Mortality Weekly Report, 64*(17), 469–478.

Dominguez-Villegas, R. (2017). *Strengthening Mexico's protection of Central American unaccompanied minors in transit*. Washington, DC: Migration Policy Institute.

Espinoza, L., Hall, I. H., & Hu, X. (2012). Diagnoses of HIV infection among Hispanics/Latinos in 40 States and Puerto Rico, 2006–2009. *Journal of Acquired Immune Deficiency Syndromes, 60*(2), 205–213.

Fenelon, A., Chinn, J. J., & Anderson, R. N. (2017). A comprehensive analysis of the mortality experience of hispanic subgroups in the United States: Variation by age, country of origin, and nativity. *SSM Population Health, 3,* 245–254. https://doi.org/10.1016/j.ssmph.2017.01.011.

Fernandez, M., Pérez-Peña, R., & Montgomery, D. (2017, July 24). In San Antonio smuggling case, a fatal journey in a packed and sweltering truck. *New York Times.com.* https://www.nytimes.com/2017/07/24/us/san-antonio-truck-trafficking.html?emc=edit_na_20170724&nl=breaking-news&nlid=2566910&ref=cta&_r=0.

Flynn, M. A., Check, P., Eggerth, D. E., & Tonda, J. (2013). Improving occupational safety and health among Mexican immigrant workers: A binational collaboration. *Public Health Reports, 128*(Suppl 3), 33–38.

Flynn, M. A., Cunningham, T. R., Guerin, R. J., Keller, B., Chapman, L. J., Hudson, D., et al. (2015). *Overlapping vulnerabilities: The occupational safety and health of young workers in small construction firms*. Publication No. 2015-178. Washington, DC: U.S. Department of Health and Human Services, Centers for Disease Control and Prevention, National Institute for Occupational Safety and Health.

Flynn, M. A., Eggerth, D. E., & Jacobson, C. J., Jr. (2015). Undocumented status as a social determinant of occupational safety and health: The workers' perspective. *American Journal of Industrial Medicine, 58*(11), 1127–1137. https://doi.org/10.1002/ajim.22531.

Flores, A., López, G., & Radford, J. (2017). *Facts on U.S. Latinos, 2015, statistical portrait of Hispanics in the United States*. http://www.pewhispanic.org/2017/09/18/facts-on-u-s-latinos-current-data/.

Forst, L., Avila, S., Anozie, S., & Rubin, R. (2010). Traumatic occupational injuries in Hispanic and foreign born workers. *American Journal of Industrial Medicine, 53*(4), 344–351. https://doi.org/10.1002/ajim.20748.

Frasca, T. (2009). *Shaping the new response: HIV/AIDS & Latinos in the Deep South*. New York, NY: The Latino Commission on AIDS. http://www.latinoaids.org/downloads/deepsouthreport.pdf.

Galvan, F. H., Ortiz, D. J., Martinez, V., & Bing, E. G. (2008). Sexual solicitation of Latino male day laborers by other men. *Salud Pública de México, 50,* 439–446.

Galeucia, M., & Hirsch, J. S. (2016). State and local policies as a structural and modifiable determinant of HIV vulnerability among Latino migrants in the United States. *American Journal of Public Health, 106*(5), 800–807. https://doi.org/10.2105/AJPH.2016.303081.

Gibson, K. (2016, May 27). *Just how dangerous is meat and poultry packing?* MoneyWatch. https://www.cbsnews.com/news/meat-and-poultry-work-is-dangerous-but-not-all-injuries-counted/.

Goldman, N., Pebley, A. R., Creighton, M. J., Teruel, G. M., Rubalcava, L. N., & Chung, C. (2014). The consequences of migration to the United States for short-term changes in the health of Mexican immigrants. *Demography, 51*(4), 1159–1173. https://doi.org/10.1007/s13524-014-0304-y.

Grzywacz, J. G., Quandt, S. A., Early, J. T., Tapia, J., Graham, C. N., & Arcury, T A. (2004). *Leaving family for work: Ambivalence & mental health among migrant Latino farmworkers*. Working Paper 04-01. Winston-Salem, NC: Center for Latino Health Research, Department of Family and Community Medicine, Wake Forest University School of Medicine.

Guendelman, S. D., Ritterman-Weintraub, M. L., Fernald, L. C. H., & Kaufer-Horwitz, M. (2013). Weight status of Mexican immigrant women: A comparison with women in Mexico and with US-born Mexican American women. *American Journal of Public Health, 103*, 1634–1640. https://doi.org/10.2105/AJPH.2012.301171.

Guevara, E. M., & Sangaramoorthy, T. (2017). *Health and housing: The impact of substandard housing on farmworker vulnerability on Maryland's Eastern Shore*. Presentation at the 77th annual meeting of the Society for Applied Anthropology, Santa Fe, NM, March 28–April 1.

Haderxhanaj, L. T., Rhodes, S. D., Romaguera, R. A., Bloom, F. R., & Leichliter, J. S. (2015). Hispanic men in the United States: Acculturation and recent sexual behaviors with female partners, 2006-2010. *American Journal of Public Health, 105*(8), e126–e133. https://doi.org/10.2105/AJPH.2014.302524.

Hall, E., Lee, S. Y., Clark, P. C., & Perilla, J. (2016). Social ecology of adherence to hypertension treatment in Latino migrant and seasonal farmworkers. *Journal of Transcultural Nursing, 27*(1), 33–41. https://doi.org/10.1177/1043659614524788.

Hall, W. J., Chapman, M. V., Lee, K. M., Merino, Y. M., Thomas, T. W., Payne, B. K., et al. (2015). Implicit racial/ethnic bias among health care professionals and its influence on health care outcomes: A systematic review. *American Journal of Public Health, 105*(12), e60–e76. https://doi.org/10.2105/AJPH.2015.302903.

Hansen, E., & Donohoe, M. (2003). Health issues of migrant and seasonal farmworkers. *Journal of Health Care for the Poor and Underserved, 14*(2), 153–164.

Hirsch, J. S., Higgins, J., Bentley, M. E., & Nathanson, C. A. (2002). The social constructions of sexuality: Marital infidelity and sexually transmitted disease—HIV risk in a Mexican migrant community. *American Journal of Public Health, 92*, 1227–1237.

Hirsch, J. S., Meneses, S., Thompson, B., Negroni, M., Pelcastre, B., & del Rio, C. (2007). The inevitability of infidelity: Sexual reputation, social geographies, and marital hiv risk in rural Mexico. *American Journal of Public Health, 97*(6), 886–996.

Hirsch, J. S., Muñoz-Laboy, M., Nyhus, C. M., Yount, K. M., & Bauermeister, J. A. (2009). They "miss more than anything their normal life back home": Masculinity and extramarital sex among Mexican migrants in Atlanta. *Perspectives on Sexual and Reproductive Health, 41*(1), 23–32.

Holmes, S. E. (2013). *Fresh fruit, broken bodies: Migrant farmworkers in the United States*. Berkeley, CA: University of California Press.

Hunter, J. B., de Zapien, J. G., Papenfuss, M., Fernandez, M. L., Meister, J., & Giuliano, A. R. (2004). The impact of a promotora on increasing routine chronic disease prevention among women aged 40 and older at the U.S.-Mexico border. *Health Education and Behavior, 31*(4 Suppl), 18S–28S.

International Organization for Migration. (2014). *Fatal journeys: Tracking lives lost during migration*. Geneva, Switzerland: International Organization for Migration. http://www.iom.int/files/live/sites/iom/files/pbn/docs/Fatal-Journeys-Tracking-Lives-Lost-during-Migration-2014.pdf.

Jacobs, A., & Richtel, M. (2017, September 16). How big business got Brazil hooked on junk food. *NYTimes.com*. https://www.nytimes.com/interactive/2017/09/16/health/brazil-obesity-nestle.html.

Kandel, W., & Parrado, E. A. (2005). Restructuring of the US meat processing industry and new Hispanic migrant destinations. *Population and Development Review, 31*(3), 447–471. https://doi.org/10.1111/j.1728-4457.2005.00079.x.

Kangovi, S., Mitra, N., Grande, D., Huo, H., Smith, R. A., & Long, J. A. (2017). Community health worker support for disadvantaged patients with multiple chronic diseases: A randomized clinical trial. *American Journal of Public Health, 107*(10), 1660–1667. https://doi.org/10.2105/AJPH.2017.303985.

Katz, M. H. (2012). Editorial comment. HIV infection among persons born outside the United States. *Journal of the American Medical Association, 308*(6), 623–624.

Kissinger, P., Althoff, M., Burton, N., Schmidt, N., Hembling, J., Salinas, O., et al. (2013). Prevalence, patterns and predictors of substance use among Latino migrant men in a new receiving community. *Drug and Alcohol Dependency, 133*(3), 814–824. https://doi.org/10.1016/j.drugalcdep.2013.08.031.

Kissinger, P., Kovacs, S., Anderson-Smits, C., Schmidt, N., Salinas, O., Hembling, J., et al. (2012). Patterns and predictors of HIV/STI risk among Latino migrant men in a new receiving community. *AIDS and Behavior, 16*(1), 199–213.

Kissinger, P., Liddon, N., Schmidt, N., Curtin, E., Salinas, O., & Narvaez, A. (2008). HIV/STI risk behaviors among Latino migrants in New Orleans post-Hurricane Katrina disaster. *Sexually Transmitted Diseases, 35*, 924–929.

Kochhar, R., Suro, R., & Tafoya, S. (2005). *The new Latino South: The context and consequences of rapid population growth*. Washington, DC: Pew Hispanic Center.

Lara, M., Gamboa, C., Kahramanian, M. I., Morales, L. S., & Hayes Bautista, D. E. (2005). Acculturation and Latino health in the United States: A review of the literature and its sociopolitical context. *Annual Review of Public Health, 26*, 367–397.

Lopez, A. A. (2007). *The farmworkers' journey*. Berkeley, CA: University of California Press.

Loury, S., Jesse, E., & Wu, Q. (2011). Binge drinking among male Mexican immigrants in rural North Carolina. *Journal of Immigrant and Minority Health, 13*(4), 664–670.

Mancini, M. A., Salas-Wright, C. P., & Vaughn, M. G. (2015). Drug use and service utilization among Hispanics in the United States. *Social Psychiatry and Psychiatric Epidemiology, 50*(11), 1679–1689. https://doi.org/10.1007/s00127-015-1111-5.

Markides, K. S., & Coreil, J. (1986). The health of Hispanics in the Southwestern United States: An epidemiologic paradox. *Public Health Reports, 101*(3), 253–264.

Marlenga, B., Berg, R. L., Linneman, J. G., Brison, R. J., & Pickett, W. (2007). Changing the child labor laws for agriculture: Impact on injury. *American Journal of Public Health, 97*(2), 276–282.

Martínez, A. D. (2013). Reconsidering acculturation in dietary change research among Latino immigrants: Challenging the preconditions of US migration. *Ethnicity and Health, 18*(2), 115–135. https://doi.org/10.1080/13557858.2012.698254.

Martinez, O., Lee, J. H., Bandiera, F., Santamaria, E. K., Levine, E. C., & Operario, D. (2017). Sexual and behavioral health disparities among sexual minority Hispanics/Latinos: Findings from the National Health and Nutrition Examination Survey, 2001–2014. *American Journal of Preventive Medicine, 53*(2), 225–231. https://doi.org/10.1016/j.amepre.2017.01.037.

Martinez, O., Wu, E., Sandfort, T., Dodge, B., Carballo-Dieguez, A., Pinto, R., et al. (2015). Evaluating the impact of immigration policies on health status among undocumented immigrants: A systematic review. *Journal of Immigrant and Minority Health, 17*(3), 947–970. https://doi.org/10.1007/s10903-013-9968-4.

Martinez-Donate, A. P., Ejebe, I., Zhang, X., Guendelman, S., Lê-Scherban, F., Rangel, G., et al. (2017). Access to health care among Mexican migrants and immigrants: A comparison across migration phases. *Journal of Health Care for the Poor and Underserved, 28*(4), 1314–1326. https://doi.org/10.1353/hpu.2017.0116.

Massey, D. S. (Ed.). (2008). *New faces in new places: The changing geography of American immigration*. New York, NY: Russell Sage Foundation.

Massey, D. S., Durand, J., & Malone, N. J. (2002). *Beyond smoke and mirrors: Mexican immigration in an era of economic integration*. New York, NY: Russell Sage Foundation.

McCoy, V., Shehadeh, N., Rubens, M., & Navarro, C. M. (2014). Newcomer status as a protective factor among Hispanic migrant workers for HIV risk. *Frontiers in Public Health, 2*, 216. https://doi.org/10.3389/fpubh.2014.00216.

Medecins sans Frontieres. (2017). *Forced to flee Central America's northern triangle: A neglected humanitarian crisis*. Mexico City: https://www.doctorswithoutborders.org/sites/usa/files/msf_forced-to-flee-central-americas-northern-triangle.pdf.

Melo, M. A. (2017). *Exploding eyes, heart-stopping potassium levels, and drowning from the inside out: The everyday realities of emergency dialysis in South Texas*. Presentation at the 77th annual meeting of the Society for Applied Anthropology, Santa Fe, NM, March 28–April 1, 2017.

Mizuno, Y., Borkowf, C. B., Ayala, G., Carballo-Diéguez, A., & Millett, G. A. (2015). Correlates of sexual risk for HIV among US-born and foreign-born Latino men who have sex with men (MSM): An analysis from the Brothers y Hermanos study. *Journal of Immigrant and Minority Health, 17*(1), 47–55. https://doi.org/10.1007/s10903-013-9894-5.

Montealegre, J. R., Risser, J. M., Selwyn, B. J., McCurdy, S. A., & Sabin, K. (2012). Prevalence of HIV risk behaviors among undocumented Central American immigrant women in Houston, Texas. *AIDS and Behavior, 16*(6), 1641–1648.

Muñoz-Laboy, M., Hirsch, J. S., & Quipse-Lazaro, A. (2009). Loneliness as a sexual risk factor for male Mexican migrant workers. *American Journal of Public Health, 99*, 1–9.

Nápoles, A. M., Santoyo-Olsson, J., Karliner, L. S., Gregorich, S. E., & Pérez-Stable, E. J. (2015). Inaccurate language interpretation and its clinical significance in the medical encounters of Spanish-speaking Latinos. *Medical Care, 53*(11), 940–947. https://doi.org/10.1097/MLR.0000000000000422.

Newland, K. (2009). *Circular migration and human development*. Human Development Research Paper 2009/42. New York, NY: United Nations Development Programme.

O'Donnell, L., Stueve, A., Joseph, H. A., & Flores, S. (2014). Adapting the VOICES HIV behavioral intervention for Latino men who have sex with men. *AIDS and Behavior, 18*, 767–775.

Organista, K. C. (2007). Towards a structural-environmental model of risk for HIV and problem drinking in Latino labor migrants: The case of day laborers. *Journal of Ethnic and Cultural Diversity in Social Work, 16*, 95–125.

Organista, K. C., Alvarado, N., Balbutin-Burnham, A., Worby, P., & Martinez, S. (2006). An exploratory study of HIV prevention with Mexican/Latino migrant day laborers. *Journal of HIV/AIDS and Social Services, 5*(2), 89–114.

Organista, K. C., Carillo, H., & Ayala, G. (2004). HIV prevention with Mexican migrants: Review, critique, and recommendations. *Journal of Acquired Immune Deficiency Syndromes, 37*, S227–S239.

Organista, K. C., & Kubo, A. (2005). Pilot survey of HIV risk and contextual problems and issues in Mexican/Latino migrant day laborers. *Journal of Immigrant Health, 7*(4), 269–281.

Organista, K. C., Worby, P. A., Quesada, J., Arreola, S. G., Kral, A. H., & Khoury, S. (2013). Sexual health of Latino migrant day labourers under conditions of structural vulnerability. *Culture, Health & Sexuality, 15*(1), 58–72. https://doi.org/10.1080/13691058.2012.740075.

Organista, K. C., Worby, P. A., Quesada, J., Kral, A. H., Díiaz, R. M., Neilands, T. B., et al. (2012). The urgent need for structural-environmental models of HIV risk and prevention for U.S. Latino populations: The case of migrant day laborers. In K. Organista (Ed.), *HIV prevention with Latinos: theory, research, and practice* (pp. 3–24). New York, NY: Oxford University Press.

Orozco, R., Borges, G., Medina-Mora, M. E., Aguilar-Gaxiola, S., & Breslau, J. (2013). A cross-national study on prevalence of mental disorders, service use, and adequacy of treatment among Mexican and Mexican American populations. *American Journal of Public Health, 103*, 1610–1618. https://doi.org/10.2105/AJPH.2012.301169.

Painter, T. M. (1996). Space, time and rural–urban linkages in Africa. Notes for a geography of livelihoods. *African Rural and Urban Studies, 3*(1), 79–98.

Painter, T. M. (1999). Livelihood mobility and AIDS prevention in West Africa: Challenges and opportunities for social scientists. In C. Becker, J.-P. Dozon, C. Obbo, & M. Touré (Eds.), *Vivre et penser le sida en Afrique. Experiencing and understanding AIDS in Africa* (pp. 645–665). Paris: Karthala, IRD.

Painter, T. M. (2008). Connecting the dots: When the risks of HIV/STD infection appear high but the burden of infection is not known—The case of male Latino migrants in the southern United States. *AIDS and Behavior, 12,* 213–226.

Painter, T. M. (2018). Social support networks: an underutilized resource for preventing HIV and other sexually transmitted diseases among Hispanic/Latino migrants and immigrants. *The Journal of Health Care for the Poor and Underserved, 29*(1), 44–57.

Painter, T. M., Organista, K., Rhodes, S., & Sañudo, F. (2012). Interventions to prevent HIV and other sexually transmitted diseases among Latino migrants. In K. Organista (Ed.), *HIV prevention with Latinos: Theory, research, and practice* (pp. 351–381). New York, NY: Oxford University Press.

Painter, T. M., Song, E. Y., Mullins, M. M., Mann-Jackson, L., Alonzo, J., Reboussin, B. A., & Rhodes, S. D. (2019). Social support and other factors associated with HIV testing by Hispanic/Latino gay, bisexual, and other men who have sex with men in the U.S. South. *AIDS and Behavior,* e-publication ahead of print, May 17, 2019. https://doi.org/10.1007/s10461-019-02540-6.

Parrado, E. A., & Flippen, C. (2010). Community attachment, neighborhood context, and sex worker use among Hispanic migrants in Durham, North Carolina, USA. *Social Science and Medicine, 70,* 1059–1069.

Parrado, E. A., Flippen, C. A., & McQuiston, C. (2004). Use of commercial sex workers among Hispanic migrants in North Carolina: Implications for the diffusion of HIV. *Perspectives on Sexual and Reproductive Health, 36,* 150–156.

Passel, J. S., & Cohn, D. (2017). *As Mexican share declined, U.S. unauthorized immigrant population fell in 2015 below recession level.* Washington, DC: Pew Research Center. http://www.pewresearch.org/fact-tank/2017/04/25/as-mexican-share-declined-u-s-unauthorized-immigrant-population-fell-in-2015-below-recession-level/.

Quandt, S. A. (2009). Health of children and women in the farmworker community in the Eastern United States. In T. A. Arcury & S. A. Quandt (Eds.), *Latino farmworkers in Eastern United States* (pp. 173–200). New York, NY: Springer Science + Business Media.

Quesada, J., Hart, L. K., & Bourgois, P. (2011). Structural vulnerability and health: Latino migrant laborers in the United States. *Medical Anthropology, 30*(4), 339–362. https://doi.org/10.1080/01459740.2011.576725.

Rangel Gomez, M. G., Tonda, J., Zapata, G. R., Flynn, M., Gany, F., Lara, J., et al. (2017). Ventanillas de salud: A collaborative and binational health access and preventive care program. *Frontiers in Public Health, 5* (Article 151). https://doi.org/10.3389/fpubh.2017.00151.

Rhodes, S. D. (2018). HIV prevention among Latina transgender women who have sex with men: Evaluation of a locally developed intervention. Unpublished research protocol for Funding Opportunity Announcement number PS 16-003. Atlanta, GA: Centers for Disease Control and Prevention, Division of HIV.AIDS Prevention.

Rhodes, S. D., Alonzo, J., Mann, L., Song, E. Y., Tanner, A. E., Arellano, J. E., et al. (2017). Small-group randomized controlled trial to increase condom use and HIV testing among Hispanic/Latino gay, bisexual, and other men who have sex with men. *American Journal of Public Health, 107*(6), 969–976. https://doi.org/10.2105/AJPH.2017.303814.

Rhodes, S. D., Hergenrather, K. C., Aronson, R. E., Bloom, F. R., Felizzola, J., Wolfson, M., et al. (2010). Latino men who have sex with men and HIV in the rural south-eastern USA: Findings from ethnographic in-depth interviews. *Culture, Health and Sexuality, 12*(7), 797–812. https://doi.org/10.1080/13691058.2010.492432.

Rhodes, S. D., Hergenrather, K. C., Bloom, F. R., Leichliter, J. S., & Montaño, J. (2009). Outcomes from a community-based, participatory lay health advisor HIV/STD prevention intervention for recently arrived immigrant Latino men in rural North Carolina, USA. *AIDS Education and Prevention, 21*(5), (Suppl. 1), 103–108.

Rhodes, S. D., Mann, L., Simán, F. M., Song, E., Alonzo, J., Downs, M., et al. (2015). The impact of local immigration enforcement policies on the health of immigrant Hispanics/Latinos in the

United States. *American Journal of Public Health, 105*(2), 329–337. https://doi.org/10.2105/AJPH.2014.302218.

Rhodes, S. D., McCoy, T. P., Hergenrather, K. C., Vissman, A. T., Wolfson, M., Alonzo, J., et al. (2012). Prevalence estimates of health risk behaviors of immigrant Latino men who have sex with men. *Journal of Rural Health, 28*(1), 73–83. https://doi.org/10.1111/j.1748-0361.2011.00373.

Rhodes, S. D., McCoy, T. P., Vissman, A. T., DiClemente, R. J., Duck, S., Hergenrather, K. C., et al. (2011). A randomized controlled trial of a culturally congruent intervention to increase condom use and HIV testing among heterosexually active immigrant Latino men. *AIDS and Behavior, 15*(8), 1764–1775.

Robles, F. (2014, June 4). Wave of minors on their own rush to cross southwest border. *New York Times.com*. https://www.nytimes.com/2014/06/04/world/americas/wave-of-minors-on-their-own-rush-to-cross-southwest-border.html?hpw&rref=world.

Rodríguez, C. M., García, E. B., Serrano, C. G., Reyes, P. R., & De Luca, M. (2008). *El VIH y el SIDA en México al 2008: Hallazgos, tendencias y reflexions*. Mexico: Centro Nacional para la Prevencíon y Control del SIDA (CENSIDA). http://www.censida.salud.gob.mx/descargas/biblioteca/VIHSIDA_MEX2008.pdf.

Rodríguez, H., Sáenz, R., & Menjívar, C. (2008). *Latinas/os in the United States: Changing the face of America*. New York, NY: Springer.

Rodriguez-Lainz, A., McDonald, M., Penman-Aguilar, A., & Barrett, D. H. (2016). Getting data right–and righteous–to improve Hispanic or Latino Health. *Journal of Healthcare, Science and the Humanities, 6*(2), 60–83.

Rosenblum, M. R., & Ruiz Soto, A. G. (2015). *An analysis of unauthorized immigrants in the United States by country and region of birth*. Washington, DC: Migration Policy Institute. http://www.migrationpolicy.org/research/analysis-unauthorized-immigrants-united-states-country-and-region-birth.

Ross, J., Felsen, U. R., Cunningham, C. O., Patel, V. V., & Hanna, D. B. (2017). Outcomes along the HIV care continuum among undocumented immigrants in clinical care. *AIDS Research and Human Retroviruses, 33*(10), 1038–1044. https://doi.org/10.1089/AID.2017.0015.

Salgado de Snyder, N., Gonzalez-Vazquez, T., Infante-Xibille, C., Marquez-Serrano, M., Pelcastre-Villafuerte, B., & Servan-Mori, E. E. (2010). Servicios de salud en la Mixteca: utilizacion y condicion de afiliacion en hogares de migrantes y no-migrantes a EU. *Salud Pública de México, 52*(5), 424–431.

Sánchez, J., De La Rosa, M., & Serna, C. A. (2013). Project Salud: Efficacy of a community-based HIV prevention intervention for Hispanic migrant workers in south Florida. *AIDS Education and Prevention, 25*, 363–375.

Sanchez, M., De La Rosa, M., Blackson, T. C., Sastre, F., Rojas, P., Li, T., et al. (2014). Pre- to post-immigration alcohol use trajectories among recent Latino immigrants. *Psychology of Addictive Behaviors, 28*(4), 990–999. https://doi.org/10.1037/a0037807.

Sanchez, M. A., Hernández, M. T., Hanson, J. E., Vera, A., Magis Rodriguez, C., Ruiz, J., et al. (2012). The effect of migration on HIV high-risk behaviors among Mexican migrants. *Journal of Acquired Immune Deficiency Syndromes, 61*(5), 610–617.

Sapkota, S., Kohl, H. W., 3rd, Gilchrist, J., McAuliffe, J., Parks, B., England, B., et al. (2006). Unauthorized border crossings and migrant deaths: Arizona, New Mexico, and El Paso, Texas, 2002–2003. *American Journal of Public Health, 96*(7), 1282–1287.

Seabury, S. A., Terp, S., & Boden, L. I. (2017). Racial and ethnic differences in the frequency of workplace injuries and prevalence of work-related disability. *Health Affairs, 36*(2), 266–273. https://doi.org/10.1377/hlthaff.2016.1185.

Shedlin, M. G., Decena, C. U., & Oliver-Velez, D. (2005). Initial acculturation and HIV risk among new Hispanic immigrants. *Journal of the National Medical Association, 97*, 32S–37S.

Singh, G. K., Rodriguez-Lainz, A., & Kogan, M. D. (2013). Immigrant health inequalities in the United States: Use of eight major national data systems. *ScientificWorldJournal*, Published on line Oct. 27. https://doi.org/10.1155/2013/512313.

Sowell, R. L., Holtz, C. S., & Velasquez, G. (2008). HIV infection returning to Mexico with migrant workers: An exploratory study. *Journal of the Association of Nurses in AIDS Care, 19*, 267–282.

Stepler, R., & Lopez, M. H. (2016). *U.S. Latino population growth and dispersion has slowed since onset of the great recession*. Washington, DC: Pew Research Center. http://www.pewhispanic.org/2016/09/08/latino-population-growth-and-dispersion-has-slowed-since-the-onset-of-the-great-recession/.

Summers, P., Quandt, S. A., Talton, J. W., Galván, L., & Arcury, T. A. (2015). Hidden farmworker labor camps in North Carolina: An indicator of structural vulnerability. *American Journal of Public Health, 105*(12), 2570–2575. https://doi.org/10.2105/AJPH.2015.302797.

Taylor, E. V., Vaidyanathan, A., Flanders, W. D., Murphy, M., Spencer, M., & Noe, R. S. (2018). Differences in heath-related mortality by citizenship status: United States, 2005–2014. *American Journal of Public Health, 108*(S2), S131–S136.

Thomson, M. D., & Hoffman-Goetz, L. (2009). Defining and measuring acculturation: A systematic review of public health studies with Hispanic populations in the United States. *Social Science and Medicine, 69*, 983–991.

Torres, J. M., & Wallace, S. P. (2013). Migration circumstances, psychological distress, and self-rated physical health for Latino immigrants in the United States. *American Journal of Public Health, 103*(9), 1619–1627. https://doi.org/10.2105/AJPH.2012.301195.

Tuckman, J. (2014, August 23). Migrants risk life and limb to reach the US on train known as the Beast. *The Guardian.com*. https://www.theguardian.com/world/2014/aug/23/migrants-mexico-train-the-beast-fleeing-poverty.

United States (U.S.) Census Bureau. (2014). *2014 national population projections, Table 10: Projections of the population by sex, Hispanic origin, and race for the United States: 2015–2060*. http://www.census.gov/population/projections/data/national/2014/summarytables.html.

U.S. Census Bureau. (2016). *Annual estimates of the resident population by sex, age, race, and Hispanic origin for the United States and States: April 1, 2010–July 1, 2015*. Release date: June. http://factfinder.census.gov/faces/tableservices/jsf/pages/productview.xhtml?src=bkmk.

U.S. Department of Labor. (2016). *Findings from the National Agricultural Workers Survey (NAWS) 2013–2014: A demographic and employment profile of United States farmworkers*. Research Report No. 12. https://www.doleta.gov/agworker/pdf/NAWS_Research_Report_12_Final_508_Compliant.pdf.

U.S. Department of Labor. (2017). *Foreign-born workers: Labor force characteristics—2016*. News Release. USDL-17-0618, May 18. https://www.bls.gov/news.release/pdf/forbrn.pdf.

U.S. Government Accountability Office (2016). *Workplace safety and health. Additional data Needed to address continued hazards in the meat and poultry industry*. GAO-16-337. Washington, DC: U.S. Government Accountability Office. http://www.gao.gov/assets/680/676796.pdf.

Valverde, E. E., DiNenno, E. A., Schulden, J. D., Oster, A., & Painter, T. (2016). Sexually transmitted infection diagnoses among Hispanic immigrant and migrant men who have sex with men in the United States. *International Journal of STD and AIDS, 27*(13), 1162–1169.

Valverde, E. E., Painter, T., Heffelfinger, J. D., Schulden, J. D., Chavez, P., & DiNenno, E. A. (2015). Migration patterns and characteristics of sexual partners associated with unprotected sexual intercourse among Hispanic immigrant and migrant women in the United States. *Journal of Immigrant and Minority Health, 17*(6), 1826–1833. https://doi.org/10.1007/s10903-014-0132-6.

Vargas Bustamante, A., Fang, H., Garza, J., Carter-Pokras, O., Wallace, S. P., Rizzo, J. A., et al. (2012). Variations in healthcare access and utilization among Mexican immigrants: the role of documentation status. *Journal of Immigrant and Minority Health, 4*(1), 146–155. https://doi.org/10.1007/s10903-010-9406-9.

Viadro, C. I., & Earp, J. A. L. (2000). The sexual behavior of married Mexican immigrant men in North Carolina. *Social Science and Medicine, 50*, 723–735.

Viruell-Fuentes, E. A., Miranda, P. Y., & Abdulrahim, S. (2012). More than culture: Structural racism, intersectionality theory, and immigrant health. *Social Science and Medicine, 75*(12), 2099–2106. https://doi.org/10.1016/j.socscimed.2011.12.037.

Walton, A. L., LePrevost, C., Wong, B., Linnan, L., Sanchez-Birkhead, A., & Mooney, K. (2017). Pesticides: Perceived threat and protective behaviors among Latino farmworkers. *Journal of Agromedicine, 22*(2), 140–147. https://doi.org/10.1080/1059924X.2017.1283278.

Warren, R., & Kerwin, D. (2017). The 2,000 mile wall in search of a purpose: Since 2007 visa overstays have outnumbered undocumented border crossers by a half million. *Journal on Migration and Human Security, 5*(1), 124–136.

Wiewel, E. W., Torian, L. V., Hanna, D. B., Bocour, A., & Shepard, C. W. (2015). Foreign-born persons diagnosed with HIV: Where are they from and where were they infected? *AIDS and Behavior, 19*(5), 890–898. https://doi.org/10.1007/s10461-014-0954-1.

Wingood, G. M., DiClemente, R. J., Villamizar, K., Er, D. L., DeVarona, M., Taveras, J., et al. (2011). Efficacy of a health educator-delivered HIV prevention intervention for Latina women: A randomized controlled trial. *American Journal of Public Health, 101*(12), 2245–2252. https://doi.org/10.2105/AJPH.2011.300340.

Worby, P. A., Organista, K. C., Kral, A. H., Quesada, J., Arreola, S., & Khoury, S. (2014). Structural vulnerability and problem drinking among Latino migrant day laborers in the San Francisco Bay Area. *Journal of Health Care for the Poor and Underserved, 25*(3), 1291–1307. https://doi.org/10.1353/hpu.2014.0121.0.

World Bank. (2017). *Brief. Migration and remittances data, annual remittances data (updated as of Apr. 2017)*, Inflows, Table: remittancedatainflowsapr2017.xls. Washington, DC: The World Bank. http://www.worldbank.org/en/topic/migrationremittancesdiasporaissues/brief/migration-remittances-data.

Zong, J., & Batalova, J. (2017). *Spotlight: Frequently requested statistics on immigrants and immigration in the United States*. Migration Information Source, Migration Policy Institute. http://www.migrationpolicy.org/article/frequently-requested-statistics-immigrants-and-immigration-united-states.

Chapter 9
The Status of Latinx Occupational Health

Sara A. Quandt and Thomas A. Arcury

Abstract Latinx workers comprise more than 16% of the total US workforce and are overrepresented in some industries including construction, agriculture/forestry/fishing/hunting, and leisure/hospitality. In this chapter, we review the industries and occupations that disproportionately employ Latinx workers, outline the rates of fatal and nonfatal injuries within these industries and occupations, highlight several key features of the work context to understand hazards and injury risks, describe conceptual approaches to studying Latinx worker health, and examine successful strategies to research and intervention. We also provide research and intervention needs and priorities of Latinx workers in the USA.

Keywords Latinx · Worker health · Occupational health · Industry · Hazard

Latinx Workers: Focused on Hazardous Jobs

Latinx workers comprised 16.3% of the total US workforce 16 years and older in 2014, and projections put this figure at 19.8% by 2024 (Toossi, 2015). This group of workers is diverse in terms of origin and ethnicity, with the largest proportion (63%) claiming Mexican heritage (Bureau of Labor Statistics [BLS], 2016b). A higher proportion of Latinx men are employed compared with the total population of men (76% vs. 69%), and the proportion of Latinx women employed is slightly less (56% vs. 57%). The Latinx workforce 25 years and older has a strikingly lower educational attainment profile, with 28% having less than a high school diploma, compared with White (8%) and African-American (8%) workers. For those with bachelor's degree or higher, the pattern is reversed, with only 19% of the Latinx workforce having a

---

S. A. Quandt (✉)
Department of Epidemiology and Prevention, Wake Forest School of Medicine,
Winston-Salem, NC 27157, USA
e-mail: squandt@wakehealth.edu

T. A. Arcury
Department of Family and Community Medicine, Wake Forest School of Medicine, Medical Center Boulevard, Winston-Salem, NC 27157, USA

college degree compared with 39% and 28% of the White and African-American populations, respectively.

Industry and Occupation

Despite comprising about one in six workers, Latinx workers are overrepresented in several industries. Construction, agriculture/forestry/fishing/hunting, and leisure/hospitality have the greatest overrepresentation with 27.3%, 23.1%, and 22.3% of workers being Latinx (BLS, 2015, 2016b).

Although Latinx workers are employed across the occupational spectrum, more are concentrated in occupations that are dangerous (BLS, 2016b). Compared with the general US worker population 16 years and older, Latinx men are underrepresented in management and professional occupations (17.8% vs. 35.5%) and overrepresented in service occupations (19.9% vs. 14.2%), including food preparation (7.6% vs. 4.7%), and building and grounds cleaning and maintenance (8.1% vs. 4.3%). They are also overrepresented in natural resources, construction and maintenance occupations (26.7% vs. 16.5%). A similar pattern is found among Latinx women, who are particularly concentrated in service occupations, relative to the total population of women workers (31.8% vs. 21.1%).

Rates of Fatal and Nonfatal Injuries

Overall, Latinx persons account for fatal work-related injuries in excess of their proportion in the US workforce. In 2015, for example, among 4836 total work-related deaths, 903 occurred in Latinx workers (18.7%). At 4.0 per 100,000 full-time equivalent workers, this rate was the highest for any racial/ethnic group for whom the Bureau of Labor Statistics calculates rates (BLS, 2016a).

In contrast, the rate of nonfatal occupational injuries resulting in days away from work is lower among Latinx workers. For 2015, their days away from work accounted for only 12% of the cases reported nationally (BLS, 2016c). However, this figure should be interpreted with caution, as race/ethnicity was not reported in 40% of cases compiled by the BLS (BLS, 2016c), and the concentration of Latinx workers in jobs with few benefits may result in their taking less time off for injuries.

Concentration in Dangerous Jobs

Latinx workers are concentrated in some of the most dangerous jobs held by US workers: agriculture, construction, meat and poultry processing, restaurant and food service, domestic services, and day labor. Occupational injury, illness, and mortality are high in these industries, leading to excess morbidity and mortality among Latinx workers compared with all workers. Several factors underlie these rates, including the existence of significant hazards, limited occupational safety regulations, limited enforcement of existing regulations, and the contingent and nonstandard aspects of work.

Agriculture. Latinx workers make up the majority of farmworkers in the US. In 2014, the National Agricultural Workers Survey found that 73% of US crop workers were born in Mexico or Central America and about half were undocumented (Gabbard, 2015). These hired laborers are responsible for much of the hand labor required to produce food crops, as well as nonfood crops, such as tobacco. Although some agricultural tasks are mechanized, most pruning, weeding, and harvesting of fruits and vegetables are still done by hand. This hand labor can range from stooping and bending to pick strawberries to climbing ladders to harvest oranges and apples (Arcury & Marín, 2009). Latinx farmworkers have more recently become the dominant source of labor on dairy farms as dairy operations have consolidated and the demand for milk has increased with the popularity of processed products such as yogurt. In contrast to many field jobs, dairy work is year-round (Baker & Chappelle, 2012).

Pesticides present a significant hazard in the agricultural workplace. Agricultural industry workers experience acute pesticide-related illness and injury at rates 37 times higher than workers in other industries (Calvert et al., 2016). This rate is likely an underestimate, as Latinx farmworkers are likely to not report pesticide-related illness and injury because of fear of job loss, limited English skills, and lack of access to health care (Prado, Mulay, Kasner, Bohes, & Calvert, 2017). A minority of farmworkers typically mix and apply pesticides; however, they risk airborne drift from applications in adjacent fields (which can result in acute pesticide poisoning) and continuous low-level exposure to dislodgeable pesticide residues on plants, tools, and soil (which has been linked to eventual neurodegenerative disease, cancer, and reproductive problems) (Arcury & Quandt, 2009). Despite the introduction of nonpersistent pesticides that degrade quickly in the environment, most farmworkers monitored are found to have pesticide metabolites in their bodies (Arcury et al., 2016, 2017). Most research has focused on insecticides in several pesticide classes (carbamates, organophosphorus pesticides), but there is growing evidence for herbicides (e.g., glyphosate) that are now being applied at high levels to crops genetically modified to resist the herbicide (Vandenberg et al., 2017).

Heat exposure presents another significant hazard to farmworkers. The combination of heat, humidity, direct sun exposure, physical exertion, and the long sleeves and long pants of protective clothing places workers at risk for heat illness even when environmental temperatures are not extreme. Dangers of heat exposure are expected to increase with rising atmospheric temperatures (Keifer et al., 2016). In data compiled for occupational heat-related mortality for 1992–2006, crop workers accounted for 16% of deaths (0.39 per 100,000 workers), a rate almost 20 times higher than that for all other US workers. North Carolina had the highest mortality rate, and more than three-quarters of cases were male immigrants from Mexico and South and Central America (CDC, 2008). Heat exposure has been implicated in putting workers at risk for traumatic injuries, possibly through reduced postural stability and mental concentration (Spector, Krenz, & Blank, 2016). Farmworker housing, which generally lacks air-conditioning and in which heat indices can climb to dangerous levels, also puts workers at risk after hours (Quandt, Wiggins, Chen, Bischoff, & Arcury, 2013).

Musculoskeletal injuries are common among farmworkers as a result of carrying heavy loads of produce and stooping (May, 2009). Additional risks are frequently crop-specific. For example, workers harvesting tobacco are affected by green tobacco sickness, poisoning from nicotine absorbed through the skin (Arcury et al., 2003; Quandt, Arcury, Preisser, Bernert, & Norton, 2001). The symptoms of nausea, vomiting, headache, and dizziness can lead to dehydration (exacerbated by heat stress) and falls. Workers in citrus and stone fruit industries risk falls and eye injuries from work in trees (Luque et al., 2007).

The risks to Latinx farmworkers are exacerbated by the terms of their employment. Most are contingent and hired only for the limited time labor is needed. The frequent use of piece rate wages, where workers are paid per unit of produce picked rather than by the hour, has been implicated in heat-related illness (Spector et al., 2015) and falls (Salazar, Keifer, Negrete, Estrada, & Snyder, 2005). This system encourages workers to forego water or rest breaks, to work through unsafe conditions, and to work too quickly.

Construction. The construction industry, both commercial and residential, relies on Latinx labor, particularly in specific job types. For example, 51.2% of roofers, 49.3% of painters, and 45.5% of construction laborers are Latinx (BLS, 2016b). The proportion of Latinx workers in this industry increased rapidly during the 1990s and into the 2000s (Dong, Wang, & Daw, 2010), as the construction industry itself expanded. Significant hazards in construction include falls, trauma from tools such as nail guns, musculoskeletal injuries from vibration and awkward postures, and suffocation in cave-ins.

Latinx work-related deaths are concentrated in construction (CDC, 2008), and foreign-born Latinx construction workers are fatally injured at more than twice the rate of their US-born counterparts in the same jobs (Dong & Platner, 2004). This high rate may, in part, be related to their concentration in specific jobs with high risk for injury (e.g., falls in commercial construction iron-working and residential construction roofing), as well as miscommunication caused by language differences and failure to demand protections because of lack of documentation (Flynn, Eggerth, & Jacobson, 2015). Working for smaller construction companies that have less oversight for safety features also places workers at risk (Welton et al., 2017). About half of fatal falls in construction occur among workers for companies with 10 or fewer workers (CPWR, 2013).

Meat and poultry processing. Vertical integration of the meat and poultry processing industries and relocation of the latter to southern states with limited union presence has produced demand for increased numbers of low-cost laborers. Immigrant workers, the majority of whom are Latinx, have filled this need (Striffler, 2005; Griffith, 2012). Nationwide, 33.8% of animal slaughtering and processing workers are Latinx (BLS, 2017).

Some of these workers are employed in concentrated animal-feeding operations (CAFOs). These workers include (for poultry) "catchers" who enter CAFOs with as many as 50,000 birds and hand-catch them, experiencing cuts, scratches, and clouds of manure dust (Quandt, Arcury-Quandt, et al., 2013). The largest number of Latinx workers is employed in the processing plants where large numbers of animals are dismembered at rapid speed in an assembly line. Workers are at risk for musculoskeletal injuries, particularly from the repetitive motion of performing the same task over and over again (Leibler & Perry, 2017; Rosenbaum et al., 2013; Sagransky et al., 2012; Cartwright et al., 2012). These include tasks such as lifting carcasses of birds onto overhead hooks (affecting shoulders and hands) and cutting and trimming meat to produce value-added deboned meat (affecting wrists and hands). A combination of high-line speeds and limited number of workers produces fast-paced, high-intensity work. Working conditions on the line produce fall hazards (wet, greasy surfaces), allow such little time for breaks that workers have reported wearing adult diapers, and, if machines become clogged, increase the possibility of amputations as workers attempt to unclog them (Nevin, Bernt, & Hodgson, 2017).

Domestic services. Almost half of hotel room cleaners and residential maids are Latinx; most are women. Tasks performed by these workers include dusting, vacuuming, scrubbing bathrooms, changing linens and making beds, cleaning mirrors, and emptying trash. These tasks expose workers to multiple hazards. Musculoskeletal disorders result from bending, pushing heavy carts, and making beds. Bed-making has become increasingly hazardous as hotels move to the use of thick mattresses and elaborate linens. Traumatic injuries result from slips, trips, and falls. Respiratory illnesses and skin reactions are common from cleaning products. Room cleaners are exposed to infections from biologic waste and blood-borne pathogens found on broken glass and needles. These hazards are exacerbated by time pressure, as room quotas are often standardized across the industry. According to data tallied from OSHA injury logs for five full-service hotel chains, the highest rate of injury among all hotel jobs was for room cleaners; the highest rates were for women, with 10.6 injuries per 100 worker-years (Buchanan et al., 2010).

Day laborers. The population of Latinx day laborers is largely composed of undocumented men who work in the informal economy, where health and safety protections may be minimal and their likelihood of wage theft or other forms of exploitation are greater than in the formal employment sector. Precise numbers of day laborers are impossible to find; estimates range from 250,000 to 750,000 workers (McDevitt, 2010; Rathod, 2016). Such workers provide flexibility to employers whose need for labor fluctuates; day laborers often find work in home construction, lawn maintenance, and restaurant cooking. Day laborers tend to materialize in large numbers when needed for cleanup after natural disasters. An estimated 10,000–20,000 appeared for recovery work from Hurricane Katrina in New Orleans, as resident workers had been displaced from the city (McDevitt, 2010).

These workers are often more marginalized, socially isolated, and chronically stressed than other workers (Galvin, Wohl, Carlos, & Chen, 2015), and it appears that a larger proportion engage in unhealthy drinking and risk behaviors related to human immunodeficiency virus (HIV) and sexually transmitted infections (Ornelas, Allen,

Vaughan, Williams, & Negi, 2015; Organista & Kubo, 2005). Some day laborers are homeless and subject to violence. They often lack basic safety equipment and may not receive safety training on the job. The fact that they compete daily for work against other day laborers reinforces the notion that they are never indispensable on the job. Such an attitude is likely tied to greater risk taking and limited ability to protest unsafe or abusive work conditions (Walter, Bourgois, Loinaz, & Schillinger, 2002).

Common Features of the Work Context Link to Common Health Issues

Across the Latinx labor force, several key features of the work context stand out as a way to understand hazards and injury risks. These features include holding some of the riskiest jobs in dangerous industries and doing contingent work (temporary, often part-time jobs) on nonstandard schedules at low pay. Within industries, Orrenius and Zavodny (2009) showed that Latinx immigrant workers, particularly men and younger workers, hold jobs associated with higher injury rates. They argue that it is more meaningful to look at occupations than to simply look at industries. Their results indicate that injuries and fatalities increase as the ability to speak English and years of formal education decline.

The rise in the number of immigrant workers has paralleled the increased use of contingent workers since the late 1990s. Contingent work may be outsourced from employers to contracting agencies. Large companies find it financially beneficial to have such agencies maintain a pool of available workers and to do the hiring, firing, and paying of these workers. Most such workers get few benefits such as health insurance or paid sick leave. Their wages can be kept lower than those of workers hired directly by the company. Some workers are paid "piece rate"; that is, by the job, rather than hourly. The companies are protected from risk of hiring undocumented workers or of providing Workers' Compensation, if injuries occur. Such contingent work for Latinx workers is common in manufacturing, including meat and poultry processing, janitorial services, and personal care services. Workers are often kept from protesting conditions by being told that other willing workers are available to take their jobs.

Latinx workers are numerous in industries that are subject to limited occupational safety regulations. For example, agriculture has had few specific safety regulations, following from the tradition of "agricultural exceptionalism" built into the federal labor laws of the 1930s. Specifically, farm laborers are excluded from the National Labor Relations Act of 1935, which provides for worker organizing and collective bargaining, and the Fair Labor Standards Act, which provides for minimum wage, overtime, and child-labor protections (Wiggin, 2009). Specific hazards, such as pesticide exposure, have weak protections that place much of the responsibility for safety on workers themselves. Risk for heat illness, a hazard for many outdoor and some indoor workers, is starting to be addressed in some states (e.g., California and Washington), but not in others.

Latinx workers are also common in industries that have limited enforcement of existing regulations and in which safety training and safety equipment are often not provided. These industries include residential construction and domestic services.

These conditions of employment of workers who are often undocumented and speak limited English create a situation in which workers are encouraged to work quickly and to work long hours, disregarding safety. They must work even when sick or injured because they do not have health insurance or paid time off. They are discouraged from reporting unsafe or exploitative situations. Such a situation plays into cultural stereotypes, so that men, in particular, are pressured to show their masculinity by working hard and providing for their families, which often means working extended hours and ignoring risks.

Across industries, common health conditions are reported. Musculoskeletal injuries are common in construction, agriculture, and the service industry. Exposures to pesticides and other chemicals occur in agriculture, landscaping, and janitorial services. Repetitive-motion injuries, such as carpal tunnel syndrome, are common in construction, poultry and meat processing, and other manufacturing. Traumatic injuries are reported in industries such as poultry processing, where time pressure results in workers taking risks to fix machinery without proper safeguards.

According to mental health data, the combined stress of job conditions, low income, marginalization, and threats of deportation results in high levels of depression and anxiety for Latinx workers, and in manifestation of some culture-based syndromes such as *susto* and *nervios* (Grzywacz, 2009). Substance abuse, particularly binge drinking, has been reported in Latinx workers across industries, particularly among men.

Conceptual Approaches to Studying Latinx Worker Health

Several conceptual approaches provide frameworks for understanding how work affects the health of Latinx persons and for designing interventions that can improve their occupational safety. These frameworks include the organization of work model (Sauter et al., 2002; Landsbergis, Grzywacz, & LaMontagne, 2014); the demand-control-support model (Karasek, 1979; Snyder, Krauss, Chen, Finlinson, & Huang, 2008); work safety culture (Cooper, 2000); and work safety climate (Zohar, 1980, 2010). In addition, Kleinman's Explanatory Models of Illness (1980, 1988) provides an ethnomedical framework for delineating what workers believe are the causes and consequences of occupational injuries and illness and ways to prevent them; and the social science approach of structural vulnerability helps show worker health as a product of workers' position in the social hierarchy and its power relationships (Leatherman, 2005; Quesada et al., 2011).

Sauter et al.'s (2002) organization of work model includes three levels: external context (economic, legal, political, technologic, and demographic forces at the national and international level); organizational context (management structure, supervisory practices, production methods, and human resource policies), and work context (job characteristics such as work scheduling and piece rate or hourly wage practices). External context is particularly important for Latinx workers, as immigration policy and legal documentation to work provide the context that dictates the type of work available to them. The external context is also important because of limitations in the way policy is applied in some industries that employ many Latinx workers, such as agriculture (Wiggins, 2009).

The job demand-control-support model provides a framework for examining the association of work organization factors from the organizational and work contexts with health among Latinx workers (Karasek, 1979, Snyder et al., 2008; Arcury, Grzywacz, Chen, Mora, & Quandt, 2014). This model posits that jobs with greater physical and psychologic demands or stressors will result in poorer health. However, jobs with greater control or decision latitude can result in better health and can offset the effects of demand leading to poor health. Lastly, support of peers and supervisors, including perceived safety climate (how workers perceive supervisors value safety over production), reduces occupational injury and buffers the effects of job demands (Johnson & Hall, 1988; Luchman & González-Morales, 2013). Work organization (particularly job demands) is associated with health outcomes that are particularly prevalent in immigrant workers, such as musculoskeletal and neurologic problems (Arcury, Grzywacz, et al., 2014, Arcury, Cartwright, et al., 2014; Lang, Ochsmann, Kraus, & Lang, 2012).

Research using the organization of work and demand-control-support models has largely focused on white-collar workers, but several recent efforts have expanded the use of these models to address the occupational safety and health of low-income, minority, and immigrant workers. Landsbergis et al. (2014) provide an analysis of the literature to illuminate how work organization results in health disparities. Grzywacz et al. (2013) consider how the organization of work in the agricultural, forestry, and fishing sector affect the occupational safety and health of immigrant workers.

Work safety culture is an important aspect of workplace safety (Cooper, 2000). On the basis of Bandura's (1986) theory of reciprocal determinism, Cooper (2000) argues that safety culture includes behavioral, situational, and psychologic elements, thereby encompassing many different aspects of the work environment. Behavioral elements include observable safety and risk behaviors. Situational elements include safety management programs and actions. Psychologic elements include subjective assessments of safety. Work safety climate, a worker's perceptions of how an employer values safety over production (Zohar, 1980, 2010), is a subjective assessment of safety that has been used in analyses of Latinx occupational health and safety, including workers employed in agriculture (Arcury, O'Hara, et al., 2012; Arcury, Kearney, Rodriguez, Arcury, & Quandt, 2015; Kearney, Rodriguez, Arcury, Quandt, & Arcury, 2015; Swanberg, Clouser, Browning, Westneat, & Marsh, 2013), construction (Arcury, Mills, et al., 2012, Arcury, Summers, et al., 2015; Ochsner et al., 2012; Shrestha & Menzel, 2014), and manufacturing (Arcury, Grzywacz, et al., 2012; Grzywacz et al., 2012). Several analyses have focused on the work safety climate of

Latinx women (Arcury, Grzywacz, et al., 2014; Arcury, Trejo, et al., 2015; Rodriguez et al., 2016).

The Explanatory Models of Illness (Kleinman 1980, 1988) provides a framework for delineating worker beliefs to inform occupational safety and health programs to be culturally appropriate. This approach has been used to understand Latinx workers' understanding of pesticide exposure (Quandt, Austin, Arcury, Summers, & Saavedra, 1999), carpel tunnel syndrome (Arcury, Mora, & Quandt, 2015), and falls from roofs (Arcury, Summers, et al., 2014). Analyses of these cultural data inform culturally appropriate occupational safety and health programs (Quandt, Arcury, Austin, & Cabrera, 2001). Although some analyses indicate that workers' models of illness are at odds with those of occupational health clinicians (e.g., Quandt, Arcury, Austin, & Saavedra, 1998), other analyses indicate that workers have an accurate understanding of the causes of occupational illness and injury (e.g., Arcury, Mora, et al., 2015, Arcury, Summers, et al., 2014), suggesting that improved health and safety require changes in the organization of work and work safety culture.

Structural vulnerability is a social science-based framework that places worker health and illness in the broader context of the social hierarchy. It highlights the political-economic and cultural and institutional sources of both psychologic and physical distress experienced by workers (Leatherman, 2005). These Latinx workers, by virtue of their documentation status, skin color, and language limitations, experience both subtle and overt discrimination, which both relegates them to so-called 3-D (dangerous, dirty, demanding) jobs and constrains their health and safety-related behavioral choices. The structural vulnerability approach to worker health and safety has been used most frequently by anthropologists. Although much of this research has focused on day laborers (e.g., Walter, Bourgois, & Loinaz, 2004) who represent the confluence of multiple social inequalities, ideas of structural vulnerability have also been used to frame the occupational health risks of indigenous farmworkers (Holmes, 2013), migrant farmworkers (Heine, Quandt, & Arcury, 2017), dairy workers (Sexsmith, 2016), and poultry catchers and production line workers (Mora, Arcury, & Quandt, 2016).

Successful Research and Intervention for Latinx Workers

Research and intervention with Latinx workers face major obstacles. Foremost among these obstacles is a lack of access to the places that these Latinx persons work. Limits to workplace access result from the same factors that increase the occupational health risks these workers face. They seldom have employment with union protection, their jobs are often contingent, they often have nonstandard work schedules, they often have multiple jobs, they change jobs frequently, they often lack documentation, they often have limited formal educational attainment, and they fear job loss if they participate in research or intervention projects. Workers do not want to antagonize their employers, and employers seldom want workers to participate in any activity that might limit productivity or place the employer at risk for sanction, should they not be in compliance with any regulation or law.

Research and intervention with Latinx workers often require that participants be found and involved in their communities rather than at the worksite. This requirement makes it difficult to recruit or involve a sufficient number of individuals working in a single industry or in a single occupation. For example, seldom are there specific neighborhoods where only workers of a single employer live. This was once the case with company towns, but such environments resulted in even greater control over the lives of workers. Although farmworker housing was traditionally provided by growers in barracks or old dwellings on farms, farmworkers today often find housing off the farm in nearby towns or cities. It is almost impossible to conduct a controlled test of an intervention in which workers from specific worksites are compared. Not having workplace access also makes the collection of data on specific working circumstances or behaviors impossible; for example, measuring the effects of a workstation on the development of carpal tunnel syndrome in a factory or meat-processing plant is not possible when one cannot measure the workstation and the line speed; similarly, measuring actual availability and use of personal protective equipment by roofers to prevent falls from roofs requires collection of worksite data.

Community-based participatory research (CBPR) provides an important approach to address this dilemma (Arcury, Austin, Quandt, & Saavedra, 1999; Arcury & Quandt, 2017). CBPR has been widely used with Latinx workers, whether with specific groups of workers (Farquhar et al., 2008; Quandt et al., 2006), or when addressing specific health issues (Rhodes, Hergenrather, Bloom, Leichliter, & Montaño, 2009). CBPR allows investigators to collaborate with worker service providers and advocacy groups to locate those with a specific occupation or who are employed in a specific industry; this has been accomplished with Latinx farmworkers (Arcury & Quandt, 2017; Salvatore et al., 2015; McCauley et al., 2013; Flocks, Monaghan, Albrecht, & Bahena, 2007; Thompson et al., 2003), forestry workers (Campe, Hoare, Hagopian, & Keifer, 2011); poultry processing workers (Quandt et al., 2006), chicken catchers (Quandt, Arcury-Quandt, et al., 2013), construction workers (Ochsner et al., 2012), and day laborers (Ochsner et al., 2008). In addition to individuals with specific occupations or employed in specific industries, CBPR allows investigators to conduct research or interventions about work safety or workers' rights with all of the residents of vulnerable communities, no matter what their specific occupation or specific industry. Such programs have addressed wage theft (Quandt et al., 2008) and carpal tunnel syndrome (Quandt et al., 2004) among low-wage Latinx workers in North Carolina.

Lay health advisors (*promotoras de salud*) are an important approach for conducting research and intervention with Latinx workers (Rhodes, Foley, Zometa, & Bloom, 2007). Migrant Health Program Salud (MHP Salud) (http://mhpsalud.org/portfolio/) has developed a substantial set of resources for lay health advisor programs with Latinx workers. Often integrated into CBPR projects, lay health advisors have proven to be successful in addressing the occupational health and safety of Latinx construction and day laborers (Ochsner et al., 2008, 2012; Williams, Ochsner, Marshall, Kimmel, & Martino, 2010), farmworkers (McCauley et al., 2013; Liebman, Juárez, Leyva, &

Corona, 2007; Flocks et al., 2007; Arcury, Marín, Snively, Hernández-Pelletier, & Quandt, 2009; Quandt, Grzywacz, et al., 2013; Luque, Mason, Reyes-Garcia, Hinojosa, & Meade, 2011; Salvatore et al., 2015), forestry workers (Bush et al., 2014), and poultry processing workers (Marín et al., 2009; Grzywacz et al., 2009). Lay health advisors have also been used to improve HIV prevention among Latinx workers (Rhodes et al., 2009).

Social marketing has also been a framework for research and education to improve occupational health and safety behavior among Latinx workers. Also, integrated into CBPR projects, social marketing has been used with Latinx construction workers (Menzel & Shrestha, 2012) and agricultural workers (Flocks et al., 2001; Tovar-Aguilar et al., 2014).

Although CBPR provides a framework for integrating Latinx workers into occupational health and safety research and health education approaches such as lay health advisors and social marketing, this research and intervention is limited in the extent to which it can improve the occupational health of Latinx workers and other vulnerable worker communities. These approaches have had little effect on the organization of work these workers encounter. Organizing efforts that result in changes in the organization through changes in industry standards or governmental regulations are needed.

Workers Centers are one mechanism to address structural changes needed to improve the occupational safety and health of Latinx workers (Fine, 2006). In addition to providing safety education and other services for Latinx and other vulnerable workers, Workers Centers are often engaged in community organizing and union organizing to support changes in the way work is organized, the regulations that are implemented, and the ways in which regulations are enforced. At least three networks of Workers Centers are active: (1) National Day Laborer Organizing Network; (2) Interfaith Worker Justice; and (3) Food Chain Workers Alliance. Other organizations are also active in addressing the organization of work for Latinx workers; for example, the Coalition of Immokalee Workers (Florida) (http://www.ciw-online.org/) has been instrumental in developing the Fair Food Program to ensure fair treatment of farmworkers (no slavery, protection from sexual harassment) and to increase pay to a living wage (Fair Food Program, 2015).

Research and Intervention Needs and Priorities for Latinx Workers

Several occupational health and safety research and intervention priorities are apparent for the protection of Latinx workers. First among these is the documentation of immediate and long-term occupational health outcomes among these workers. Intervention development must be based on such research. This research should emphasize innovative designs to help delineate any long-term effects of occupational exposures on workers and the members of their families. This research could examine the subclinical effects of occupational exposure; for example, Quandt and colleagues measured subclinical differences in olfaction (Quandt et al., 2016; Quandt, Walker, Talton, Chen, & Arcury, 2017) and cholinesterase depression (Quandt, Pope, Chen, Summers, & Arcury, 2015) to delineate potential neurologic effects of pesticide exposure among Latinx farmworkers.

Although research at the places where Latinx workers are employed is needed, access to such workplaces is limited because of the limited power of these workers (e.g., lack of union representation, limited documentation leading to fear of job loss). The lack of workplace access also makes it difficult to develop, implement, and evaluate interventions to improve workplace safety and reduce occupational injury and illness. Again, innovative design, such as CBPR approaches and working with Worker Centers (Forst et al., 2013; Quandt et al., 2006), can provide access to workers for research and safety interventions outside of the workplace. This research should focus on how work is organized and on work safety culture.

Research has focused on a few occupational groups and on a limited number of outcomes. Research and intervention with workers in agriculture, construction, and manufacturing need to continue. Research should also be implemented with Latinx workers in other industries, particularly the service industries (hotel cleaners, restaurant workers, home cleaners, and lawn maintenance), and forestry (Bush et al., 2014; Campe et al., 2011).

Research is needed on the effects of work on workers' families. Research on how workplace exposures can result in contamination of homes and exposures for family members, referred to as para-occupational exposure, has been limited largely to farmworker exposure to agricultural pesticides. This research has documented substantial agricultural pesticide exposure in farmworkers' homes (Quandt et al., 2004; Quirós-Alcalá et al., 2011) and that family members, particularly children, experience substantial pesticide doses (Arcury, Grzywacz, Barr, Tapia, Chen, & Quandt, 2007; Lambert et al., 2005; Thompson, Griffith, Barr, Coronado, Vigoren, & Faustman, 2014). This exposure results in considerable neurobehavioral health effects for children in farmworker families (Bouchard et al., 2011; Rowe et al., 2016; Stein et al., 2016), as well as affecting pulmonary function (Raanan et al., 2016).

Documenting the intersection of work and domestic roles among Latinx women is important for the development of interventions (Eggerth, Delaney, Flynn, & Jacobson, 2012; Rodriguez et al., 2016). Latinx women experience demanding domestic roles and an unequal division of household work (Guendelman, Malin, Herr-Harthorn, & Vargas, 2001), resulting in work-family conflict. Their extraordinary domestic work burdens and the resulting work-family conflict affect their mental and physical health.

Lastly, research to validate the efficacy of occupational health and safety policy and regulations is needed. When regulations exist, their efficacy is often in doubt. For example, the U S Environmental Protection Agency (EPA) has regulations that are meant to protect migrant and seasonal farmworkers from pesticide exposure; these regulations are called the Worker Protection Standard (WPS) (www.epa.gov/pesticide-worker-safety/agricultural-worker-protection-standard-wps). After a 20-year struggle, a revised WPS was implemented in 2017. However, no evaluation of the earlier WPS was ever conducted by the US EPA, US Department of Agriculture, US Department of Labor, or any state agency. Research by academic researchers found that the earlier WPS was never fully implemented and that the agencies charged with enforcement were understaffed (Arcury, Quandt, Austin, Preisser, & Cabrera, 1999). Further research documented that farmworkers continued to be exposed frequently to pesticides and that this exposure was at high levels (Arcury, Grzywacz, et al., 2009; Arcury et al., 2010). The current revision of the WPS has no provision for evaluation and no additional resources for enforcement. Therefore, it is likely to have limited value in reducing worker pesticide exposure. Analyses by academic and advocacy researchers will continue to find instances of the regulations not being implemented, and they will document that farmworkers continue to be exposed to pesticides frequently and at high levels.

Similar results have been reported for federal regulations applied to migrant farmworkers' housing (Arcury, Weir, et al., 2012; Vallejos et al., 2011) and field sanitation (Whalley et al., 2009). Latinx construction workers report that Workers' Compensation regulations are also not applied (Arcury, Summers, et al., 2014). The same is likely true for occupational health and safety regulations in other industries that employ large numbers of Latinx workers. The empirical questions that need to be considered are: What occupational health and safety regulations have been developed? Are existing occupational health and safety regulations implemented? and Do existing occupational health and safety regulations have the desired effects?

References

Arcury, T. A., Austin, C. K., Quandt, S. A., & Saavedra, R. (1999). Enhancing community participation in a public health project: Farmworkers and agricultural chemicals in North Carolina. *Health Education & Behavior, 26*, 563–578.

Arcury, T. A., Cartwright, M. S., Chen, H., Rosenbaum, D. A., Walker, F. O., Mora, D. C., et al. (2014). Musculoskeletal and neurological injuries associated with work organization among immigrant Latino women manual workers in North Carolina. *American Journal of Industrial Medicine, 57*, 468–475.

Arcury, T. A., Chen, H., Laurienti, P. J., Howard, T. D., Barr, D. B., Mora, D. C., et al. (2017). Farmworker and nonfarmworker Latino immigrant men in North Carolina have high levels of specific pesticide urinary metabolites. *Archives of Environmental & Occupational Health, 16*, 1–9.

Arcury, T. A., Grzywacz, J. G., Anderson, A. M., Mora, D. C., Carrillo, L., Chen, H., et al. (2012). Personal protective equipment and work safety climate among Latino poultry processing workers in western North Carolina, USA. *International Journal of Occupational and Environmental Health, 18*, 320–328.

Arcury, T. A., Grzywacz, J. G., Barr, D. B., Tapia, J., Chen, H., & Quandt, S. A. (2007). Pesticide urinary metabolite levels of children in eastern North Carolina farmworker households. *Environmental Health Perspectives, 115*, 1254–1260.

Arcury, T. A., Grzywacz, J. G., Chen, H., Mora, D. C., & Quandt, S. A. (2014). Work organization and health among immigrant women: Latina manual workers in North Carolina. *American Journal of Public Health, 104*, 2445–2452.

Arcury, T. A., Grzywacz, J. G., Chen, H., Vallejos, Q. M., Galván, L., Whalley, L. E., et al. (2009). Variation across the agricultural season in organophosphorus pesticide urinary metabolite levels for Latino farmworkers in eastern North Carolina: Project design and descriptive results. *American Journal of Industrial Medicine, 52,* 539–550.

Arcury, T. A., Grzywacz, J. G., Talton, J. W., Chen, H., Vallejos, Q. M., Galván, L., et al. (2010). Repeated pesticide exposure among North Carolina migrant and seasonal farmworkers. *American Journal of Industrial Medicine, 53,* 802–813.

Arcury, T. A., Kearney, G. D., Rodriguez, G., Arcury, J. T., & Quandt, S. A. (2015). Work safety culture of youth farmworkers in North Carolina: A pilot study. *American Journal of Public Health, 105,* 344–350.

Arcury, T. A., Laurienti, P. J., Chen, H., Howard, T. D., Barr, D. B., Mora, D. C., et al. (2016). Organophosphate pesticide urinary metabolites among Latino immigrants: North Carolina farmworkers and non-farmworkers compared. *Journal of Occupational and Environmental Medicine, 58,* 1079–1086.

Arcury, T. A., & Marín, A. J. (2009). Latino/ farmworkers and farm work in the eastern United States: The context for health, safety, and justice. In T. A. Arcury & S. A. Quandt (Eds.), *Latino farmworkers in the eastern United States: Health, safety, and justice* (pp. 15–36). New York: Springer.

Arcury, T. A., Marín, A., Snively, B. M., Hernández-Pelletier, M., & Quandt, S. A. (2009). Reducing farmworker residential pesticide exposure: Evaluation of a lay health advisor intervention. *Health Promotion Practice, 10,* 447–455.

Arcury, T. A., Mills, T., Marin A. J., Summers, P., Quandt, S. A., Rushing, J., ... Grzywacz, J. G. (2012). Work safety climate and safety practices among immigrant Latino residential construction workers. *American Journal of Industrial Medicine, 55,* 736–745.

Arcury, T. A., Mora, D. C., & Quandt, S. A. (2015). "...you earn money by suffering pain:" Beliefs about carpal tunnel syndrome among Latino poultry processing workers. *Journal of Immigrant and Minority Health, 17,* 791–801.

Arcury, T. A., O'Hara, H., Grzywacz, J. G., Isom, S., Chen, H., & Quandt, S. A. (2012). Work safety climate, musculoskeletal discomfort, working while injured, and depression among migrant farmworkers in North Carolina. *American Journal of Public Health, 102,* S272–S278.

Arcury, T. A., & Quandt, S. A. (2009). Pesticide exposure among farmworkers and their families in the eastern United States: Matters of safety and environmental justice. In T. A. Arcury & S. A. Quandt (Eds.), *Latino farmworkers in the eastern United States: Health, safety, and justice* (pp. 103–129). New York: Springer.

Arcury, T. A., & Quandt, S. A. (2017). Community-based participatory research and occupational health disparities: Pesticide exposure among immigrant farmworkers. In F. Leong, D. Eggerth, D. Chang, M. Flynn, K. Ford, & R. Martinez R (Eds.), *Occupational health disparities: Improving the well-being of ethnic and racial minority workers* (pp. 89–112). Washington, DC: APA Press.

Arcury, T. A., Quandt, S. A., Austin, C. K., Preisser, J., & Cabrera, L. F. (1999). Implementation of US-EPA's Worker Protection Standard training for agricultural laborers: An evaluation using North Carolina data. *Public Health Reports, 114,* 459–468.

Arcury, T. A., Quandt, S. A., Preisser, J. S., Bernert, J. T., Norton, D., & Wang, J. (2003). High levels of transdermal nicotine exposure produce green tobacco sickness in Latino farmworkers. *Nicotine & Tobacco Research, 5,* 315–321.

Arcury, T. A., Summers, P., Carrillo, L., Grzywacz, J. G., Quandt, S. A., & Mills, T. H. (2014). Occupational safety beliefs among Latino residential roofing workers. *American Journal of Industrial Medicine, 57,* 718–725.

Arcury, T. A., Summers, P., Rushing, J., Grzywacz, J. G., Mora, D. C., Quandt, S. A., ... Mills, T. H. (2015). Work safety climate, personal protection use, and injuries among Latino residential roofers. *American Journal of Industrial Medicine, 58,* 69–76.

Arcury, T. A., Trejo, G., Suerken, C. K., Grzywacz, J. G., Ip, E. H., & Quandt, S. A. (2015). Work and health among Latina mothers in farmworker families. *Journal of Occupational and Environmental Medicine, 57,* 292–299.

Arcury, T. A., Weir, M., Chen, H., Summers, P., Pelletier, L. E., Galván, L., ... Quandt, S. A. (2012). Migrant farmworker housing regulation violations in North Carolina. *American Journal of Industrial Medicine, 55,* 191–204.

Baker, D., & Chappelle, D. (2012). Health status and needs of Latino dairy farmworkers in Vermont. *Journal of Agromedicine, 17,* 277–287.

Bandura, A. (1986). *Social foundations of thought and action: A social cognitive theory.* Englewood Cliffs, NJ: Prentice-Hall.

Bouchard, M. F., Chevrier, J., Harley, K. G., Kogut, K., Vedar, M., Calderon, N., ... Eskenazi, B. (2011). Prenatal exposure to organophosphate pesticides and IQ in 7-year-old children. *Environmental Health Perspectives, 119,* 1189–1195.

Buchanan, S., Vossenas, P., Krause, N., Moriarty, J., Frumin, E., Shimek, J., et al. (2010). Occupational injury disparities in the US hotel industry. *American Journal of Industrial Medicine, 53,* 116–125.

Bureau of Labor Statistics, US Department of Labor. (2016a). *Census of fatal occupational injuries (CFOI) 2015,* released December 16, 2016. https://www.bls.gov/iif/oshcfoi1.htm#2015.

Bureau of Labor Statistics, US Department of Labor. (2016b). Labor force characteristics by race and ethnicity, 2015. *BLS Reports, Report 1062,* September, 2016. http://www.bls.gov/opub/reports/race-and-ethnicity/2015/home.htm.

Bureau of Labor Statistics, US Department of Labor. (2016c). *Nonfatal occupational injuries and illnesses requiring days away from work, 2015,* released November 10, 2016. https://www.bls.gov/iif/oshcdnew.htm.

Bureau of Labor Statistics, US Department of Labor. (2017). *Labor force statistics from Current Population Survey, 2016.* Last modified date: February 8, 2017. https://www.bls.gov/cps/cpsaat18.htm.

Bureau of Labor Statistics, US Department of Labor [BLS]. (2015). Hispanics and Latinos in industries and occupations. *TED: The Economics Daily,* October 9. http://www.bls.gov/opub/ted/2015/s-and-latinos-in-industries-and-occupations.htm.

Bush, D. E., Wilmsen, C., Sasaki, T., Barton-Antonio, D., Steege, A. L., & Chang, C. (2014). Evaluation of a pilot promotora program for Latino forest workers in southern Oregon. *American Journal of Industrial Medicine, 57,* 788–799.

Calvert, G. M., Beckman, J., Prado, J. B., Bojes, H., Schwartz, A., Mulay, P., et al. (2016). Acute occupational pesticide-related illness and injury—United States, 2007–2011. *MMWR Morbidity and Mortality Weekly Report, 63,* 11–16.

Campe, J., Hoare, L., Hagopian, A., & Keifer, M. (2011). Using community-based methods and a social ecological framework to explore workplace health and safety of bloqueros on the Olympic Peninsula. *American Journal of Industrial Medicine, 54,* 438–449.

Cartwright, M. S., Walker, F. O., Blocker, J. N., Schulz, M. R., Arcury, T. A., Grzywacz, J. G., et al. (2012). The prevalence of carpal tunnel syndrome in Latino poultry-processing workers and other Latino manual workers. *Journal of Occupational and Environmental Medicine, 54,* 198–201.

Center for Construction Research and Training. (2013). *The construction chart book: The US construction industry and its workers* (5th ed.). Silver Spring, MD: CPWR.

Centers for Disease Control and Prevention [CDC]. (2008). Heat-related deaths among crop workers—United States, 1992–2006. *MMWR. Morbidity and Mortality Weekly Report, 57,* 649–653.

Cooper, M. D. (2000). Towards a model of safety culture. *Safety Science, 36,* 111–136.

Dong, X., & Platner, J. W. (2004). Occupational fatalities of construction workers from 1992 to 2000. *American Journal of Industrial Medicine, 45,* 45–54.

Dong, X. S., Wang, X., & Daw, C. CPWR Data Center. (2010). Fatal and nonfatal injuries among construction workers. *CPWR Data Brief, 2,* 1–19. http://www.cpwr.com/pdfs/_Data_Brief3.pdf.

Eggerth, D., Delaney, S., Flynn, M., & Jacobson, J. (2012). Work experiences of Latina immigrants: A qualitative study. *Journal of Career Development, 39,* 13–30.

Fair Food Program. (2015). *Fair Food Program 2015 Annual Report.* http://www.fairfoodprogram.org/.

Farquhar, S., Samples, J., Ventura, S., Davis, S., Abernathy, M., McCauley, L., ... Shadbeh, N. (2008). Promoting the occupational health of indigenous farmworkers. *Journal of Immigrant and Minority Health, 10,* 269–280.

Fine, J. (2006). *Worker centers: Organizing communities at the edge of the dream.* Ithaca, NY: Cornell University Press.

Flocks, J., Clarke, L., Albrecht, S., Bryant, C., Monaghan, P., & Baker, H. (2001). Implementing a community-based social marketing project to improve agricultural worker health. *Environmental Health Perspectives, 109*(Suppl 3), 461–468.

Flocks, J., Monaghan, P., Albrecht, S., & Bahena, A. (2007). Florida farmworkers' perceptions and lay knowledge of occupational pesticides. *Journal of Community Health, 32,* 181–194.

Flynn, M. A., Eggerth, D. E., & Jacobson, C. J., Jr. (2015). Undocumented status as a social determinant of occupational safety and health: The workers' perspective. *American Journal of Industrial Medicine, 58,* 1127–1137.

Forst, L., Ahonen, E., Zanoni, J., Holloway-Beth, A., Oschner, M., Kimmel, L., et al. (2013). More than training: Community-based participatory research to reduce injuries among construction workers. *American Journal of Industrial Medicine, 56,* 827–837.

Gabbard, S. (2015). *Changing trends in crop agriculture and migrant crop workers.* Presented at the Interstate Migrant Education Council Symposium, October 2015, Clearwater, FL. https://www.doleta.gov/naws/pages/research/presentations.cfm.

Galvin, F. H., Wohl, A. R., Carlos, J. A., & Chen, Y. T. (2015). Chronic stress among Latino day laborers. *Journal of Behavioral Sciences, 37,* 75–89.

Griffith, D. (2012). Labor recruitment and immigration in the Eastern North Carolina food industry. *International Journal of Sociology of Agriculture and Food, 19,* 102–118.

Grzywacz, J. G. (2009). Mental health among farmworkers in the Eastern United States. In T. A. Arcury & S. A. Quandt (Eds.), *Latino farmworkers in the eastern United States: Health, safety, and justice* (pp. 153–172). New York: Springer.

Grzywacz, J. G., Arcury, T. A., Marín, A., Carrillo, L., Coates, M. L., Burke, B., et al. (2009). Using lay health promoters in occupational health: Outcome evaluation in a sample of Latino poultry processing workers. *New Solutions, 19,* 449–466.

Grzywacz, J. G., Arcury, T. A., Mora, D., Anderson, A., Chen, H., Rosenbaum, D. A., ... Quandt, S. A. (2012). Work organization and musculoskeletal health: Clinical findings among immigrant Latino workers. *Journal of Occupational and Environmental Medicine, 54,* 995–1001.

Grzywacz, J. G., Lipscomb, H. J., Casanova, V., Neis, B., Fraser, C., Monaghan, P., et al. (2013). Organization of work in the agricultural, forestry, and fishing sector in the US Southeast: Implications for immigrant workers' occupational safety and health. *American Journal of Industrial Medicine, 56,* 925–939.

Guendelman, S., Malin, C., Herr-Harthorn, B., & Vargas, P. N. (2001). Orientations to motherhood and male partner support among women in Mexico and Mexican-origin women in the United States. *Social Science and Medicine, 52,* 1805–1813.

Heine, B., Quandt, S. A., & Arcury, T. A. (2017). *Aguantamos*: Limits to Latino migrant farmworker agency in North Carolina labor camps. *Human Organization, 76,* 240–250.

Holmes, S. M. (2013). *Fresh fruit, broken bodies: Migrant farm workers in the United States.* Berkeley, CA: University of California Press.

Johnson, J. V., & Hall, E. M. (1988). Job strain, work place social support, and cardiovascular disease: A cross-sectional study of a random sample of the Swedish working population. *American Journal of Public Health, 78,* 1336–1342.

Karasek, R. A., Jr. (1979). Job demands, job decision latitude, and mental strain: Implications for job. *Administrative Science Quarterly, 24,* 285–308.

Kearney, G. D., Rodriguez, G., Arcury, J. T., Quandt, S. A., & Arcury, T. A. (2015). Work safety climate, safety behaviors, and occupational injuries of youth farmworkers in North Carolina. *American Journal of Public Health, 105,* 1336–1343.

Keifer, M., Rodríguez-Guzmán, J., Watson, J., van Wendel de Joode, B., Mergler, D., & da Silva, A. S. (2016). Worker health and safety and climate change in the Americas: Issues and research needs. *Revista Panamericana de Salud Pública, 40,* 192–197.

Kleinman, A. (1980). *Patients and healers in the context of culture.* Berkeley, CA: University of California Press.

Kleinman, A. (1988). *Illness narratives: Suffering, healing and the human condition.* New York: Basic Press.

Lambert, W. E., Lasarev, M., Muniz, J., Scherer, J., Rothlein, J., Santana, J., et al. (2005). Variation in organophosphate pesticide metabolites in urine of children living in agricultural communities. *Environmental Health Perspectives, 113,* 504–508.

Landsbergis, P. A., Grzywacz, J. G., & LaMontagne, A. D. (2014). Work organization, job insecurity, and occupational health disparities. *American Journal of Industrial Medicine, 57,* 495–515.

Lang, J., Ochsmann, E., Kraus, T., & Lang, J. W. (2012). Psychosocial work stressors as antecedents of musculoskeletal problems: A systematic review and meta-analysis of stability-adjusted longitudinal studies. *Social Science and Medicine, 75,* 1163–1174.

Leatherman, T. (2005). A space of vulnerability in poverty and health: Political-ecology and biocultural analysis. *Ethos, 33,* 46–70.

Leibler, J. H., & Perry, M. J. (2017). Self-reported occupational injuries among industrial beef slaughterhouse workers in the Midwestern United States. *Journal of Occupational and Environmental Hygiene, 14,* 23–30.

Liebman, A. K., Juárez, P. M., Leyva, C., & Corona, A. (2007). A pilot program using promotoras de salud to educate farmworker families about the risk from pesticide exposure. *Journal of Agromedicine, 12,* 33–43.

Luchman, J. N., & González-Morales, M. G. (2013). Demands, control, and support: A meta-analytic review of work characteristics interrelationships. *Journal of Occupational Health Psychology, 18,* 37–52.

Luque, J. S., Mason, M., Reyes-Garcia, C., Hinojosa, A., & Meade, C. D. (2011). Salud es vida: Development of a cervical cancer education curriculum for promotora outreach with Latina farmworkers in rural Southern Georgia. *American Journal of Public Health, 101,* 2233–2235.

Luque, J. S., Monaghan, P., Contreras, R. B., August, E., Baldwin, J. A., Bryant, C. A., et al. (2007). Implementation evaluation of a culturally competent eye injury prevention program for citrus workers in a Florida migrant community. *Progress in Community Health Partnerships, 1,* 359–369.

Marín, A., Carrillo, L., Arcury, T. A., Grzywacz, J. G., Coates, M. L., & Quandt, S. A. (2009). Ethnographic evaluation of a lay health promoter program to reduce occupational injuries among Latino poultry processing workers. *Public Health Reports, 124*(suppl. 1), 36–43.

McCauley, L., Runkle, J. D., Samples, J., Williams, B., Muniz, J. F., Semple, M., et al. (2013). Oregon indigenous farmworkers: Results of promotor intervention on pesticide knowledge and organophosphate metabolite levels. *Journal of Occupational and Environmental Medicine, 55,* 1164–1170.

McDevitt, J. (2010). Compromise is complicity: Why there is no middle road in the struggle to protect day laborers in the United States. *ABA Journal of Labor & Employment Law, 26,* 101–121.

Menzel, N. N., & Shrestha, P. P. (2012). Social marketing to plan a fall prevention program for Latino construction workers. *American Journal of Industrial Medicine, 55,* 729–735.

Mora, D. C., Arcury, T. A., & Quandt, S. A. (2016). Good job, bad job: Occupational perceptions among Latino poultry workers. *American Journal of Industrial Medicine, 59,* 877–886.

Nevin, R. L., Bernt, J., & Hodgson, M. (2017). Association of poultry processing industry exposures with reports of occupational finger amputations: Results of an analysis of OSHA Severe Injury Report (SIR) data. *Journal of Occupational and Environmental Medicine, 59,* e159–e163.

Ochsner, M., Marshall, E., Kimmel, L., Martino, C., Cunningham, R., & Hoffner, K. (2008). Immigrant Latino day laborers in New Jersey: Baseline data from a participatory research project. *New Solutions, 18,* 57–76.

Ochsner, M., Marshall, E. G., Martino, C., Pabelón, M. C., Kimmel, L., & Rostran, D. (2012). Beyond the classroom: A case study of immigrant safety liaisons in residential construction. *New Solutions, 22,* 365–386.

Organista, K. C., & Kubo, A. (2005). Pilot survey of HIV risk and contextual problems and issues of Mexican/Latino migrant day laborers. *Journal of Immigrant Health, 7,* 269–281.

Ornelas, I. J., Allen, C., Vaughan, C., Williams, E. C., & Negi, N. (2015). Vida PURA: A cultural adaptation of screening and brief intervention to reduce unhealthy drinking among Latino day laborers. *Substance Abuse, 36,* 264–271.

Orrenius, P. A., & Zavodny, M. (2009). Do immigrants work in riskier jobs? *Demography, 3,* 535–551.

Prado, J. B., Mulay, P. R., Kasner, E. J., Bojes, H. K., & Calvert, G. M. (2017). Acute pesticide-related illness among farmworkers: Barriers to reporting to public health authorities. *Journal of Agromedicine, 22,* 395–405.

Quandt, S. A., Arcury, T. A., Austin, C. K., & Cabrera, L. F. (2001). Preventing occupational exposure to pesticides: Using participatory research with Latino farmworkers to develop an intervention. *Journal of Immigrant Health, 3,* 85–96.

Quandt, S. A., Arcury, T. A., Austin, C. K., & Saavedra, R. (1998). Farmworker and farmer perceptions of farmworker agricultural chemical exposure in North Carolina. *Human Organization, 57,* 359–368.

Quandt, S. A., Arcury, T. A., Preisser, J. S., Bernert, J. T., & Norton, D. (2001). Environmental and behavioral predictors of salivary cotinine in Latino tobacco workers. *Journal of Occupational and Environmental Medicine, 43,* 844–852.

Quandt, S. A., Arcury-Quandt, A. E., Lawlor, E. J., Carrillo, L., Marín, A. J., Grzywacz, J. G., et al. (2013). 3-D jobs and health disparities: The health implications of Latino chicken catchers' working conditions. *American Journal of Industrial Medicine, 56,* 206–215.

Quandt, S. A., Austin, C. K., Arcury, T. A., Summers, M., & Saavedra, R. (1999). Agricultural chemical training materials for farmworkers: Review and annotated bibliography. *Journal of Agromedicine, 6,* 3–24.

Quandt, S. A., Grzywacz, J. G., Marín, A., Carrillo, L., Coates, M. L., Burke, B., et al. (2006). Illnesses and injuries reported by Latino poultry workers in western North Carolina. *American Journal of Industrial Medicine, 49,* 343–351.

Quandt, S. A., Grzywacz, J. G., Talton, J. W., Trejo, G., Tapia, J., D'Agostino, R. B., Jr., … Arcury, T. A. (2013). Evaluating the effectiveness of a lay health promoter-led community-based participatory pesticide safety intervention with farmworker families. *Health Promotion Practice, 14,* 425–432.

Quandt, S. A., Lane, C. M., Grzywacz, J. G., Marín, A., Carrillo, L., Coates, M. L., & Arcury, T. A. (2004). *La historia de María. [Maria's story].* [Flip chart]. Winston-Salem, NC: Wake Forest School of Medicine.

Quandt, S. A., Lane, C. M., Grzywacz, J. G., Marín, A., Carrillo, L., Coates, M. L., & Arcury, T. A. (2008). *Javier no recibe sup ago. [Javier doesn't get paid].* [Flip chart]. Winston-Salem, NC: Wake Forest School of Medicine.

Quandt, S. A., Pope, C. N., Chen, H., Summers, P., & Arcury, T. A. (2015). Longitudinal assessment of blood cholinesterase activities over 2 consecutive years among Latino nonfarmworkers and pesticide-exposed farmworkers in North Carolina. *Journal of Occupational and Environmental Medicine, 57,* 851–857.

Quandt, S. A., Walker, F. O., Talton, J. W., Chen, H., & Arcury, T. A. (2017). Olfactory function in Latino farmworkers over 2 years: Longitudinal exploration of subclinical neurological effects of pesticide exposure. *Journal of Occupational and Environmental Medicine, 59,* 1148–1152.

Quandt, S. A., Walker, F. O., Talton, J. W., Summers, P., Chen, H., McLeod, D. K., et al. (2016). Olfactory function in Latino farmworkers: Subclinical neurological effects of pesticide exposure in a vulnerable population. *Journal of Occupational and Environmental Medicine, 58,* 248–253.

Quandt, S. A., Wiggins, M. F., Chen, H., Bischoff, W. E., & Arcury, T. A. (2013). Heat index in migrant farmworker housing: Implications for rest and recovery from work-related heat stress. *American Journal of Public Health, 103,* e24–e26.

Quesada, J., Hart, L. K., & Bourgois, P. (2011). Structural vulnerability and health: Latino migrant laborers in the United States. *Medical Anthropology, 30,* 339–362.

Quirós-Alcalá, L., Bradman, A., Nishioka, M., Harnly, M. E., Hubbard, A., McKone, T. E., et al. (2011). Pesticides in house dust from urban and farmworker households in California: An observational measurement study. *Environmental Health, 10,* 19.

Raanan, R., Balmes, J. R., Harley, K. G., Gunier, R. B., Magzamen, S., Bradman, A., et al. (2016). Decreased lung function in 7-year-old children with early-life organophosphate exposure. *Thorax, 71,* 148–153.

Rathod, J. M. (2016). Danger and dignity: Immigrant day laborers and occupational risk. *Seton Hall Law Review, 46,* 813–882.

Rhodes, S. D., Foley, K. L., Zometa, C. S., & Bloom, F. R. (2007). Lay health advisor interventions among s/Latinos: A qualitative systematic review. *American Journal of Preventive Medicine, 33,* 418–427.

Rhodes, S. D., Hergenrather, K. C., Bloom, F. R., Leichliter, J. S., & Montaño, J. (2009). Outcomes from a community-based, participatory lay health adviser HIV/STD prevention intervention for recently arrived immigrant Latino men in rural North Carolina. *AIDS Education and Prevention, 21*(5 Suppl), 103–108.

Rodriguez, G., Trejo, G., Schiemann, E., Quandt, S. A., Daniel, S. S., Sandberg, J. C., et al. (2016). Latina workers in North Carolina: Work organization, domestic responsibilities, health, and family life. *Journal of Immigrant and Minority Health, 18,* 687–696.

Rosenbaum, D. A., Grzywacz, J. G., Chen, H., Arcury, T. A., Schulz, M. R., Blocker, J. N., et al. (2013). Prevalence of epicondylitis, rotator cuff syndrome, and low back pain in Latino poultry workers and manual laborers. *American Journal of Industrial Medicine, 56,* 226–234.

Rowe, C., Gunier, R., Bradman, A., Harley, K. G., Kogut, K., Parra, K., et al. (2016). Residential proximity to organophosphate and carbamate pesticide use during pregnancy, poverty during childhood, and cognitive functioning in 10-year-old children. *Environmental Research, 150,* 128–137.

Sagransky, M. J., Pichardo-Geisinger, R. O., Muñoz-Ali, D., Feldman, S. R., Mora, D. C., & Quandt, S. A. (2012). Pachydermodactyly from repetitive motion in poultry processing workers: A report of 2 cases. *Archives of Dermatology, 148,* 925–928.

Salazar, M. K., Keifer, M., Negrete, M., Estrada, F., & Synder, K. (2005). Occupational risk among orchard workers: A descriptive study. *Family & Community Health, 28,* 239–252.

Salvatore, A. L., Castorina, R., Camacho, J., Morga, N., López, J., Nishioka, M., et al. (2015). Home-based community health worker intervention to reduce pesticide exposures to farmworkers' children: A randomized-controlled trial. *Journal of Exposure Science & Environmental Epidemiology, 25,* 608–615.

Sauter, S. L., Brightwell, W. S., Colligan, M. J., Hurrell, J. J., Katz, T. M., LeGrande, D. E., … Tetrick, L. E. (2002). *The changing organization of work and the safety and health of working people: Knowledge gaps and research directions.* DHHS (NIOSH) Publication, 2002-116. Cincinnati, OH: National Institute for Occupational Safety and Health.

Sexsmith, K. (2016). Exit, voice, constrained loyalty, and entrapment: Migrant farmworkers and the expression of discontent on New York dairy farms. *Citizenship Studies, 20,* 311–325.

Shrestha, P. P., & Menzel, N. N. (2014). Construction workers and assertiveness training. *Work, 49,* 517–522.

Snyder, L. A., Krauss, A. D., Chen, P. Y., Finlinson, S., & Huang, Y.-H. (2008). Occupational safety: Application of the job demand-control-support model. *Accident Analysis and Prevention, 40,* 1713–1723.

Spector, J. T., Bonauto, D. K., Sheppard, L., Busch-Isaksen, T., Calkins, M., Adams, D., et al. (2016). A case-crossover study of heat exposure and injury risk in outdoor agricultural workers. *PLoS ONE, 11,* e0164498.

Spector, J., Krenz, J., & Blank, K. (2015). Risk factors for heat-related illness in Washington crop workers. *Journal of Agromedicine, 20,* 349–359.

Stein, L. J., Gunier, R. B., Harley, K., Kogut, K., Bradman, A., & Eskenazi, B. (2016). Early childhood adversity potentiates the adverse association between prenatal organophosphate pesticide exposure and child IQ: The CHAMACOS cohort. *Neurotoxicology, 56,* 180–187.

Striffler, S. (2005). *Chicken: The dangerous transformation of America's favorite food.* New Haven, CT: Yale University Press.

Swanberg, J. E., Clouser, J. M., Browning, S. R., Westneat, S. C., & Marsh, M. K. (2013). Occupational health among Latino horse and crop workers in Kentucky: The role of work organization factors. *Journal of Agromedicine, 18,* 312–325.

Thompson, B., Coronado, G. D., Grossman, J. E., Puschel, K., Solomon, C. C., Islas, I., … Fenske, R. A. (2003). Pesticide take-home pathway among children of agricultural workers: Study design, methods, and baseline findings. *Journal of Occupational and Environmental Medicine, 45,* 42–53.

Thompson, B., Griffith, W. C., Barr, D. B., Coronado, G. D., Vigoren, E. M., & Faustman, E. M. (2014). Variability in the take-home pathway: Farmworkers and non-farmworkers and their children. *Journal of Exposure Science & Environmental Epidemiology, 24,* 522–531.

Toossi, M. (2015). Labor force projections to 2024. *Monthly Labor Review,* December. http://www.bls.gov/opub/mlr/2015/article/labor-force-projections-to-2024.htm.

Tovar-Aguilar, J. A., Monaghan, P. F., Bryant, C. A., Esposito, A., Wade, M., … Ruiz, O. (2014). Improving eye safety in citrus harvest crews through the acceptance of personal protective equipment, community-based participatory research, social marketing, and community health workers. *Journal of Agromedicine, 19,* 107–116.

Vallejos, Q. M., Quandt, S. A., Grzywacz, J. G., Isom, S., Chen, H., … Galván, L. (2011). Migrant farmworkers' housing conditions across an agricultural season in North Carolina. *American Journal of Industrial Medicine, 54,* 533–544.

Vandenberg, L. N., Blumberg, B., Antoniou, M. N., Benbrook, C. M., Carroll, L., … Colborn, T. (2017). Is it time to reassess current safety standards for glyphosate-based herbicides? *Journal of Epidemiology and Community Health, 71,* 613–618.

Walter, N., Bougois, P., Loinaz, H. M., & Schillinger, D. (2002). Social context of work injury among undocumented day laborers in San Francisco. *Journal of General Internal Medicine, 17,* 221–229.

Walter, N., Bourgois, P., & Loinaz, H. M. (2004). Masculinity and undocumented labor migration: Injured Latino day laborers in San Francisco. *Social Science and Medicine, 59,* 1159–1168.

Welton, M., DeJoy, D., Castellanos, M. E., Ebell, M., Shen, Y., & Robb, S. (2017). Ethnic disparities of perceived safety climate among construction workers in Georgia, 2015. *Journal of Racial and Ethnic Health Disparities.* https://doi.org/10.1007/s40615-017-0394-5. [Epub ahead of print].

Whalley, L. E., Grzywacz, J. G., Quandt, S. A., Vallejos, Q. M., Walkup, M., Chen, H., … Arcury, T. A. (2009). Migrant farmworker field and camp safety and sanitation in eastern North Carolina. *Journal of Agromedicine, 14,* 421–436.

Wiggins, M. (2009). Farm labor and the struggle for justice in the Eastern United States fields (pp. 201–220). In T. A. Arcury & S. A. Quandt (Eds.), *Latino farmworkers in the eastern United States: Health, safety, and justice* (pp. 201–220). New York: Springer.

Williams, Q., Jr., Ochsner, M., Marshall, E., Kimmel, L., & Martino, C. (2010). The impact of a peer-led participatory health and safety training program for Latino day laborers in construction. *Journal of Safety Research, 41,* 253–261.

Zohar, D. (1980). Safety climate in industrial organizations: Theoretical and applied implications. *Journal of Applied Psychology, 65,* 96–102.

Zohar, D. (2010). Thirty years of safety climate research: Reflections and future directions. *Accident Analysis and Prevention, 42,* 1517–1522.

Chapter 10
The Health and Well-Being of Latinx Sexual and Gender Minorities in the USA: A Call to Action

Scott D. Rhodes, Lilli Mann-Jackson, Jorge Alonzo, Jonathan C. Bell, Amanda E. Tanner, Omar Martínez, Florence M. Simán, Timothy S. Oh, Benjamin D. Smart, Jesus Felizzola and Ronald A. Brooks

Abstract Latinx sexual and gender minority (SGM) persons, specifically lesbian, gay, bisexual, transgender, queer, and intersex (LGBTQI) persons, experience profound health disparities based on multiple factors, including their ethnicity/race, sexual orientation, gender identity, and immigration status. Although the terms SGM and LGBTQI arc often used as umbrella terms, the communities and populations described by these terms are deeply varied. Currently, SGM persons are increasingly open and visible in the USA and many other parts of the world, and a modest body of knowledge on the health and well-being of some SGM subgroups currently exists. However, there are profound gaps in this emerging knowledge base. Specifically, we know very little about the health and well-being of Latinx SGM persons in the USA. In this chapter, we define some of the key terms often used to describe communities and populations of SGM, highlight some of the health disparities experienced by Latinx SGM populations, and outline critical research needs and priorities to improve the health and well-being of Latinx SGM populations.

S. D. Rhodes (✉) · L. Mann-Jackson · J. Alonzo · J. C. Bell · B. D. Smart
Department of Social Sciences and Health Policy, Wake Forest School of Medicine, Winston-Salem, NC, USA
e-mail: srhodes@wakehealth.edu

A. E. Tanner
Department of Public Health Education, University of North Carolina Greensboro, Greensboro, NC, USA

O. Martínez
School of Social Work, Temple University, Philadelphia, PA, USA

F. M. Simán
El Pueblo, Inc., Raleigh, NC, USA

T. S. Oh
McGaw Medical Center of Northwestern University, Chicago, IL, USA

J. Felizzola
Department of Psychology, George Washington University, Washington, D.C., WA, USA

R. A. Brooks
Department of Family Medicine, UCLA David Geffen School of Medicine, Los Angeles, CA, USA

© Springer Nature Switzerland AG 2020
A. D. Martínez and S. D. Rhodes (eds.), *New and Emerging Issues in Latinx Health*, https://doi.org/10.1007/978-3-030-24043-1_10

Keywords Latinx · Gay · Bisexual · Lesbian · Transgender · Queer · Intersex · Gender minority · Sexual minority · Discrimination · Disparities

Defining Sexual Orientation and Gender Identity

Sexual orientation and gender identity are complex constructs that are highly contingent upon cultural and social contexts, which may vary by place and shift over time. Sexuality encompasses at least three critical components: sexual identity, sexual attraction, and sexual behavior. Sexual identity is an individual's own perception of their overall sexual self. For many individuals, their sexual identity, such as "lesbian", "gay", "bisexual", or "heterosexual", may seem consistent with their sexual attraction and behaviors, but for some, sexual identity may seem inconsistent with attraction and/or behavior. For example, a man whose primary sexual partner is a woman may identify as heterosexual yet may have sex with men. There are also individuals who do not identify with traditional categories of sexual orientation or who identify with other terms such as "queer" or with identities that fall outside these categories, such as pansexual or asexual.

Queer is another umbrella term for sexual and gender minority (SGM) persons who do not identify as heterosexual or cisgender (i.e., non-transgender). In the late nineteenth century, some communities and cultures began using queer as a pejorative term for people who had same-sex attraction or appeared outside traditional gender norms, usually gay men. Then in the late 1980s, SGM activists worked to claim the word, embracing the queer label as a proud rebellion and politically radical symbol in place of "lesbian", "gay", "bisexual", and "transgender".

Gender refers to the psychological, cultural, or behavioral traits that a culture associates with the female and male sex. Gender is different from the sex of a person. Transgender generally refers to persons whose gender identity, or self-concept, differs from the sex they were assigned at birth according to the physiological characteristics of their bodies; gender identity is often manifested externally as gender expression. For example, a transgender woman is a person whose sex assigned at birth was male but whose sense of self is female. It is important not to conflate sexual orientation and gender identity because they are separate constructs; for example, a transgender person may have a heterosexual, bisexual, lesbian, or gay sexual identity, or may not identify with any of these labels.

Gender identity exists across a spectrum. Some may not adhere to socially and culturally constructed norms and expectations that generally define women and men and the associated qualities of what is feminine or masculine. They may not identify exclusively as female or male; they may identify as both, neither, or a combination of the two. For example, some may identify as non-binary, queer, genderqueer, or gender fluid, as examples (Baldwin et al., 2018; Lykens, LeBlanc, & Bockting, 2018). People may also identify and express themselves more as one gender some of the time and as another gender at other times. Such variability among personal identity makes these overarching constructs inherently complex and individualized.

Intersex is a general term encompassing a variety of conditions wherein a person is born with reproductive or sexual anatomy that does not fit typical definitions of female and male, or their reproductive or sexual anatomy may correspond to a combination of both. Intersex persons may be born with sex chromosomes, external genitalia, or internal reproductive systems that are not considered "typical" for either female or male, or their reproductive or sexual anatomy may correspond to a combination of both female and male. The existence of intersex persons shows that there are not just two sexes and that classical ways of thinking about sex and gender (trying to force individuals to fit into either the female category or the male category) are socially constructed.

Challenges to Understanding the Health of SGM Persons

Understanding the health and well-being of SGM populations, including lesbian, gay, bisexual, transgender, queer, and intersex (LGBTQI) persons, is stymied by several factors. First, it is difficult for researchers to consistently define and measure sexual orientation and gender identity. As noted previously, while some persons may be consistent across the three dimensions of sexual orientation (identity, attraction, and behavior), others may not be. For example, in a recent community-based sample of Latinx gay, bisexual, and other men who have sex with men (GBMSM) and transgender persons, more than 5% self-identified as heterosexual, 23% self-identified as bisexual, and 10% reported sex with both women and men. Additionally, 6% self-identified as male-to-female transgender (Rhodes et al., 2017). Furthermore, some transgender persons may not be familiar with the language used around sexual orientation and gender identity. They may conflate sexual orientation and gender identity, as do many cisgender persons, or have language preferences, preferring either the use of the term "transgender" or the gender they identify with (i.e., "female" or "male") without using the term "transgender."

To illustrate the relevance of language, in one of a community-based participatory research (CBPR) study in the US South (Rhodes, Alonzo, et al., 2018), a Spanish-speaking Latinx participant who presented with gender characteristics typically associated with female identity (e.g., skirt, long hair, make-up, and women's shoes) did not self-identify as transgender or female despite multiple opportunities during an interviewer-administered Spanish-language quantitative assessment. After data collection was complete, the interviewer asked the participant further about the participant's understanding of what it meant to be transgender. The participant explained that in order to identify as transgender, the participant would need breast implants; without surgical intervention, the participant explained they were "transvestite."

It is important to carefully select the words designed to measure and understand sexual orientation and gender identity. A common approach to measuring gender identity includes assessing one's sex assignment at birth (i.e., female or male) and the gender that one currently identifies with. However, even with this approach, definitions and meanings may not be congruent across individuals, communities, or populations. Not only can sexual orientation and gender identity be difficult to operationalize, but measurement is also further complicated by time; orientation and identity may evolve over time and across the life course.

Another factor that limits an understanding of SGM populations is the reluctance of some individuals to identify themselves to others, including researchers, practitioners, and providers. In many cultures, sexual orientation and gender identity are very sensitive topics. SGM persons have historically faced discrimination, stigmatization, and marginalization. Thus, SGM persons are often reluctant or not willing to disclose their SGM status in particular contexts or settings. For Latinx SGM persons in the USA, discrimination, stigmatization, and marginalization may be particularly acute because of the intersecting identities known as intersectionality: being both Latinx and SGM persons. Moreover, SGM persons may have experienced violence or physical harm because of their identity.

Finally, while there are numerous studies of SGM samples, particularly within the HIV prevention, care, and treatment literature, these samples tend to be small and/or non-representative convenience samples. Unfortunately, sexual orientation and gender identity are not assessed on most national or state surveys (e.g., US Census), making it difficult to estimate the size of SGM populations and obtain an understanding of the health and well-being of SGM persons. Given the intense scrutiny, racism, and anti-immigrant sentiment and rhetoric that Latinx persons face in the USA, Latinx SGM populations may have increased rates of (1) non-participation in sampling efforts, (2) item non-response (which happens when a respondent provides some information but not all), and (3) socially desirable answers. Thus, because of the lack of precise measurement and the likelihood that Latinx SGM persons understandably can be reluctant to participate in research or share information about their sexual orientation and gender identity, what we know about their health and well-being is extremely limited.

The Health and Well-Being of Latinx SGM Persons in the USA

Epidemiology

It is estimated that about 6.1% of all Latinx persons in the USA identify as SGM persons, one of the highest rates by ethnicity/race (Kastanis & Gates, 2010; Newport, 2018); thus, there are more than three million Latinx persons in the USA who identify as SGM persons. SGM persons across all ethnic/racial groups face profound health disparities and inequities linked to discrimination, stigma, and marginalization, and to be clear, marginalization includes the denial of civil and human rights. Discrimination, stigmatization, and marginalization have been associated with high rates of psychiatric disorders, post-traumatic stress disorder (often associated with immigration), substance abuse, and suicide among Latinx SGM persons (Almeida, Johnson, Corliss, Molnar, & Azrael, 2009; Bostwick et al., 2014; O'Donnell, Meyer, & Schwartz, 2011). Experiences of violence and victimization are frequent for SGM persons and have long-lasting effects on SGM persons and communities. Personal, family, and social acceptance of sexual orientation and gender identity also affects the mental health and personal safety of SGM persons. Latinx SGM persons face disproportional challenges compared to their non-Latinx counterparts related to immigration; homelessness; discrimination, harassment, victimization, and violence; mental health disorders; suicide; tobacco, alcohol, and other drug use; obesity; cancer; and sexually transmitted infections (STIs) and HIV.

Immigration

There are up to one million immigrant SGM adults in the USA, and it is estimated that about 30% of these immigrants are undocumented (Gates, 2013). There are direct relationships between anti-immigration policies and their effects on access to health services and health outcomes among undocumented individuals. As a result of these policies, undocumented immigrants experience negative mental health outcomes, including depression, anxiety, and post-traumatic stress disorder. Undocumented Latinx SGM face multiple challenges in the USA related to decreased access to needed services and medical care, economic insecurity, and violence and harassment (Martinez et al., 2015; Rhodes et al., 2015).

Studies have also found pervasive mistreatment of SGM persons by U.S. Immigration and Customs Enforcement (ICE) or while in ICE custody (Burns, Garcia, & Wolgin, 2013). One report indicated that one in five substantiated sexual abuse and assault cases in ICE facilities involved transgender detainees, who only comprise one in 500 ICE detainees (United States Government Accountability Office, 2013). Immigration, as it relates to health and well-being, must be further studied among immigrant SGM persons.

Furthermore, the US legal system may not serve immigrant SGM persons well. Attorneys may hold biases and prejudices about SGM persons and/or may lack training on working with SGM persons, the very persons they are to serve (Yamanis et al., 2018).

Homelessness

It is well established that SGM persons are disproportionately affected by homelessness. About 1.6 million young persons experience homelessness in the USA every year, and 40% of these are SGM persons. Currently, limited data are available to describe the rates of homelessness specifically among SGM of color, including Latinx persons. However, in the few studies that have explored ethnicity and race among homeless SGM persons, homeless SGM persons tend to be disproportionately persons of color (Page, 2017).

While homeless Latinx heterosexual persons, including youth, are highly vulnerable to discrimination and victimization because of their ethnicity, homeless Latinx SGM persons are even more vulnerable than their Latinx heterosexual counterparts. This reflects the intersection and compounded effects of ethnicity/race, sexual orientation, and gender identity. At the same time, homeless Latinx SGM persons are more likely to engage in risky behaviors such as substance use and survival sex compared to their non-Latinx counterparts (Keuroghlian, Shtasel, & Bassuk, 2014; Page, 2017). These behaviors also tend to cluster with experiences of discrimination and victimization, depression, internalized homophobia and homo-negativity, and transphobia among homeless Latinx SGM persons.

Acceptance, approval, and support from family members can play a role in predicting one's likelihood of becoming homeless. Many homeless SGM youth run away from family or are rejected and forced out of their home by parents/guardians because of their sexual orientation or gender identity. They may have experienced emotional and/or financial neglect. They may also have been subjected to physical, emotional, or sexual abuse at home. Homeless SGM may fall through the cracks of "mainstream" youth services or have aged out of the foster care system (Castellanos, 2016; Kane, Nicoll, Kahn, & Groves, 2012; Ream, 2014). The situation may be compounded for some Latinx youth, including SGM youth, who are homeless or are at risk of homelessness because of issues related to their immigration status or the immigration status of family members.

Furthermore, community-based support services for Latinx SGM persons are limited, and the support that is available may seem risky to access. Latinx SGM persons may worry that it might be necessary to provide documents related to immigration status to receive services and that accessing help may lead to detention and deportation. It is important to note that being documented does not necessarily reduce concerns and increase trust and confidence in resources. It is well established that Latinx persons who are documented are still subject to assumptions about their own immigration status, may worry about the legality of their status, and/or may be connected to friends and family members who are undocumented (Rhodes et al., 2014, 2015).

Homeless Latinx SGM persons also may assume that services for homeless persons would not be welcoming to them as Latinx and as SGM persons. In fact, many organizations that serve homeless persons are not prepared to provide culturally congruent services and safe housing for Latinx and SGM persons due to language barriers and gender-segregated facilities, as examples, and some organizations turn away transgender persons seeking services (Chinchilla, 2012).

There has been a slow but steady growth of research on homelessness among SGM persons in the USA. However, much more research is needed including research that explores the intersection of ethnicity/race, sexual orientation, and gender identity as well as immigration status, and the impacts of these identities individually and synergistically on homelessness.

Discrimination, Harassment, Victimization, and Violence

Experiences of discrimination, harassment, victimization, and violence are pervasive among SGM persons, and hate crimes against Latinx and SGM communities continue to be a public health crisis in the USA. Deeply held homophobic and transphobic attitudes, often combined with a lack of adequate legal protection against discrimination on grounds of sexual orientation and gender identity, expose many SGM persons of all ages to egregious violations of their human rights. Over the past decade, the USA has made unprecedented progress toward lesbian, gay, bisexual, transgender, queer, and intersex (LGBTQI) equality; however, to date, neither the federal government nor most states have explicit statutory non-discrimination laws protecting individuals on the basis of sexual orientation and gender identity. Furthermore, it is widely recognized that non-discrimination laws do not always translate to actual fair treatment. These laws, however, can set a precedent and promote an expectation of justice that reduces victimization and violence (Thoreson, 2018; Tilcsik, 2011).

The majority of persons reporting hate crimes related to SGM status are from ethnic/racial minority groups, the largest percentage of which self-identify as Latinx (Criminal Justice Information Services Division, 2018). Incidents include verbal, online, or social media-based harassment; threats and intimidation; and physical violence. Latinx SGM youth, in particular, are common victims of verbal and physical harassment both inside and outside of school settings. Research suggests that 85% of Latinx SGM students experience verbal harassment at school; 58% feel unsafe at school because of their sexual orientation; 43% feel unsafe because of their gender identity; 27% have been physically harassed at school because of their sexual orientation; and 13% have been physically harassed at school because of their gender identity (Kane et al., 2012).

Similarly, roughly one-third of Latinx SGM youth report have been verbally harassed outside of school, compared to less than a quarter of Latinx non-SGM youth. Although 8 in 10 Latinx SGM youth overall report they have been the target of harassment due to their sexual orientation or gender identity, Latinx SGM youth have reported to be very optimistic about their futures. A critical component to the optimism these youth feel may be fueled by their belief that one day they will leave the town where they grew up and where they have experienced discrimination and start a life elsewhere (Kane et al., 2012).

While discrimination, harassment, victimization, and violence profoundly affect SGM persons in the USA, transgender persons are impacted even more heavily. In one seminal study, 26% of transgender persons reported losing a job due to anti-transgender bias; 50% reported being harassed at work; 20% reported being evicted or denied housing; and 78% of transgender students reported being harassed or assaulted (James et al., 2016). The data indicate an even more dire situation for Latinx persons who are also transgender. They are most at risk for discrimination, harassment, victimization, and violence in the USA. In the school system alone, 77% of Latinx transgender persons in grades kindergarten through 12 reported experiences of harassment; 36% reported physical assault; and 13% reported sexual assault.

Moreover, 21% of Latinx transgender students experienced harassment so severe that they left their school, and 9% were expelled due to transphobia and racism (National Center for Transgender Equality, 2012). It is important to note that perpetrators of discrimination, harassment, victimization, and violence are not just peers but also teachers and school administrators. Moreover, the lack of policies protecting SGM persons, inside and outside of school, compounds the potential for discrimination, harassment, victimization, and violence.

It is also important to acknowledge the profoundly negative impact of the statements, actions, and policies of the US federal government under President Donald Trump on the lives of Latinx SGM persons. The highly charged political climate and anti-immigrant rhetoric and actions that have been fostered in the USA provide some explanation as to why Latinx persons carry such disproportionate burden of discrimination, harassment, victimization, and violence. Between 2016 and 2017, hate crimes against ethnic/racial minorities including Latinx persons and SGM persons increased by 17% (Levin & Reitzel, 2018). Given that the Trump administration has been so openly antagonistic regarding the issue of immigration, such feelings of fear and prejudice can be reflected by the general population and lead to more acts of discrimination, harassment, victimization, and violence toward persons of color and immigrants, with Latinx SGM persons being especially targeted.

Announcements about discharging transgender service members of the US Armed Services and supporting "religious exemptions" that deny LGBT rights, as examples, only fuel further anti-LGBTQI sentiment and hostility and reduce the health and well-being of SGM persons. Anti-immigration rhetoric, including blatantly hateful speech, is prevalent under the Trump administration and has a deleterious impact on the health and well-being of Latinx SGM persons.

Mental Health

Perhaps nowhere is the impact of intersectionality more relevant than within the field of mental health. As detailed in the previous section, while SGM persons may experience discrimination and micro-aggressions due to homophobia, homo-negativity, and transphobia, ethnic/racial minorities also experience discrimination stemming from racism. An individual experiencing discrimination and aggression from being both a SGM person and an ethnic/racial minority is extremely vulnerable to poor mental health outcomes (Balsam, Molina, Beadnell, Simoni, & Walters, 2011).

There has been some limited research documenting the mental health needs and disparities of ethnic and racial minorities and for SGM, but more research at the intersection of identities is needed. A respondent-driven sampling study of adult Spanish-speaking Latinx GBMSM and transgender women in the US South estimated the prevalence of clinically significant depressive symptoms to be 74.8% (95% confidence interval [CI]: 61.9–80.2). Moderate to high internalized homo-negativity, a measure of homophobia, was 88.5% (95% CI: 83.8–93.6); and perceived day-to-day discrimination was 31.9% (95% CI: 22.7–44.7) (Rhodes et al., 2013).

Discrimination based on homophobia, transphobia, and racism can result in social isolation, low self-esteem, reduced access to healthcare services, and poor mental health outcomes. For example, in a study conducted to assess psychological distress in Latinx gay and bisexual men living in New York, Miami, and Los Angeles, 912 Latinx gay and bisexual men reported high levels of discrimination related to their minority identities, and this discrimination was linked to decreased social support and self-esteem and increased psychological symptoms of distress (Diaz, Ayala, Bein, Henne, & Marin, 2001).

Depression and anxiety among Latinx persons, like most ethnic/racial minority groups, and SGM persons are rooted in a myriad of complicated issues such as discrimination and harassment, substance use, and trauma. Notably, one of the most significant indicators of depression is family acceptance. Family acceptance has been identified as a critical need and priority among Latinx SGM youth and a barrier to "coming out" fully and obtaining the support and resources needed throughout adolescent development. In a study of psychiatric disorders among SGM youth from diverse ethnic/racial groups, SGM persons who came from Latinx families on average had worse mental health outcomes than their non-Latinx counterparts. Family rejection has been directly associated with negative mental health outcomes in adulthood, putting Latinx SGM persons at a markedly higher risk for developing depression and anxiety (Russell & Fish, 2016).

Suicide

SGM youth have higher rates of suicidal ideation, suicide attempts, and suicides than their non-SGM counterparts. Lifetime attempted suicide rates range from 10 to 40% among sexual minority persons (i.e., lesbian, gay, and bisexual) as opposed to 0.4–5.1% among sexual majority persons (i.e., heterosexual). Among SGM youth, Latinx and American Indian youth have the highest rates of suicide of all ethnic/racial groups (Bostwick et al., 2014). Although Black and White SGM youth are more likely to report suicidal ideation, Latinx SGM youth have the highest reported frequency of suicide attempts. Latinx SGM youth are more than twice as likely to attempt suicide compared to their Latinx non-SGM counterparts (Bostwick et al., 2014; O'Donnell et al., 2011).

In a large study of youth ages 11–19, female-to-male transgender adolescents reported the highest rate of attempted suicide (50.8%), followed by adolescents who identified as not exclusively male or female (41.8%), male-to-female adolescents (29.9%), and questioning adolescents (27.9%). Notable for transgender adolescents, no other sociodemographic characteristic, besides gender identity, was associated with suicide attempts (Toomey, Syvertsen, & Shramko, 2018).

Tobacco, Alcohol, and Other Drug Use

Use of tobacco products, particularly cigarettes, is highly prevalent among SGM persons in the USA. It is estimated that about 21% of SGM adults smoke compared to 15% of their non-SGM counterparts. Limited data exist on tobacco use, including cigarette smoking, among transgender persons; however, cigarette smoking prevalence is reported to be higher among transgender persons than the general population (Buchting et al., 2017).

The limited available data suggest that Latinx SGM persons have lower prevalence rates of smoking than their non-Latinx SGM counterparts (Agaku et al., 2014; Martell, Garrett, & Caraballo, 2016). However, Latinx SGM do face smoking-related risks given that the tobacco industry has prioritized growing Latinx populations and SGM as markets and has developed targeted advertising for members of these communities (American Lung Association; Office on Smoking and Health, 2018). A respondent-driven sampling study of adult Spanish language-preferring Latinx GBMSM and transgender women in the US South, which is a region with higher rates of overall tobacco use, estimated the prevalence of ever smoking to be 43.8% (95% CI: 31.0–50.1); smoking sometimes to be 36.6% (95% 29.8–48.3); and smoking every day to be 6.4% (2.0–9.8) (Rhodes et al., 2012).

In addition to tobacco, rates of other forms of substance use and abuse are high within SGM communities, including Latinx SGM communities, though more research is needed. Alcohol use has been identified as high within some studies of Latinx persons; however, as with many other health issues, studies may not be designed and implemented in a way that is as culturally congruent as necessary to obtain a full and accurate picture. For example, drinking patterns among Latinx SGM persons may reflect other trends such as "fiesta drinking" (i.e., drinking as a social activity central to social interactions and celebrations rather than as a coping strategy), which may look like high rates of drinking through our measurement tools (e.g., heavy episodic/binge drinking) (Gilbert, Perreira, Eng, & Rhodes, 2014). Other measures that take into consideration associated outcomes of drinking may be more insightful. For example, a measure of weekly drunkenness may better identify risk associated with alcohol use (Daniel-Ulloa et al., 2014; O'Brien et al., 2006). Understanding issues of substance use within Latinx SGM communities is important, and it is essential to understand how substance use affects other facets of health such as sexual behavior and sexual health.

Obesity

Obesity remains a critical public health issue in the USA because of the numerous associated health risks and consequences. Compared to their heterosexual counterparts, gay and bisexual men have a lower body mass index (BMI) and decreased odds of being overweight or obese. Among women, the relationship between orientation and weight is inverse; studies have consistently concluded that lesbian women have an increased likelihood of being overweight and obese compared with heterosexual women (Deputy & Boehmer, 2014). Furthermore, higher rates of obesity have been documented among Latinx sexual minority women than non-Latinx sexual minority women (Newlin Lew, Dorsen, Melkus, & Maclean, 2018).

Some studies also indicate that gender minority persons are more likely to be obese than their cisgender counterparts (VanKim et al., 2014). More research is needed to understand weight and obesity specifically among Latinx SGM persons.

Cancer

Behaviors such as smoking, alcohol consumption, unprotected sex, having multiple sexual partners, and having sex at earlier ages all put SGM persons at a higher risk of developing various types of cancers in later years (Rosario et al., 2014). Diagnoses of cancers including esophageal, colon, and lung are correlated with smoking and heavy drinking, behaviors which SGM persons are at increased risk of engaging in. Having multiple sex partners, having unprotected sex, and having sex at earlier ages put SGM persons at a higher risk of exposure to cancer-related pathogens like human papillomavirus (HPV). HPV is commonly contracted through anal, vaginal, and oral sex and later can lead to the development of anal, cervical, vulvar, vaginal, penile, and oropharyngeal cancers. Latinx populations, generally, also have disproportionately high rates of some types of cancer, particularly infection-related cancers such as stomach cancer, liver cancer, and cancers caused by HPV, as well as gallbladder cancer (American Red Cross, 2018). However, in spite of these elevated risks, few studies have explored the intersection of these cancer disparities among Latinx SGM.

Sexually Transmitted Infections (STIs) and HIV

The Latinx population living in the USA is severely affected by the STI and HIV epidemics. Rates of gonorrhea, chlamydia, and syphilis are two to four times higher among Latinx persons compared to non-Latinx Whites. The Latinx population has the second highest rate of AIDS diagnoses among all ethnic and racial groups, accounting for nearly 20% of the total number of new AIDS cases reported each year; that is three times the rate of new cases among non-Latinx Whites (Centers for Disease Control and Prevention, 2017).

The rate of new HIV diagnoses among GBMSM is more than 44 times that of other men. Latinx persons accounted for 24% of all HIV diagnoses among GBMSM in 2015, compared to 39 and 31% for non-Latinx Black and White GBMSM, respectively; this HIV burden is disproportionate to the percentage of GBMSM overall who are Latinx. Latinx GBMSM in the USA accounted for 85% of HIV diagnoses among Latinx men in 2015. HIV incidence among Latinx GBMSM increased by 25.4% from 2008 to 2015, while it remained relatively stable among non-Latinx Black GBMSM and decreased among White GBMSM (Centers for Disease Control and Prevention, 2017). If current HIV diagnosis rates persist, one in four Latinx GBMSM may be diagnosed with HIV during their lifetime (Hess, Hu, Lansky, Mermin, & Hall, 2016).

Additionally, while it has been estimated that up to one in four transgender women is living with HIV (Herbst et al., 2008; Lippman et al., 2015) and some studies of transgender women have found prevalence as high as 39% (Rapues, Wilson, Packer, Colfax, & Raymond, 2013), current estimates suggest that around 14% of transgender women and 3% of transgender men in the USA have HIV (Becasen, Denard, Mullins, Higa, & Sipe, 2018). Latinx transgender women are particularly affected by HIV (Habarta, Wang, Mulatu, & Larish, 2015; Kellogg, Clements-Nolle, Dilley, Katz, & McFarland, 2001; Nuttbrock et al., 2009; Rapues et al., 2013). Furthermore, it is well established that many transgender persons have higher rates of not being screened, and thus, are unaware of their HIV status (Habarta et al., 2015; Lippman et al., 2015). In fact, it is estimated that less than half of all transgender women with HIV know their status (Herbst et al., 2008). It is important to note, however, that many studies of sexual behavior and related health outcomes such as HIV are not based on representative samples. They often are based on small and/or convenience samples. Research is needed to better understand sexual health among Latinx GSM persons.

Theory, Community Engagement, and Latinx SGM Populations

Beyond the Individual

The root causes of health inequities and disparities are complex; factors at multiple levels, including biological, individual, sociocultural, neighborhood, structural, and policy, profoundly influence Latinx health and well-being. However, many of the models used to explain and intervene on inequities and disparities experienced by Latinx SGM persons are based on individual factors (i.e., intra- and interpersonal). For example, when we think of increasing the uptake of pre-exposure prophylaxis (PrEP) for HIV prevention among Latinx SGM persons, our first impulse may be to increase awareness, knowledge, and intention to use PrEP among individual Latinx persons considered to be at risk for HIV. Perhaps some, but overall very little, focus is given to the sociocultural, neighborhood, structural, and policy factors that potentially influence uptake. To make the necessary strides needed to increase PrEP uptake, it is critical to understand the role of an individual's community in influencing uptake, including but not limited to stigma; and whether access to LGBT- or Latinx-focused community organizations influence uptake, as examples. It is also important to better understand the roles that various policies play in PrEP uptake. Our research has illustrated that a security guard at a clinic, for example, can have a profoundly chilling effect on whether that clinic is visited by Latinx persons, among other populations. The use of one's preferred name and their preferred pronouns can also make a profound difference in terms of whether a community resource is viewed as friendly. In our work with immigrant Latinx transgender persons, we have seen improvements at health and medical care institutions. However, other service providers and community resources including regional Consulates have been slower to adopt inclusive policies, and the feelings of discrimination and the challenges faced in one setting by Latinx GSM persons bleed into other arenas, discouraging the use of needed resources, including PrEP access and uptake.

Moreover, policy issues such as not allowing access to driver's licenses for undocumented persons and a state's refusal to participate in Medicaid expansion profoundly influence the health of Latinx persons generally and Latinx SGM persons in particular. It may not only be the actual policy that is affecting health (e.g., not having a driver's license or not having health insurance coverage) but also the context in which that policy occurs. Not allowing undocumented persons access to driver's licenses and not expanding Medicaid, as examples, send negative messages to the entire community about perceptions and values regarding marginalized communities that can promulgate discrimination, harassment, victimization, and violence. These messages also can become internalized and affect how Latinx SGM persons feel about themselves.

Thus, explanatory models that blend theories to identify and explore the multilevel influences on Latinx SGM health are likely to be effective in guiding priorities to reduce health inequities and disparities. To create lasting change, political will must be garnered to intervene on macro-level influences (e.g., structures and policies). Health, after all, is indeed political. Thus, in addition to explanatory theories that include multiple levels of influence and theories of community organizing and social change and action must be harnessed to affect the multilevel factors that influence the health of Latinx SGM persons.

Community-Engaged Research

At the same time, theories must be blended with the real-world experiences of Latinx SGM persons and measurement for research and evaluation must align. Community-engaged research has emerged as an approach to increase health equity, reduce health disparities, and promote health by building bridges among community members, those who serve communities through service delivery and practice, and researchers. Incorporating the experiences of community members—who are experts in their lived experiences and their community's needs, priorities, and assets—and the perspectives of community organization representatives and sound science can promote deeper and more informed understandings of health-related phenomena and the identification of actions (e.g., interventions, programs, policies, and system changes) that are more relevant; culturally congruent; and likely to be effective, sustained, and scalable, if warranted (Kost et al., 2017; Rhodes, Tanner, Mann-Jackson, Alonzo, Simán, et al., 2018; Wolfson et al., 2017). Furthermore, by working in partnership *with* rather than merely working *in* communities, those applying community-engaged research approaches may strengthen a community's overall capacity to problem-solve and address subsequent community priorities beyond the current research goal. CBPR is a form of community-engaged research in which community members are equal partners sharing leadership with academic researchers throughout the entire research process (Rhodes, 2014; Rhodes, Tanner, Mann-Jackson, Alonzo, Simán, et al., 2018; Rhodes, Tanner, Mann-Jackson, Alonzo, Horridge, et al., 2018).

Research Needs and Priorities

Measurement

There are profound gaps in our understanding of the health and well-being of Latinx SGM persons. As noted, some of these gaps exist because of the lack of adequate measurement of sexual orientation and gender identity within existing epidemiologic research. The stigma and discrimination based on ethnicity/race and SGM status that many Latinx SGM persons experience also contribute to difficulty reaching these populations through research; Latinx SGM persons may not participate in research or disclose their orientations or identities. New and effective strategies for building trust with, recruiting and retaining, and collecting meaningful data from Latinx SGM persons in research studies must be developed and applied.

Bias

Furthermore, it is not beyond comprehension that funding for Latinx SGM research is stymied by unconscious bias. Bias is insidious; it is very difficult to recognize and acknowledge. Unconscious or involuntary biases include social stereotypes about certain groups, e.g., Latinx SGM persons, that individuals from outside their own conscious awareness. Mostly everyone holds unconscious beliefs about communities, populations, and subgroups, and these biases stem from one's tendency to organize and categorize "others." Unconscious bias is much more prevalent than conscious prejudice, and it is often incompatible with one's own conscious values. Thus, our lack of understanding and the health inequities and disparities that Latinx SGM experience may be related to the unconscious biases that affect how resources related to both research and practice are allocated and used. Additionally, many of the macro-level factors shaping Latinx SGM health are politically charged (e.g., immigration enforcement and transgender rights), and local, state, and national political climates may also contribute to challenges securing funding for and implementing studies to understand and address these factors.

Rigor

Furthermore, there is a profound need for data from representative samples to understand the prevalence of health behaviors and outcomes. Very little is known about the health of Latinx SGM persons outside of sexual health. Approaches such as respondent-driven sampling, as well as the addition of items to collect data on sexual orientation and gender identity on larger national surveys, can help to address these gaps. Moreover, future research must be rigorous and sound.

Multilevel Determinants

There is a need for studies that identify the unique health needs and priorities of Latinx SGM populations and the most culturally congruent strategies to arrange healthcare service access and delivery for these populations to ameliorate the health disparities they experience. Furthermore, strategies must move beyond individual-level factors influencing health and well-being and tackle some of the macro-level factors affecting Latinx SGM populations. Interventions designed to reduce disparities have focused primarily on individual factors. Rigorously evaluated, evidence-based structural interventions are needed to address multilevel structural factors that systemically lead to and perpetuate inequities (Brown et al., 2019; Rhodes, Leichliter, Sun, & Bloom, 2016).

To illustrate with an example, rather than only focusing on felt stigma among Latinx sexual minority women (e.g., Latinx lesbian women), there is a need for strategies to change the structures that contribute to stigma. Sexual minority women are often assumed to not be at risk for HPV; as a result, they tend to have lower rates of HPV vaccination and cervical cancer screening (Quinn et al., 2015). Frontline staff, nurses, and other providers need better training on meeting the needs of SGM persons. They must not assume one's health-related needs and risks, and systems must be in a place that ensures each person receives the care they need.

It is also well documented that providers are less likely to recommend HPV vaccination for Latinx adolescents (Ylitalo, Lee, & Mehta, 2013), in spite of evidence that Latinx families are more receptive and responsive to provider recommendations than non-Latinx families (Galbraith et al., 2016). These low rates of recommendation may be related to healthcare provider perceptions that Latinx parents may be less accepting of the HPV vaccination due to cultural norms related to discussing sexuality or concerns that HPV vaccination may condone early sexual activity (Galbraith et al., 2016). To be effective, training for providers and other clinic staff must move beyond workplace diversity or cultural competency workshops; instead, training should raise the consciousness of providers and other clinic staff about these disparities and their potential role in either reducing or perpetuating them and should be fundamental to the professional preparation of providers and other clinic staff.

Summary

Latinx SGM carry a high burden of morbidity and mortality across many health issues, yet their unique needs are often overlooked in research, policy, and practice. It is essential that this shifts in order to promote the overall health of persons within these vulnerable and marginalized populations. Profound gaps exist in the emerging knowledge base on the health and well-being of Latinx SGM persons, including but not limited to immigration; homelessness; discrimination, harassment, victimization, and violence; mental health disorders; suicide; tobacco, alcohol, and other drug use; obesity; cancer; and STIs and HIV. To fill these gaps, we must move beyond the individual and explore factors at multiple levels, including at the biological, individual, sociocultural, neighborhood, structural, and policy levels, that profoundly influence Latinx health and well-being. We must blend theories, apply authentic community-engaged research approaches, develop better measurement, address biases in our funding practices and prioritization, improve rigor, and address the multilevel determinants of health and well-being. This chapter is not only a summary of what we know about the health of Latinx SGM persons, but also it is a call for action for one of our most vulnerable and marginalized communities. There is much work to be done.

References

Agaku, I. T., King, B. A., Husten, C. G., Bunnell, R., Ambrose, B. K., Hu, S. S., … Day, H. R. (2014). Tobacco product use among adults–United States, 2012-2013. *MMWR Morbidity & Mortality Weekly Report, 63*(25), 542–547.

Almeida, J., Johnson, R. M., Corliss, H. L., Molnar, B. E., & Azrael, D. (2009). Emotional distress among LGBT youth: The influence of perceived discrimination based on sexual orientation. *Journal of Youth and Adolescence, 38*(7), 1001–1014.

American Lung Association. The LGBT Community: A Priority Population for Tobacco Control (Vol. Available at: https://www.lung.org/assets/documents/tobacco/lgbt-issue-brief-update.pdf). Greenwood Village, CO: American Lung Association, Smokefree Communities Project.

American Red Cross. (2018). *Cancer facts & figures for Hispanics/Latino 2018–2020.* Atlanta, GA: American Cancer Society.

Baldwin, A., Dodge, B., Schick, V. R., Light, B., Scharrs, P. W., Herbenick, D., & Fortenberry, J. D. (2018). Transgender and genderqueer individuals' experiences with health care providers: What's working, what's not, and where do we go from here? *Journal of Health Care for the Poor Underserved, 29*(4), 1300–1318.

Balsam, K. F., Molina, Y., Beadnell, B., Simoni, J., & Walters, K. (2011). Measuring multiple minority stress: The LGBT people of color microaggressions scale. *Cultural Diversity & Ethnic Minority Psychology, 17*(2), 163–174.

Becasen, J. S., Denard, C. L., Mullins, M. M., Higa, D. H., & Sipe, T. A. (2018). Estimating the prevalence of HIV and sexual behaviors among the US transgender population: A systematic review and meta-analysis, 2006–2017. *American Journal of Public Health,* e1–e8.

Bostwick, W. B., Meyer, I., Aranda, F., Russell, S., Hughes, T., Birkett, M., & Mustanski, B. (2014). Mental health and suicidality among racially/ethnically diverse sexual minority youths. *American Journal of Public Health, 104*(6), 1129–1136.

Brown, A. F., Ma, G. X., Miranda, J., Eng, E., Castille, D., Brockie, T., ... Trinh-Shevrin, C. (2019). Structural interventions to reduce and eliminate health disparities. *American Journal of Public Health, 109*(S1), S72–S78.

Buchting, F. O., Emory, K. T., Scout, Kim, Y., Fagan, P., Vera, L. E., & Emery, S. (2017). Transgender use of cigarettes, cigars, and e-cigarettes in a national study. *American Journal of Preventive Medicine, 53*(1), e1–e7.

Burns, C., Garcia, A., & Wolgin, P. E. (2013). *Living in dual shadows: LGBT undocumented immigrants*. Washington, DC: Center for American Progress.

Castellanos, H. D. (2016). The role of institutional placement, family conflict, and homosexuality in homelessness pathways among Latino LGBT youth in New York City. *Journal of Homosexuality, 63*(5), 601–632.

Centers for Disease Control and Prevention. (2017). *HIV surveillance report, 2016*. Available at: http://www.cdc.gov/hiv/library/reports/surveillance/, 28.

Chinchilla, M. (2012). Stemming the rise of latino homelessness: lessons from Los Angeles county (Vol. Available at: https://latino.ucla.edu/wp-content/uploads/2019/02/FINAL-DRAFT-02_08_19-Stemming-the-Rise-of-Homelessness.pdf). Los Angeles, CA: Latino Policy & Politics Initative.

Criminal Justice Information Services Division, U. D. o. J. (2018). Hate crime statistics, 2017 (pp. Available at: https://ucr.fbi.gov/hate-crime/2017/resource-pages/hate-crime-summary). Washington, DC: US Department of Justice, Federal Bureau of Investigation.

Daniel-Ulloa, J., Reboussin, B. A., Gilbert, P. A., Mann, L., Alonzo, J., Downs, M., & Rhodes, S. D. (2014). Predictors of heavy episodic drinking and weekly drunkenness among immigrant Latinos in North Carolina. *American Journal of Mens Health, 22*(8), 339–348.

Deputy, N. P., & Boehmer, U. (2014). Weight status and sexual orientation: Differences by age and within racial and ethnic subgroups. *American Journal of Public Health, 104*(1), 103–109.

Diaz, R. M., Ayala, G., Bein, E., Henne, J., & Marin, B. V. (2001). The impact of homophobia, poverty, and racism on the mental health of gay and bisexual Latino men: Findings from 3 US cities. *American Journal of Public Health, 91*(6), 927–932.

Galbraith, K. V., Lechuga, J., Jenerette, C. M., Moore, L. A., Palmer, M. H., & Hamilton, J. B. (2016). Parental acceptance and uptake of the HPV vaccine among African-Americans and Latinos in the United States: A literature review. *Social Science and Medicine, 159*, 116–126.

Gates, G. J. (2013). *LGBT adult immigrants in the United States*. Los Angeles, CA: The Williams Insititute.

Gilbert, P. A., Perreira, K., Eng, E., & Rhodes, S. D. (2014). Social stressors and alcohol use among immigrant sexual and gender minority Latinos in a nontraditional settlement state. *Substance Use and Misuse, 49*(11), 1365–1375.

Habarta, N., Wang, G., Mulatu, M. S., & Larish, N. (2015). HIV testing by transgender status at centers for disease control and prevention-funded sites in the United States, Puerto Rico, and US Virgin Islands, 2009–2011. *American Journal of Public Health, 105*(9), 1917–1925.

Herbst, J. H., Jacobs, E. D., Finlayson, T. J., McKleroy, V. S., Neumann, M. S., & Crepaz, N. (2008). Estimating HIV prevalence and risk behaviors of transgender persons in the United States: A systematic review. *AIDS Behavior, 12*(1), 1–17.

Hess, K., Hu, X., Lansky, A., Mermin, J., & Hall, I. (2016). *Estimating the lifetime risk of a diagnosis of HIV infection in the United States*. Paper presented at the Conference on Retroviruses and Opportunistic Infections (CROI) Boston, MA.

James, S. E., Herman, J. L., Rankin, S., Keisling, M., Mottet, L., & Anafi, M. (2016). *The report of the 2015 U.S. transgender survey*. Washington, DC: National Center for Transgender Equality.

Kane, R., Nicoll, A. E., Kahn, E., & Groves, S. (2012). *Supporting and caring for our Latino LGBT youth*. Washington, DC: Human Rights Campaign.

Kastanis, A., & Gates, G. J. (2010). LGBT Latino/a Individuals and Latino/a Same-Sex Couples (pp. Available at: https://williamsinstitute.law.ucla.edu/wp-content/uploads/Census-2010-Latino-Final.pdf). Los Angeles, CA: Williams Institute, UCLA School of Law.

Kellogg, T. A., Clements-Nolle, K., Dilley, J., Katz, M. H., & McFarland, W. (2001). Incidence of human immunodeficiency virus among male-to-female transgendered persons in San Francisco. *Journal of Acquired Immune Deficiency Syndrome, 28*(4), 380–384.

Keuroghlian, A. S., Shtasel, D., & Bassuk, E. L. (2014). Out on the street: A public health and policy agenda for lesbian, gay, bisexual, and transgender youth who are homeless. *American Journal of Orthopsychiatry, 84*(1), 66–72.

Kost, R. G., Leinberger-Jabari, A., Evering, T. H., Holt, P. R., Neville-Williams, M., Vasquez, K. S., ... Tobin, J. N. (2017). Helping basic scientists engage with community partners to enrich and accelerate translational research. *Academic Medicine, 92*(3), 374.

Levin, B., & Reitzel, J. D. (2018). *Report to the nation: Hate crimes rise in US cities and counties in the time of division & foreign interference*. Compilation of Official Data (38 Jurisdictions) (Vol. Available at: https://csbs.csusb.edu/sites/csusb_csbs/files/2018%20Hate%20Final%20Report%205-14.pdf). San Bernardino: Center for the Study of hate and Extremism, California State University, San Bernardino.

Lippman, S. A., Moran, L., Sevelius, J., Castillo, L. S., Ventura, A., Treves-Kagan, S., & Buchbinder, S. (2015). Acceptability and feasibility of HIV self-testing among transgender women in San Francisco: A mixed methods pilot study. *AIDS Behavior, 20*(4), 928–938.

Lykens, J. E., LeBlanc, A. J., & Bockting, W. O. (2018). Healthcare experiences among young adults who identify as genderqueer or nonbinary. *LGBT Health, 5*(3), 191–196.

Martell, B. N., Garrett, B. E., & Caraballo, R. S. (2016). Disparities in adult cigarette smoking—United States, 2002–2005 and 2010–2013. *MMWR Morbidity Mortality Weekly Report, 65*(30), 753–758.

Martinez, O., Wu, E., Sandfort, T., Dodge, B., Carballo-Dieguez, A., Pinto, R., ... Chavez-Baray, S. (2015). Evaluating the impact of immigration policies on health status among undocumented immigrants: A systematic review. *Journal of Immigrant and Minority Health, 17*(3), 947–970.

National Center for Transgender Equality. (2012). *Injustice at every turn: A look at Latino/a respondents in the national transgender discrimination survey*. Washington, DC: National Center for Transgender Equality.

Newlin Lew, K., Dorsen, C., Melkus, G. D., & Maclean, M. (2018). Prevalence of obesity, prediabetes, and diabetes in sexual minority women of diverse races/ethnicities: Findings from the 2014–2015 BRFSS surveys. *Diabetes Education, 44*(4), 348–360.

Newport, F. (2018). *In the U.S., estimate of LGBT population rises to 4.5%* (pp. Available at: https://news.gallup.com/poll/234863/estimate-lgbt-population-rises.aspx). Gallup.

Nuttbrock, L., Hwahng, S., Bockting, W., Rosenblum, A., Mason, M., Macri, M., & Becker, J. (2009). Lifetime risk factors for HIV/sexually transmitted infections among male-to-female transgender persons. *Journal of Acquired Immune Deficiency Syndrome, 52*(3), 417–421.

O'Brien, M. C., McCoy, T. P., Champion, H., Mitra, A., Robbins, A., Teuschlser, H., ... DuRant, R. H. (2006). Single question about drunkenness to detect college students at risk for injury. *Academic Emergency Medicine, 13*(6), 629–636.

O'Donnell, S., Meyer, I. H., & Schwartz, S. (2011). Increased risk of suicide attempts among Black and Latino lesbians, gay men, and bisexuals. *American Journal of Public Health, 101*(6), 1055–1059.

Office on Smoking and Health, N. C. f. C. D. P. a. H. P. (2018). *Hispanics/Latinos and tobacco use* (Vol. Available at: https://www.cdc.gov/tobacco/disparities/hispanics-latinos/index.htm). Atlanta, GA: Centers for Disease Control and Prevention.

Page, M. (2017). Forgotten youth: Homeless LGBT youth of color and the Runaway and Homeless Youth Act. *Northwestern Journal of Law & Social Policy, 12*(2), 17–45.

Quinn, G. P., Sanchez, J. A., Sutton, S. K., Vadaparampil, S. T., Nguyen, G. T., Green, B. L., ... Schabath, M. B. (2015). Cancer and lesbian, gay, bisexual, transgender/transsexual, and queer/questioning (LGBTQ) populations. *CA: A Cancer Journal for Clinicians, 65*(5), 384–400.

Rapues, J., Wilson, E. C., Packer, T., Colfax, G. N., & Raymond, H. F. (2013). Correlates of HIV infection among transfemales, San Francisco, 2010: Results from a respondent-driven sampling study. *American Journal of Public Health, 103*(8), 1485–1492.

Ream, G. L. (2014). Homeless lesbian, gay, bisexual and transgender (LGBT) youth in New York City: Insights from the field. *Child Welfare, 93*(2), 7–22.

Rhodes, S. D. (2014). Authentic engagement and community-based participatory research for public health and medicine. In S. D. Rhodes (Ed.), *Innovations in HIV prevention research and practice through community engagement* (pp. 1–10). New York, NY: Springer.

Rhodes, S. D., Alonzo, J., Mann Jackson, L., Tanner, A. E., Vissman, A. T., Martinez, O., ... Reboussin, B. A. (2018). Selling the product: Strategies to increase recruitment and retention of Spanish-speaking Latinos in biomedical research. *Journal of Clinical and Translational Science, 2*(3), 147–155.

Rhodes, S. D., Alonzo, J., Mann, L., Song, E., Tanner, A. E., Arellano, J. E., ... Painter, T. M. (2017). Small-group randomized controlled trial to increase condom use and HIV testing among Hispanic/Latino gay, bisexual, and other men who have sex with men. *American Journal of Public Health, 107*(6), 969–976.

Rhodes, S. D., Leichliter, J. S., Sun, C. J., & Bloom, F. R. (2016). The HoMBReS and HoMBReS Por un Cambio interventions to reduce HIV disparities among immigrant Hispanic/Latino men. *MMWR. Morbidity and Mortality Weekly Report, 65*(1), 51–56.

Rhodes, S. D., Mann, L., Alonzo, J., Downs, M., Abraham, C., Miller, C., ... Reboussin, B. A. (2014). CBPR to prevent HIV within ethnic, sexual, and gender minority communities: Successes with long-term sustainability. In S. D. Rhodes (Ed.), *Innovations in HIV prevention research and practice through community engagement* (pp. 135–160). New York, NY: Springer.

Rhodes, S. D., Mann, L., Simán, F. M., Song, E., Alonzo, J., Downs, M., ... Hall, M. A. (2015). The impact of local immigration enforcement policies on the health of immigrant Hispanics/Latinos in the United States. *American Journal of Public Health, 105*(2), 329–337.

Rhodes, S. D., Martinez, O., Song, E. Y., Daniel, J., Alonzo, J., Eng, E., ... Reboussin, B. (2013). Depressive symptoms among immigrant Latino sexual minorities. *American Journal of Health Behavior, 37*(3), 404–413.

Rhodes, S. D., McCoy, T. P., Hergenrather, K. C., Vissman, A. T., Wolfson, M., Alonzo, J., ... Eng, E. (2012). Prevalence estimates of health risk behaviors of immigrant Latino men who have sex with men. *Journal of Rural Health, 28*(1), 73–83.

Rhodes, S. D., Tanner, A. E., Mann-Jackson, L., Alonzo, A., Simán, F. M., Song, E. Y., ... Aronson, R. E. (2018). Promoting community and population health in public health and medicine: A stepwise guide to initiating and conducting community-engaged research. *Journal of Health Disparities Research and Practice, 11*(3), 16–31.

Rhodes, S. D., Tanner, A. E., Mann-Jackson, L., Alonzo, J., Horridge, D. N., Van Dam, C. N., ... Andrade, M. (2018). Community-engaged research as an approach to expedite advances in HIV prevention, care, and treatment: A call to action. *AIDS Education and Prevention, 30*(3), 243–253.

Rosario, M., Corliss, H. L., Everett, B. G., Reisner, S. L., Austin, S. B., Buchting, F. O., & Birkett, M. (2014). Sexual orientation disparities in cancer-related risk behaviors of tobacco, alcohol, sexual behaviors, and diet and physical activity: pooled Youth Risk Behavior Surveys. *American Journal of Public Health, 104*(2), 245–254.

Russell, S. T., & Fish, J. N. (2016). Mental health in lesbian, gay, bisexual, and transgender (LGBT) youth. *Annual Review of Clinical Psychology, 12,* 465–487.

Thoreson, R. (2018). *"All We Want is Equality": Religious exemptions and discrimination against LGBT people in the United States*. New York, NY: Human Rights Watch.

Tilcsik, A. (2011). Pride and prejudice: Employment discrimination against openly gay men in the United States. *American Journal of Sociology, 117*(2), 586–626.

Toomey, R. B., Syvertsen, A. K., & Shramko, M. (2018). Transgender adolescent suicide behavior. *Pediatrics, 142*(4), e20174218.

United States Government Accountability Office. (2013). *Immigration detention: Additional actions could strengthen DHS efforts to address sexual abuse*. Washington, DC: United States Government Accountability Office.

VanKim, N. A., Erickson, D. J., Eisenberg, M. E., Lust, K., Simon Rosser, B. R., & Laska, M. N. (2014). Weight-related disparities for transgender college students. *Health Behavior Policy Review, 1*(2), 161–171.

Wolfson, M., Wagoner, K. G., Rhodes, S. D., Egan, K. L., Sparks, M., Ellerbee, D., … Yang, E. (2017). Coproduction of research questions and research evidence in public health: The study to prevent teen drinking parties. *Biomed Research International, 2017*, 3639596.

Yamanis, T. J., Zea, M. C., Rame Montiel, A. K., Barker, S. L., Diaz-Ramirez, M. J., Page, K. R., … Rathod, J. (2018). Immigration legal services as a structural HIV intervention for Latinx sexual and gender minorities. *Journal of Immigrant & Minority Health, Nov*, 1–8.

Ylitalo, K. R., Lee, H., & Mehta, N. K. (2013). Health care provider recommendation, human papillomavirus vaccination, and race/ethnicity in the US National Immunization Survey. *American Journal of Public Health, 103*(1), 164–169.

Part II
Communities, Systems, and Structures

Chapter 11
Health Insurance Reform and the Latinx Population

Mark A. Hall and Lilli Mann-Jackson

Abstract This chapter addresses how health insurance reform—principally through the Patient Protection and Affordable Care Act (ACA)—has affected the Latinx population in the USA. Described first are issues that this population faced in obtaining insurance coverage before implementation of the ACA in 2014. Then, details are given on how the ACA improves insurance coverage for Latinx persons but also on how it falls short in achieving universal coverage. The chapter concludes with a brief discussion of the uncertain future of the ACA and health insurance reform.

Keywords Affordable care act · Healthcare coverage · Health insurance reform · Latinx population

Health insurance is essential to have adequate access to health care in the USA, for obvious reasons. Numerous studies have documented that uninsured people are much less likely to have a usual source of care and much more likely to not obtain needed care—both because providers are more reluctant to serve those who have difficulty paying and because people are less likely to seek care when they cannot afford to pay for it. Although a so-called safety net of providers willing to treat patients regardless of their ability to pay is available, it is very spotty in many places and has significant gaps in most places, especially for specialist care (Hall, 2013).

The Latinx population in the USA historically has had less insurance coverage than the general US population. Prior to the Affordable Care Act (ACA), a third of Latinx persons younger than 65 years were uninsured, which was almost twice the 18% uninsured rate for the general population (Garrett & Gangopadhyaya, 2016). As a consequence, the Latinx population has reported facing more barriers to health care than the general population. In 2011, the proportion of adults who reported being able to get medical care when needed was 10 percentage points lower in the Latinx population than in the overall population (73% vs. 83%), and only 60% of Latinx

M. A. Hall
Wake Forest University School of Law, Winston-Salem, NC, USA

M. A. Hall · L. Mann-Jackson (✉)
Department of Social Sciences and Health Policy, Wake Forest School of Medicine, Winston-Salem, NC, USA
e-mail: Lmann@wakehealth.edu

© Springer Nature Switzerland AG 2020
A. D. Martínez and S. D. Rhodes (eds.), *New and Emerging Issues in Latinx Health*, https://doi.org/10.1007/978-3-030-24043-1_11

239

persons reported having a personal physician, compared with 78% of adults overall (State Health Access Data Assistance Center, 2017).

Sources of Insurance

Adults younger than 65 years have two basic sources of insurance: private health insurance, which is obtained mainly through work as an employee benefit, and Medicaid, the government program that covers some people who live below the poverty level. Private health insurance as a workplace benefit is available mainly to people employed full-time by large employers—those with 200 or more full-time employees. Within that segment, almost all employers (98%) offer health insurance. In contrast, less than half (46%) of the smallest employers—those with fewer than 10 full-time workers—offer health insurance benefits, and only 61% of employers with 10–24 workers do so. Employers in the southern and western parts of the USA are less likely (52–54%) to offer health insurance (regardless of employer size) than elsewhere (58–63%). Further, health insurance is less often a fringe benefit among employers engaged in retail sales (43%), agriculture and construction (50%), manufacturing (52%), and the service sector (59%) (Kaiser Family Foundation, 2016).

Although the rate of full-time employment for Latinx persons (73% in 2011) is similar to that for non-Latinx persons (80%), only 56% of Latinx workers in 2010 had a job that offered insurance (compared with 73% of employed non-Latinx White persons and 76% of employed non-Latinx Black persons) (Janicki, 2013). This discrepancy is largely because Latinx persons tend to have the kinds of jobs that less frequently offer health insurance. For example, more than half (53%) of Latinx persons (Kaiser Commission on Medicaid and the Uninsured, 2013a), and an even higher proportion of foreign-born Latinx persons (Stepler & Brown, 2016), work in agriculture, the service sector, or construction. Also, Latinx persons tend to have lower-paying jobs; indeed, among full-time workers, they have the lowest earnings of any racial or ethnic group (Stepler & Brown, 2016). Thus, Latinx persons often cannot afford insurance when it is offered (Kaiser Commission on Medicaid and the Uninsured, 2013a). Accordingly, in 2011, 28.3% of Latinx adults reported receiving employer-based insurance, compared with 44.6% of the US population overall (Mendes, 2012).

When working persons do not have health insurance benefits, they may seek to buy private health insurance individually, rather than as part of a group. Before the ACA's reform of health insurance markets, individual health insurance could be difficult to obtain and afford. When health insurers were not selling to large groups, they screened individuals for their existing and previous health conditions to determine their likely health care costs. Based on this information, insurers either declined to cover those likely to incur high costs or they charged them significantly more for coverage. Also, prior to the ACA, insurers would exclude any so-called pre-existing conditions from the coverage that they sold to individuals or small groups. Also, insurers would exclude key areas of coverage that drew predictably higher costs, such as maternity care, treatment of human immunodeficiency virus infection, and behavioral health care. Thus, even if people could qualify and afford coverage, it often did not cover what they most needed it for. Thus, only about 6% of the population saw it as worthwhile to buy individual insurance before the implementation of the ACA.

Medicaid, the public program for persons with low income, is operated by state governments but jointly funded by the federal government. Accordingly, Medicaid has some common features across states, but it also differs substantially from state to state. The minimum federal standards require states to cover people who live below the poverty level only if they fall into defined categories of need, such as children, pregnant women, and persons with disabilities. Moreover, states may choose, within limits, what income level is required to qualify within each eligible category. Although a number of states are more generous in that they cover pregnant women and children well above the poverty level, or cover parents or able-bodied adults without dependents below the poverty level, many states adhere to, or do not go much beyond, the minimum federal categorical requirements or they impose especially low-income limits.

In addition, federally funded Medicaid does not cover undocumented immigrants. Even for permanent residents (green card holders), adults must have permanent resident status for five years before they become eligible (unless they are pregnant). States that want to expand their Medicaid programs to cover undocumented immigrants must do so entirely without federal funds; accordingly, no state has done so for adults, and only a few, such as California, have comprehensive Medicaid for undocumented children (California Department of Health Care Services, 2017).

Potentially, Medicaid is especially important for Latinx persons because such a substantial portion of them live below the poverty level: 23.5%, compared with 15% of the general population (Stepler & Brown, 2016). However, because of Medicaid's eligibility restrictions, fewer than half (45%) of Latinx persons living below the poverty level were covered before the ACA (Kaiser Commission on Medicaid and the Uninsured, 2011). Given that around half of Latinx adults are foreign-born (Stepler & Brown, 2016), these low levels of coverage may be due in part to immigration-related barriers, as only 15% of noncitizens had Medicaid or other public insurance coverage, compared with 21% of US-born citizens (Kaiser Commission on Medicaid and the Uninsured, 2013b). However, Medicaid played a more substantial role in providing insurance for Latinx children, covering half of Latinx children overall, and almost two-thirds (63%) of low-income Latinx children (Kaiser Commission on Medicaid and the Uninsured, 2011).

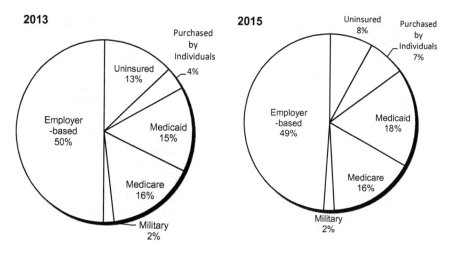

Fig. 11.1 Insurance coverage before and after implementation of the ACA. *Source* Authors' computations based on US census data

The Affordable Care Act

Basic Provisions

The ACA is a sprawling piece of legislation that does many things, often in complicated ways, but at its core, it can be usefully understood in two ways: what it does and what it does not do (Hall & Lord, 2014). Starting with the latter, the ACA, despite its name, does not make health care more affordable in terms of what providers, hospitals, drug companies, etc. charge. The ACA addresses only health insurance, not health care, strictly speaking. Insurance, of course, makes care much more affordable, and the ACA makes insurance more affordable; hence its name. However, contrary to false impressions, the ACA does not take over the entire healthcare system.

Within the realm of insurance, it further helps to understand that the ACA only slightly changed how people obtained insurance before and after the ACA (Fig. 11.1). About half of the population continues to receive private insurance through employer groups. The ACA requires larger employers (defined as those with 50 or more workers) to pay a fee if they do not offer insurance. This fee was instituted to discourage employers from dropping insurance, but the requirement does not actually constitute an employer mandate, as employers can decide whether to offer coverage or pay the fee, which is substantially less than the cost of insurance. Most employers that previously offered coverage continue to do so, and thus the ACA affected few people with group insurance.

In addition, before the implementation of the ACA, almost a third of the population was covered by public insurance—either Medicare for individuals who are older than 65 or are disabled or Medicaid for the poor. This proportion also did not change much under the ACA, except that Medicaid coverage expanded, as will be described. The ACA improved Medicare benefits in several important ways (e.g., increased coverage for prescription medications and preventive services), but basic eligibility for Medicare remains the same (covering anyone who has received disability payments for two years, or who is 65 years old and paid [or his or her spouse paid] the payroll tax for at least 10 years).

The ACA fundamentally changed Medicaid by expanding beyond the defined categories of people in need. No longer is Medicaid focused mainly on what category of need people with low income fall into and whether they meet state-specific income levels. Before the ACA, many states, for instance, provided no or very limited coverage to nondisabled adults without dependent children, and states varied a great deal in the income levels required for other categories of need. Under the ACA, the federal government pays most (90%) of the cost for states to expand their Medicaid programs to cover every legal resident younger than 65 years up to 138% of the poverty level, regardless of whether he or she falls into a defined category of need. In 2018, that level (in all states except Alaska and Hawaii, which are higher) was $16,753 for a single person, $22,715 for a couple, and $34,638 for a family of four (or higher for larger families).

The ACA, as written, requires states to expand the Medicaid programs as described. However, in *National Federation of Independent Business v. Sebelius* (2012), the Supreme Court ruled that this expansion mandate violates states' rights under the Constitution. Accordingly, states are free to decline the ACA's generous federal funding for expansion. Although doing so deprives residents of the substantial health and economic benefits that their tax dollars are still paying for, as of October 2018, 17 states have not adopted Medicaid expansion (Kaiser Family Foundation, 2018).

These states refuse Medicaid expansion largely because of ideological or political opposition to the ACA. Some observers also see a racial component to this opposition because many of these 17 nonexpanding states also opposed federal civil rights laws in the 1960s, on purported grounds of states' rights (Hall, 2014). Whatever the explanation, the Latinx population is especially disadvantaged by non-expansion because these refusing states are concentrated in the South and Southwest, where much of the new immigrant population lives (Kochhar, Suro, & Tafoya, 2005). Indeed, seven of the 10 states that have had the fastest growing Latinx populations since 2000 are non-expansion states (Alabama, North Carolina, North Dakota, South Carolina, South Dakota, Tennessee, and Virginia) (Stepler & Lopez, 2016).

The segment showing the most change under the ACA is that covering the individual market and the uninsured (Fig. 11.1). The individual market doubled in size under the ACA, for several reasons. The ACA fundamentally changes how health insurance is designed and sold. First, insurers no longer may discriminate based on health status or predicted risk; instead, they must cover all applicants, for a comprehensive set of so-called essential health benefits, at average community rates.

Second, the federal government subsidizes the cost of individual insurance for those who are not eligible for either Medicaid or an employer plan. Subsidies are designed so that a Silver plan (one that covers 70% of medical costs on average) will not cost more than 10% of household income for people who earn four times the poverty level, down to 2% of income for people near the poverty level. No subsidies are available for people earning more than four times the poverty level, even if their insurance costs more than 10% of income.

Third, individual coverage is now sold through online insurance exchanges that are run by either the federal government (healthcare.gov) or states (e.g., California, Colorado, Illinois, Massachusetts, and New York). Those who claim a subsidy must use the new exchanges; others may do so as well or may continue to buy directly from insurers. These exchanges are designed to produce price-competitive markets by requiring insurers to package their coverage in more standardized ways that facilitate comparison shopping. The ACA also funds or encourages a network of enrollment navigators to assist people in making their insurance choices.

In a broad perspective, the ACA does not accomplish universal insurance. At best, it was expected to reduce the number of uninsured people by about half. Thus, both political sides criticize the ACA. From a liberal perspective, many people would still prefer a single-payer approach, such as "Medicare for all," because it would be more comprehensive and would be less dependent on profit-based private markets.

Social progressives are also concerned that the ACA does nothing to expand coverage for undocumented immigrants, who still remain ineligible for Medicaid and who also are not eligible to purchase insurance through the subsidized exchanges (only through the unsubsidized market). Basic humanitarian considerations, supported by existing laws, compel treatment of at least emergency conditions and active labor regardless of citizenship status. Thus, providing access to primary care would also seem to make good sense on simple cost-efficiency grounds, in order to reduce emergency care costs. Plus, primary care can address infectious disease, substance abuse, prenatal care, and other matters that have broad public health importance. These arguments have not been strong enough, however, to make the case for public funding of comprehensive insurance for all noncitizens.

Despite these limitations, the ACA achieves a singular accomplishment, for all citizens and noncitizens alike: universal insurability. No longer may insurers turn anyone down, refuse to cover what a person needs, or charge a person an extraordinarily higher fee because of a pre-existing health condition. In short, under the ACA, no one is at risk of ever again becoming uninsurable.

The ability to get coverage at any point in one's life is a fundamental human protection that is widely cherished. This guarantee allows people to change jobs, pursue new careers, or make other major life decisions without worrying about how doing so might affect their basic ability to keep or obtain health insurance for themselves or family members. Thus, the ACA's guarantee of universal insurability is freedom-promoting for everyone, even those who do not benefit immediately from its specific funding and programs.

Effects of ACA on Coverage of Latinx Persons

The ACA has been a boon for coverage for many Latinx persons. Overall, the ACA reduced the proportion of adults younger than 65 years without insurance from 22% in 2010 to 13% by 2015 (Avery, Finegold, & Whitman, 2016). The proportionate reduction has been noticeably greater for the Latinx population, however. Before the ACA, 33% of Latinx adults younger than 65 years were uninsured, but by 2015, this number had dropped by 12% points, compared with a 9 point decrease for the US adult population overall (Garrett & Gangopadhyaya, 2016).

The ACA glass is only half-full for the Latinx population. Despite having a much greater gain in coverage, this population remains the racial/ethnic group with the highest proportion of uninsured, with 21% of adults younger than 65 years lacking coverage in 2015, compared with 11% for the overall population, 13% for the black population, and 10% for other racial minority groups combined (Garrett & Gangopadhyaya, 2016). As a result, despite their gains in coverage, Latinx persons now make up a greater proportion of the uninsured than they did before health care reform. In fact, by 2016, Latinx persons represented almost as large a segment (40%) of uninsured adults as did White persons (41%) (Collins, Gunja, Doty, & Beutel, 2016).

The ACA's limited coverage of non-citizens is a major reason that Latinx persons still struggle to obtain coverage. Non-citizens now make up fully half of the Latinx adults younger than 65 years who are uninsured, and almost two-thirds (62%) of uninsured Latinx persons are ineligible for financial assistance under the ACA (Artiga, Ubri, Foutz, & Damico, 2016). The impact on Latinx persons is particularly great in states that chose not to expand Medicaid. Among those states, 37% of Latinx adults younger than 65 years remained uninsured in 2015, compared with 23% among expansion states (Avery et al., 2016).

Latinx persons who continue to lack coverage must turn to safety-net providers for care. As they did before the ACA, hospitals must continue to screen all individuals who come to the emergency room to determine whether they have a condition that needs urgent treatment. Also, the ACA now requires non-profit hospitals to have more clearly developed and announced policies for treating individuals without emergency treatment needs who are in financial need.

Although the ACA reduced the number of uninsured people overall, and thus relieved some of the burden on safety-net providers, in another way, the ACA, in combination with some states' decisions to not expand Medicaid, have decreased financial support for safety-net institutions (Hall & Rosenbaum, 2012). Because the ACA assumed Medicaid would expand, it reduced a segment of Medicaid payments to hospitals designed to compensate hospitals that serve a disproportionate share of uninsured people. By law, this reduction in disproportionate share remains in place, even in states that have not expanded Medicaid. Thus, in those states, hospitals struggle more than in the past to continue serving uninsured individuals.

For primary care, however, uninsured people, including Latinx persons, often turn to community health centers. Centers that are federally qualified must offer comprehensive primary care services in a fashion that constitutes a so-called medical home.

The ACA substantially increased funding for these clinics so that they would have the capacity to treat newly insured people, but these clinics also accept individuals regardless of the ability to pay and regardless of citizenship status. The ACA has further enhanced access to care at hospitals and clinics by requiring that they better accommodate people who do not speak English (Department of Health and Human Services, n.d.). However, at the same time, other safety-net primary care providers, such as free clinics, have expressed concerns that the misperception that there are few remaining uninsured persons will result in reduced volunteerism by providers and support from the public and private funders and individual donors (Swan & Foley, 2016).

In these various ways, overall the ACA has improved both insurance coverage and access to care for Latinx persons. The ACA's coverage expansion has improved health care access for all racial and ethnic groups (Schmittdiel et al., 2017; Sommers, Gunja, Finegold, & Musco, 2015), but more so for the Latinx population than for the general population (Chen, Vargas-Bustamante, Mortensen, & Ortega, 2016). For example, the percentage of Latinx adults with a personal physician increased two percentage points (from 60 to 62%) between 2011 and 2015, compared with an increase of less than a percentage point for US adults overall. In addition, the percentage of Latinx adults who reported they could get medical care when needed increased by six percentage points (from 72.6 to 78.3%), compared with a three-percentage-point increase in general (State Health Access Data Assistance Center, 2017).

Latinx persons still face substantial disparities in access, however. On most key measures (e.g., forgoing necessary medical care because of costs, having had an emergency department visit in the past 12 months, not having had a primary care visit in the past 12 months, and not having a usual place to go for medical care), they still lag significantly behind White persons (Alcalá, Chen, Langellier, Roby, & Ortega, 2017; Castañeda & Diaz, 2017), and constitute a disproportionately large share of those who remain uninsured (Collins et al., 2016). Although some Latinx persons are ineligible for subsidized coverage because of immigration status, that is not the case for most. Instead, the barriers they face are largely informational. A substantial portion of Latinx persons reports being unaware of their eligibility for coverage under the ACA, especially among those who speak primarily Spanish (Castañeda & Diaz, 2017; Doty, Gunja, Collins, & Beutel, 2016). Also, eligible Latinx persons who live in households of mixed immigration status may be fearful of pursuing coverage out of concern about exposing family members who may be undocumented (Alsan & Yang, 2018). These observations suggest that tailored efforts are required to reach out to eligible Latinx persons who remain uninsured, in order to inform them and to assist with enrollment (Arcury et al., 2017).

The Uncertain Future

The ACA was President Obama's signature piece of domestic legislation. Many people consider it to be an important achievement in advancing equitable access to care. In addition to increasing access to insurance, it increased what insurance covers, including important aspects of reproductive health, such as contraception. Also, predictions that providers would refuse to see people with coverage through the ACA or that, somehow, ACA plans would provide care of inferior quality, have found no supporting evidence.

However, the ACA has also been controversial. Many people opposed the law's original requirement (since repealed) to pay a tax if they do not purchase affordable coverage. Moreover, a segment of the population, composed mainly of younger healthy men, now must pay much more than before for their insurance, because it now covers more than before (including maternity care), and insurers no longer vary rates based on gender or health condition.

Because the ACA is so complex, people tend to focus on different aspects in forming their views of its merits. Accordingly, these views tend to divide along political lines, with most Democrats having a favorable opinion and most Republicans having a negative one (Gramlich, 2016). Many Republicans, including President Donald Trump, have run for office over the past few years based on a pledge to repeal the ACA. Once President Trump took office and the Republican Party retained control of Congress, it was widely assumed that the ACA's days were numbered.

The Trump administration found it more difficult than expected to repeal the ACA, however. After the public realized that the ACA may actually be repealed, people became more focused on the benefits it offers, which were at risk of being sacrificed. Therefore, Republicans in Congress have vowed not just to repeal the law but to replace it with a different approach to health insurance reform that they believe will work better and be less costly. It became quickly evident, however, that Republican leaders had not previously formulated the specifics of how a new approach might be achieved, in ways that would easily gain the support of a majority in Congress. The lack of a viable alternative that is both as popular and cheaper reflects the fact that some of the law's most popular provisions are also its most expensive.

The core of the ACA's reform consists of regulatory provisions and subsidy provisions. The regulatory provisions tell the insurance industry how to sell its products and what they must cover. The subsidy provisions make health insurance more affordable or they fund Medicaid for people who cannot afford private insurance. To make insurance less expensive, Congress could roll back the regulations that require insurers to cover all essential health benefits and to accept all applicants at average community rates, regardless of their health status. But people would then be excluded or charged more if they have pre-existing conditions, and insurance might not cover areas of treatment that are most important to them.

One possible remedy for these market shortcomings is to create so-called high-risk pools that cover people who are excluded from or priced out of a less regulated market. These pools would need to be heavily subsidized, however, in order to be effective. Most healthcare costs are incurred by the small percentage of people who have extraordinarily expensive conditions. For instance, the top 5% most expensive patients each year account for fully half of all health care spending (National Institute for Health Care Management Foundation, 2012); thus, if high-risk pools covered only that part of the population, they would cost tens of billions of dollars, and they would need to cover even more than that in order to make less regulated insurance truly affordable (Hall, 2017).

Instead, Congress could retain most of the ACA's regulatory provisions but seek to alter how it subsidizes comprehensive coverage. Rather than paying for a percentage of the premium based on a person's income, the federal government could give people tax credits to offset the costs they incur. Uniform tax credits would give people the same financial assistance regardless of their income. Thus, the tax credits would have to be very generous in order for low-income people to afford insurance, which would end up subsidizing the middle class much more than the ACA currently does. Instead, if uniform tax credits are set only at the level needed by the middle class, those with lower income will be priced out of the market. It is difficult to strike the right balance without using a sliding scale approach, but a sliding scale is more complicated to administer.

Potential reforms to Medicaid are also crucial. Replacement of the ACA is highly likely to withdraw the federal government's more generous funding of an expanded Medicaid that offered to cover everyone living near the poverty level. Instead, Congress could return to its previous funding formula, allowing states to decide what level of Medicaid eligibility they want to provide for different categories of people. However, a return to the past is unlikely. Instead, Congress has considered changing federal funding for Medicaid to more of a so-called block grant program than an entitlement program. An entitlement program guarantees a specified level of benefits for a defined eligible population. In contrast, a block grant program caps the amount of funding, but leaves states with more choice over how to spend their allocation.

This block granting can be done in different ways (Rudowitz, 2017), but, no matter how it is done, there is a concern that the effect will be to reduce federal support for Medicaid and also reduce the minimum areas of coverage that states must fund in order to receive federal support.

These issues affect everyone in the USA, but they are especially crucial to the Latinx population, given that this population makes up a disproportionate percentage of the uninsured and faces greater barriers to health care access because of poverty, language, and immigration status. At the time of writing (August 2018), these issues remain unresolved in Congress. Although it is difficult to forecast how Congress will move ahead, it is unlikely that health insurance reform will maintain the same form it took under the ACA. But, it is also highly unlikely that the country will simply return to the way things were before 2014. Thus, we are left in the peculiar position of being unable to imagine even the rough outlines of how things will change, yet knowing that substantial change is inevitable.

References

Alcalá, H. E., Chen, J., Langellier, B. A., Roby, D. H., & Ortega, A. N. (2017). Impact of the Affordable Care Act on health care access and utilization among Latinos. *Journal of the American Board of Family Medicine, 30*(1), 52–62. https://doi.org/10.3122/jabfm.2017.01.160208.

Alsan, M., & Yang, C. (2018). *Fear and the Safety Net: Evidence from Secure Communities* (NBER Working Paper No. 24731). Cambridge, MA: National Bureau of Economic Research. Retrieved from http://www.nber.org/papers/w24731.

Arcury, T. A., Jensen, A., Mann, M., Sandberg, J. C., Wiggins, M. F., Talton, J. W., … Quandt, S. A. (2017). Providing health information to Latino farmworkers: The case of the Affordable Care Act. *Journal of Agromedicine*. https://doi.org/10.1080/1059924X.2017.1319314.

Artiga, S., Ubri, P., Foutz, J., & Damico, A. (2016). *Health coverage by race and ethnicity: Examining changes under the ACA and the remaining uninsured* (Issue Brief). Menlo Park, CA: Kaiser Family Foundation. Retrieved from http://files.kff.org/attachment/Issue-Brief-Health-Coverage-by-Race-and-Ethnicity-Examining-Changes-Under-the-ACA-and-the-Remaining-Uninsured.

Avery, K., Finegold, K., & Whitman, A. (2016). *Affordable Care Act has led to historic, widespread increase in health insurance coverage* (ASPE Issue Brief). Washington, DC: Department of Health and Human Services. Retrieved from https://aspe.hhs.gov/system/files/pdf/207946/ACAHistoricIncreaseCoverage.pdf.

California Department of Health Care Services. (2017). SB 75: Full scope Medi-Cal for all children. Retrieved May 9, 2017, from http://www.dhcs.ca.gov/services/medi-cal/eligibility/Pages/sb-75.aspx.

Castañeda, X., & Diaz, V. (2017). *Access to healthcare for Latinos in the United States* (Fact Sheet). UC-Mexico Initiative, Health Working Group. Retrieved from https://hiaucb.files.wordpress.com/2017/04/access-to-healthcare-for-latinos-english.pdf.

Chen, J., Vargas-Bustamante, A., Mortensen, K., & Ortega, A. N. (2016). Racial and ethnic disparities in health care access and utilization under the Affordable Care Act. *Medical Care, 54*(2), 140–146. https://doi.org/10.1097/MLR.0000000000000467.

Collins, S. R., Gunja, M. Z., Doty, M. M., & Beutel, S. (2016). *Who are the remaining uninsured and why haven't they signed up for coverage? Findings from the Commonwealth Fund Affordable Care Act Tracking Survey, February–April 2016* (Issue Brief). New York, NY: The Commonwealth Fund. Retrieved from http://www.commonwealthfund.org/publications/issue-briefs/2016/aug/who-are-the-remaining-uninsured.

Department of Health and Human Services. (n.d.). Section 1557: Ensuring meaningful access for individuals with limited English proficiency. Retrieved May 8, 2017, from https://www.hhs.gov/sites/default/files/1557-fs-lep-508.pdf.

Doty, M. M., Gunja, M. Z., Collins, S. R., & Beutel, S. (2016, August 18). Latinos and Blacks have made major gains under the Affordable Care Act, but inequalities remain. Retrieved May 8, 2017, from http://www.commonwealthfund.org/publications/blog/2016/aug/latinos-blacks-major-gains-under-aca.

Garrett, B., & Gangopadhyaya, A. (2016). *Who gained health insurance coverage under the ACA, and where do they live?* Washington, DC: Urban Institute. Retrieved from http://www.urban.org/sites/default/files/publication/86761/2001041-who-gained-health-insurance-coverage-under-the-aca-and-where-do-they-live.pdf.

Gramlich, J. (2016). Views of health care law break sharply along partisan lines. Retrieved May 8, 2017, from http://www.pewresearch.org/fact-tank/2016/10/27/health-care-law-partisan-divide/.

Hall, M. A. (2013). Organizing uninsured safety-net access to specialist physician services. *Journal of Health Care for the Poor and Underserved, 24*(2), 741–752. https://doi.org/10.1353/hpu.2013.0076.

Hall, M. A. (2014). States' decisions not to expand Medicaid. *North Carolina Law Review, 92*(5), 1459–1480.

Hall, J. P. (2017). High-risk pools for people with preexisting conditions: A refresher course. Retrieved May 8, 2017, from http://www.commonwealthfund.org/publications/blog/2017/mar/high-risk-pools-preexisting-conditions.

Hall, M. A., & Lord, R. (2014). Obamacare: What the Affordable Care Act means for patients and physicians. *BMJ (Clinical Research Edition), 349*, g5376.

Hall, M. A., & Rosenbaum, S. (Eds.). (2012). *The health care safety net in a post-reform world*. New Brunswick, N.J.: Rutgers University Press.

Janicki, H. (2013). *Employment-based health insurance: 2010* (Household Economic Studies No. P70-134). Washington, DC: U.S. Census Bureau. Retrieved from https://www.census.gov/prod/2013pubs/p70-134.pdf.

Kaiser Commission on Medicaid and the Uninsured. (2011). *Medicaid's role for Hispanic Americans* (No. 8189). Washington, DC: Kaiser Family Foundation. Retrieved from https://kaiserfamilyfoundation.files.wordpress.com/2013/01/8189.pdf.

Kaiser Commission on Medicaid and the Uninsured. (2013a). *Health coverage for the Hispanic population today and under the Affordable Care Act* (No. 8432). Washington, DC: Kaiser Family Foundation. Retrieved from https://kaiserfamilyfoundation.files.wordpress.com/2013/04/84321.pdf.

Kaiser Commission on Medicaid and the Uninsured. (2013b). *Key facts on health coverage for low-income immigrants today and under the Affordable Care Act* (Brief No. 8279-02). Washington, DC: Kaiser Family Foundation. Retrieved from https://kaiserfamilyfoundation.files.wordpress.com/2013/03/8279-02.pdf.

Kaiser Family Foundation. (2016). 2016 Employer Health Benefits Survey. Retrieved May 8, 2017, from http://kff.org/health-costs/report/2016-employer-health-benefits-survey/.

Kaiser Family Foundation. (2018). Status of State Action on the Medicaid Expansion Decision. KFF State Health Facts, updated September 11, 2018. Retrieved on October 25, 2018, from https://www.kff.org/health-reform/slide/current-status-of-the-medicaid-expansion-decision/.

Kochhar, R., Suro, R., & Tafoya, S. (2005). *The new Latino south: The context and consequences of rapid population growth*. Washington, DC: Pew Research Center. Retrieved from http://www.pewhispanic.org/2005/07/26/the-new-latino-south/.

Mendes, E. (2012). Fewer Americans have employer-based health insurance. Retrieved May 8, 2017, from http://www.gallup.com/poll/152621/Fewer-Americans-Employer-Based-Health-Insurance.aspx.

National Institute for Health Care Management Foundation. (2012). *The Concentration of Health Care Spending* (Data Brief). Washington, DC: National Institute for Health Care Management. Retrieved from https://www.nihcm.org/pdf/DataBrief3%20Final.pdf.

Rudowitz, R. (2017). *5 key questions: Medicaid block grants & per capita caps* (Issue Brief). Menlo Park, CA: Kaiser Family Foundation. Retrieved from http://kff.org/medicaid/issue-brief/5-key-questions-medicaid-block-grants-per-capita-caps/.

Schmittdiel, J. A., Barrow, J. C., Wiley, D., Ma, L., Sam, D., Chau, C. V., et al. (2017). Improvements in access and care through the Affordable Care Act. *The American Journal of Managed Care, 23*(3), e95–e97.

Sommers, B. D., Gunja, M. Z., Finegold, K., & Musco, T. (2015). Changes in self-reported insurance coverage, access to care, and health under the Affordable Care Act. *Journal of the American Medical Association, 314*(4), 366–374. https://doi.org/10.1001/jama.2015.8421.

State Health Access Data Assistance Center. (2017). State Health Compare. Retrieved May 8, 2017, from http://statehealthcompare.shadac.org/.

Stepler, R., & Brown, A. (2016). Statistical portrait of Hispanics in the United States. Retrieved May 8, 2017, from http://www.pewhispanic.org/2016/04/19/statistical-portrait-of-hispanics-in-the-united-states/.

Stepler, R., & Lopez, M. H. (2016). *U.S. Latino population growth and dispersion has slowed since onset of the Great Recession.* Washington, DC: Pew Research Center. Retrieved from http://www.pewhispanic.org/2016/09/08/latino-population-growth-and-dispersion-has-slowed-since-the-onset-of-the-great-recession/.

Swan, G. A., & Foley, K. L. (2016). The perceived impact of the Patient Protection and Affordable Care Act on North Carolina's free clinics. *North Carolina Medical Journal, 77*(1), 23–29. https://doi.org/10.18043/ncm.77.1.23.

Chapter 12
Immigration Enforcement Policies and Latinx Health: State of Knowledge

Nolan Kline and Heide Castañeda

Abstract In recent years, immigration enforcement policies have exacerbated Latinx immigrants' health-related vulnerabilities and threatened the health and well-being of entire communities, including US-born citizen children in mixed-status families. Accordingly, the relationship between health, immigration status, and immigration enforcement has become an important public health issue in the USA, necessitating long-term attention to immigration policies and their impacts. This chapter examines how local and state governments' enforcement of immigration policies are related to health by presenting the conceptual and theoretical approaches used to conduct this research and inform interventions. We end by identifying future research priorities and intervention needs.

Keywords Immigrant · Immigration enforcement · Migration · Migrant health · Latinx populations

Population

The Latinx population in the USA is a diverse group and includes persons with varied citizenship and immigration status. Depending on nationality, age, form of entry into the USA, family ties, and government classification (e.g., childhood arrival, refugee, guest worker, or victim of a crime), immigration status brings with it a number of associated sets of rights and entitlements as well as limitations. There may also be several immigration status configurations in one family; for example, Latinx children born in the USA may have citizen, refugee, undocumented, or legal permanent resident parents.

Unauthorized or undocumented status is arguably the most stigmatized and is associated with few political and social entitlements. Because of their immigration

N. Kline (✉)
Department of Anthropology, Rollins College, Winter Park, FL, USA
e-mail: nkline@rollins.edu

H. Castañeda
Department of Anthropology, University of South Florida, Tampa, FL, USA

© Springer Nature Switzerland AG 2020
A. D. Martínez and S. D. Rhodes (eds.), *New and Emerging Issues in Latinx Health*, https://doi.org/10.1007/978-3-030-24043-1_12

status, undocumented immigrants are prohibited from participating in publicly funded health entitlement programs such as Medicaid and Medicare (Kullgren, 2003; Siddiqi, Zuberi, & Nguyen, 2009) and are also excluded from purchasing health insurance through exchanges created through the Patient Protection and Affordable Care Act (ACA) (Wallace et al., 2013). Undocumented immigrants are also likely to lack employer-provided health insurance (Carrasquillo, Carrasquillo, & Shea, 2000; Goldman, Smith, & Sood, 2005), even though they often engage in forms of labor with heightened risks of occupational injury (Gany, Novo, Dobslaw, & Leng, 2014). With significant constraints in accessing services, many immigrants with a precarious legal status have no regular source for health care beyond emergency rooms, public health clinics, or charitable care organizations (Derose, Bahney, Lurie, & Escarce, 2009; Ortega et al., 2007).

Beyond issues of access, however, immigration status also plays a role in health outcomes. For example, immigration status can mediate whether some immigrants receive primary and secondary prevention services for a number of cancers, which may drive existing cancer disparities between the Latinx population and other populations (Miranda et al., 2017). Immigration status is also associated with outcomes related to HIV infection, as undocumented Latinx persons are more likely than White, Black, or documented Latinx persons to begin HIV care when AIDS is at an advanced stage, which results in lower survival rates (Dang, Giordano, & Kim, 2012). When undocumented immigrants are insured, however, HIV-related clinical outcomes are similar to those of documented immigrants (Ross, Felsen, Cunningham, Patel, & Hanna, 2017). Furthermore, the risk for poor occupational health outcomes is higher among undocumented immigrants than among documented populations (Hall & Greenman, 2015), which, along with immigration and labor policy, can influence long-term disability trajectories (Mueller & Bartlett, 2017). Overall, as existing evidence suggests, immigration status is a form of vulnerability linked to poor health outcomes (Castañeda et al., 2015; Flynn, Eggerth, & Jacobson, 2015).

In recent years, immigration enforcement policies have exacerbated undocumented Latinx immigrants' health-related vulnerabilities and threatened the health and well-being of entire communities, including US-born citizen children in mixed-status families. There are an estimated 11 million undocumented Latinx immigrants in the USA (Warren, 2016), and 4.5–5.5 million children have at least one undocumented parent (Dreby, 2015; Zayas & Bradlee, 2014). Accordingly, the relationship between health, undocumented status, and immigration enforcement has become an important public health issue in the USA. Immigration-related health concerns persist on national and local levels and, depending on political priorities, may vary in severity at any moment in time, necessitating long-term attention to immigration policies and their impacts.

Immigration Enforcement Policies

A variety of immigration enforcement policies influencing Latinx health exist at federal, state, and local levels. At the federal level, security measures along the US-Mexico border have had an impact on the health of undocumented immigrants by making their entry riskier and more likely to result in death. Increases in the number of officers along the US-Mexico border, militarization, extensions of the existing wall, and augmented surveillance technology (such as sensors, drones, and blimps) have all led to riskier crossing attempts and increases in the number of injuries and deaths along the border. Such amplified enforcement efforts have escalated the serious physical dangers associated with border crossing since the mid-1990s (Cornelius, 2001; Trevino, 1998), resulting in a growing number of deaths due to exposure, injury, and dehydration, and increasing risks for interpersonal violence and sexual assault during border crossings (Cornelius, 2001; Falcon, 2001; Slack & Whiteford, 2011). Attentive to these changes, scholars have argued that the newly militarized US-Mexico border, replete with armed officers carrying combat equipment, has made entry into the country more life-threatening than ever before (De León, 2015; Doty, 2011; Falcon, 2001; Nevins, 2007). The consequences of pushing migration routes away from urban areas and into more desolate locations are no accident; rather, it is a strategic measure by the federal government as part of its Prevention through Deterrence Program—an effort to discourage migrants from crossing into the USA from Mexico by using the environmental conditions that are dangerous and may result in death for some (De León, 2015). These efforts represent a racially driven logic of excluding migrants from Mexico and Central and South America, in particular. Such efforts are an extension of historical efforts of excluding immigrants based on race (Fairchild, 2004; Ngai, 2014), but militarized border enforcement and the Prevention through Deterrence Program additionally incorporate the natural environment into enforcement efforts.

Beyond the border, federal immigration laws have had health-related consequences for undocumented immigrants throughout the interior of the USA. These laws include the REAL ID Act, Section 287(g) of the Immigration and Nationality Act (INA) of 1996, and the Secure Communities Program. Combined, these laws have created distrust of local authorities or increased fears of apprehension, whereas others, such as the Deferred Action for Childhood Arrivals (DACA) Program, perpetuate forms of vulnerability and do little to advance immigrants' health needs.

The Real ID Act, passed in 2005, established security standards for issuing driver's licenses and other forms of identification (Department of Homeland Security, 2016). Based on recommendations from the 9/11 Commission to increase surveillance of the resident population, the Real ID Act effectively excludes undocumented immigrants from obtaining a driver's license by requiring that applicants provide evidence of lawful status (National Conference of State Legislatures, 2016). The Act sets a legislative standard that states must follow unless they make their own provisions, and to date, only 12 states and the District of Columbia have passed legislation permitting undocumented immigrants to obtain driver's licenses (National Conference of State

Legislatures, 2016). By curtailing access to a license, the Act has an impact on work opportunities, access to health care, and overall mobility for individual immigrants and their families. Moreover, not having a driver's license—or having a license conspicuously identifying the holder as undocumented or the recipient of DACA, as some states currently do—can make undocumented immigrants more easily identifiable to local law enforcement officials granted enforcement authority through INA Section 287(g) and the Secure Communities Program.

Section 287(g) permits state and local law enforcement officers to enter into memorandums of agreement with federal authorities to enforce immigration laws. Through deputizing local officers as federal agents, 287(g) grants local police access to federal immigration databases, provides them authority to interrogate and arrest anyone believed to have violated immigration laws, and gives them power to detain anyone suspected of having an unauthorized status (American Immigration Council, 2012). Similarly, the Secure Communities Program uses agreements with local and federal authorities to provide access to federal fingerprint databases. Through this program, after an arrest, fingerprints are assessed through immigration and criminal databases to determine potential matches. If an arrestee's fingerprint is matched with that of a noncitizen, including a lawfully present resident (see, e.g.: Aguilasocho, Rodwin, & Ashar, 2012), Immigration and Customs Enforcement (ICE) officials are notified and can initiate deportation proceedings. Concerns that Secure Communities will result in higher-than-expected rates of deportations for minor infractions and misdemeanors—such as driving without a license (Thompson & Cohen, 2014)—led the Obama administration to replace it with the Priority Enforcement Program (Johnson, 2014), which purportedly focused on immigrants who had been convicted of serious crimes. The Trump administration, however, reinstated Secure Communities through an Executive Order, despite evidence challenging its effectiveness in lowering local crime rates (Miles & Cox, 2014).

Combined, 287(g), Secure Communities, the Priority Enforcement Program, and the Real ID Act operate by increasing the likelihood of an undocumented immigrant being arrested for not having a driver's license, and such an arrest can ultimately result in their removal from the country. In practice, these laws make roadways and other public spaces sites of possible detection, arrest, and deportation (Coleman, 2007). With public spaces becoming associated with apprehension, federal immigration enforcement efforts have a direct impact on immigrants' willingness to seek health services or participate in community-based health programs (Alexander & Fernandez, 2014; Hardy et al., 2012).

Federal immigration enforcement efforts heighten the deportability of undocumented immigrants, but in recent years, some undocumented immigrants have become eligible for temporary reprieves from deportation through deferred-action initiatives. Announced in 2012, DACA has deferred deportation and provided work authorization for immigrants who are younger than 31 years and have no serious criminal convictions, if they have lived in the USA continuously since 2007 and since at least age 16 (Zayas & Bradlee, 2014). DACA provides two years of deportation relief and can be renewed. Rather than a form of legal residency status, it instead provides a form of prosecutorial discretion whereby the federal government agrees to delay processing an individual's deportation. Since its inception, DACA has faced a variety of critiques from both immigrant rights activists and proponents of stricter immigration control policies and faces an uncertain future.

Such short-term, limited deportation reprieves are highly precarious and subject to simple revocation, demonstrating how they are insufficient responses to an otherwise stringent immigration enforcement regime. Although better than no reprieve at all, programs like DACA require individuals to live with precarity and in perpetual liminality (Menjívar, 2006). Furthermore, such reprieves cannot entirely counteract the negative consequences of harsh immigration laws that persons may encounter earlier in the life course, such as neglected preventive health care and an inability to seek out treatment for chronic illnesses. In fact, the lifelong, cumulative effects of undocumented status will emerge later in the life course as people move into midlife and older age (Suárez-Orozco, Yoshikawa, Teranishi, & Suárez-Orozco, 2011).

In addition to existing federal enforcement efforts, individual states have enacted immigration policies focusing on enforcement and restrictions to social services. Among some of the most well known are those colloquially referred to as "show me your papers" laws, which grant police officers permission to request proof of legal status from anyone suspected of being undocumented. States laws allow for localized immigration enforcement to occur without training or input from federal agencies; these laws have passed in Arizona, Georgia, North Carolina, Alabama, and Texas and have been considered in several other states. Immigration-enforcement laws at the state level are often coupled with statutes focused on restricting access to entitlements, such as banning undocumented immigrants from attending public colleges and universities (Chavez, Soriano, & Oliverez, 2007; Holley-Walker, 2011), proposals to prevent DACA recipients from obtaining driver's licenses (see, e.g., Senate Bill 404 in Georgia), and legislative efforts to punish sanctuary cities from resisting collusion with federal enforcement activities. Although oversight of immigration enforcement has historically been reserved for the federal level, state legislation represents a growing trend in the devolution of immigration enforcement to local levels (Coleman, 2012).

Within individual states, municipalities and counties are also becoming sites of immigration enforcement through local police practices and in ways that can have a direct impact on Latinx immigrants' health. For instance, some local governments use police roadblocks and checkpoints to target Latinx drivers and trigger the kinds of state immigration enforcement procedures discussed earlier (Kline, 2019; Stuesse & Coleman, 2014). One local enforcement practice that affects people living along the US-Mexico border, in particular, is the fixed Border Patrol checkpoints. Within a 100-mile zone between the border and the US interior, agents have extra-constitutional powers, including the operation of immigration checkpoints. Residents in these zones are subject to additional surveillance and often describe feeling "trapped," as they are often unable to travel to other parts of the state (Castañeda & Melo, 2019; Núñez & Heyman, 2007). This surveillance produces a sense of total enclosure and immobility that can affect their ability to access health services, especially specialty care (e.g., for cancer, burns, or organ transplantation) (Castañeda & Melo, 2014).

Conversely, some municipal, county, and state governments have explicitly countered hostile policy climates. For example, some municipalities, such as San Francisco, have joined the so-called sanctuary city movement, wherein local governments resist assisting federal immigration enforcement (Marrow, 2012). Furthermore, San Francisco grants undocumented immigrants city identification cards and all residents under the age of 18, regardless of immigration status, are eligible for publicly subsidized health insurance (Marrow, 2012). San Francisco and other cities are legally able to not comply with federal immigration enforcement efforts because local governments have historically had the authority to govern their own populations and can exercise a number of powers unless state legislatures restrict them (Pham & Van, 2010; Rodriguez, 2008; Villazor, 2010), as the Texas legislature did in 2017. Moreover, some local governments opt out of cooperation with federal immigration enforcement efforts because of concerns about the negative impact on immigrants' well-being, communities' relationship with law enforcement, and financial concerns about channeling local resources to federal efforts (Pham, 2005). Like municipalities, some county governments have resisted immigration enforcement efforts by initiating inclusive identification programs, which can mitigate undocumented immigrants' risks of detection and deportation (LeBrón et al., 2018), and have considered creating aid programs for undocumented residents (Stanton, 2017). Similarly, states have countered hostile immigration policies through proposals to expand eligibility for public services. California, for example, passed legislation that would have allowed undocumented immigrants to participate in health insurance exchanges created through the ACA, but the state ultimately halted this effort once the Trump administration took office (Ibarra & Terhune, 2017).

Despite these examples of inclusive policies, some state and federal governments have challenged sanctuary city policies and other efforts to resist harsh immigrant policing regimes through proposals to withhold funding from cities where local police do not cooperate with federal immigration officials. For example, Texas Senate Bill 4, which passed in 2017, is largely articulated as a ban on sanctuary cities and mandates local jail cooperation with ICE, including punitive measures for law enforcement officials who fail to comply with the statute (Bernal, 2017). Beyond legislative efforts, procedural and administrative efforts to punish perceived sanctuary governments have gained momentum, including efforts to withhold funds from local governments that limit cooperation with immigration enforcement authorities and in some cases, demanding that some local governments return dispersed funds (Taylor, 2017). Efforts to tie funds for social services to immigration enforcement efforts underscore potential broad, health-related implications on state and local governments that rely on federal grants to fund numerous programs and services that have a direct impact on the health of numerous populations.

Health Impacts

In the aggregate, immigration enforcement policies perpetuate health disparities (Philbin et al., 2018), exacerbate existing health-related vulnerabilities related to immigration status, and create new health concerns for some Latinx immigrants. For example, a state-level policy analysis of mental health morbidity in the Latinx population demonstrated an association between number of poor mental health days and exclusionary immigration policies, specifically finding significantly higher rates of poor mental health days among Latinx persons compared with non-Latinx persons (Hatzenbuehler et al., 2017). Furthermore, enforcement efforts affect individual health behaviors and interpersonal relationships and potentially promote ethnic bias that can translate to poor care or experiences of discrimination in health service settings.

Aggressive immigration regimes have an impact on a variety of individual health behaviors and perceptions of racism and discrimination. For example, following Arizona's 2010 immigration enforcement law, Senate Bill 1070, some Latinx persons reported increased overall feelings of fear, limited mobility, and diminished trust in law enforcement (Hardy et al., 2012). In practice, these feelings resulted in some immigrants being less likely to seek care in what they perceived to be a more aggressive climate than in the past and created new health concerns such as emotional distress (Hardy et al., 2012). Similarly, following the passage of Alabama's sweeping immigration enforcement law, The Alabama Taxpayer and Citizen Protection Act; House Bill 56, Latinx women reported perceived mistreatment by clinical staff, fears of not being able to have their foreign-born children treated in clinical settings, and limited access to care because of the law's provisions (White, Yeager, Menachemi, & Scarinci, 2014).

Health-related impacts of federal initiatives such as the 287(g) program mirror the consequences of state immigration legislation. In 287(g) counties in North Carolina, immigration enforcement policies have shaped undocumented immigrants' distrust of staff at public and private health agencies and resulted in their inability or unwillingness to access or use health services for which they were eligible (Alexander & Fernandez, 2014; Rhodes et al., 2015). Furthermore, some immigrants reported that enforcement "promoted racial profiling and discrimination, including in health care settings" (Rhodes et al, 2015), and among police officers on roadways. Perceived racial discrimination ultimately led some Latinx immigrants to avoid driving, even when there was a medical emergency. Given the feelings of discrimination and risk of apprehension by police, it is unsurprising that undocumented immigrants also reported enforcement policies and driver's license restrictions as new barriers to seeking care, not seeking medical and mental health services when needed, and having late and inadequate prenatal care (Rhodes et al., 2015).

In addition to these individual impacts, enforcement also affects the health and well-being of undocumented immigrants' family members (Castañeda & Melo, 2014). Assessments of state and federal laws have shown how immigration enforcement policies may result in parents fearing discovery of their documentation status when they take their children to health services, resulting in circumstances where children did not receive necessary treatment (Rhodes et al., 2015). Instead, families find alternate sources of care, including self-diagnosis and self-treatment (Rhodes et al., 2015). Common strategies include sharing prescription medicines, using imported and unregulated pharmaceutical products, taking folk remedies more regularly, and using unlicensed medical and dental providers (Castañeda, 2016). The full extent of consequences of immigration enforcement may therefore not yet be known, especially among children and nonpregnant women, whose care may be made more precarious (White et al., 2014).

Just as continuous immigration enforcement efforts may have an impact on undocumented immigrants' health, so too might be more fleeting enforcement initiatives, such as immigration raids or temporary checkpoints. Immediately following a raid, immigrants have reported higher stress levels and lower self-rated health scores (Lopez et al., 2017). Moreover, research done after a 2008 immigration raid in Postville, Iowa—the largest raid in US history—showed a relationship between the raid and maternal health outcomes (Novak, Geronimus, & Martinez-Cardoso, 2017). The risk of low birth rate for infants born to Latinx women was higher after the raid than the year prior, while no changes in birth weight were found among infants born to non-Latinx women. The findings highlight that racialized stressors related to immigration enforcement extend beyond immigrants and extend the impact on US-born Latinx persons (Novak et al., 2017). Furthermore, findings suggest that immigration enforcement events create both long-term and short-time exposures that result in deleterious health outcomes and require additional empirical and theoretical attention.

Lastly, the detrimental impact of deportation and detention on family and community health cannot be overstated. Detention and deportation disrupt family relationships by producing economic and psychosocial stressors for family members and altering relationships between parents and children with precarious legal statuses (Valdez, Padilla, & Valentine, 2013). Furthermore, children whose parents have been deported or detained are more likely than children without a deported parent to experience a host of social concerns and mental health problems, including decreased school performance, depression, anxiety, aggression, and conduct issues (Allen, Cisneros, & Tellez, 2015; Brabeck, Lykes, & Cristina Hunter, 2014; Suárez-Orozco, Todorova, & Louie, 2002). Among some of the most marginalized subgroups of undocumented immigrants, such as farmworkers, family separation heightens existing financial and health-related vulnerabilities, resulting in worsened housing conditions and greater barriers to accessing health services than nonseparated workers (Ward, 2010).

More broadly, deportation directly affects communities and can have a negative impact on immigrants' social capital, resulting in potential isolation due to fears of deportation and racial profiling (Valdez et al., 2013). In some circumstances, deportation concerns may increase social capital and result in immigrants sharing information and legal resources, and financially assisting one another (Valdez et al., 2013), indicating that additional research may be needed to understand the mechanisms that alter social capital. Concerns over deportation also heighten some undocumented immigrants' distrust of law enforcement and other authorities, eroding relationships between communities and police officers (Hacker et al., 2011). Accordingly, fears of deportation work in concert with increased presence of law enforcement officers, heightened surveillance activity, criminalization of minor infractions such as driving without a license, and combinations of actions and policies to cumulatively form an elevated sense of immigrant policing (Kline, 2017).

Relevant Theoretical Approaches

Understanding the impacts of immigration enforcement on undocumented immigrants' well-being requires adopting a variety of available multilevel theoretical approaches and also pushing the boundaries of existing models. Well-known individual-level frameworks examine the relationship between health outcomes and enforcement policies and police practices. Tracing the connections between health behaviors and mediating factors such as police presence and feelings of discrimination will continue to be useful, drawing from behavioral frameworks such as the theory of reasoned action (Fishbein, 1979), for example, to understand how immigration enforcement might shape intention to seek health services based on beliefs of potential outcomes, such as being arrested. Similarly, interpersonal approaches examining social support in a harsh immigration climate are useful in understanding how social networks, family relationships, and provider interactions play a role in mental health conditions, health outcomes related to stress (such as cardiovascular disease and delivery of low-birth-weight children), care for chronic conditions, and seeking health services. Additionally, given research on how enforcement affects perceptions of anti-immigrant political climates and trust of law enforcement, future research should adopt community-level theoretical perspectives such as diffusion of innovation, which examines how specific ideas, practices, and concepts become adopted, especially through the use of change agents (Greenberg, 2006). Diffusion of innovation may be useful in examining existing efforts to improve the relationship between law enforcement and immigrant communities and considering how such efforts can be applied in other contexts. This perspective can also be applied to understanding how immigration perspectives in both sanctuary cities and aggressive enforcement locations gain acceptance and spread to other sites.

Assessing the complex relationship between immigration enforcement and health also requires adopting theoretical perspectives that emphasize systemic factors. Such perspectives include systems science or systems thinking (Leischow & Milstein, 2006; Luke & Stamatakis, 2012), ecologic models (Stokols, 1992), and the political economy of health (Brenner, 1995), which permit theorizing relationships among social phenomena and political process that influence poor health. Furthermore, perspectives emphasizing both the acute and long-term effects of immigration enforcement are needed, and a life course approach to understanding immigration policies and health may be especially appropriate. System perspectives assessing the consequences of immigration enforcement through the life course would allow for a deeper understanding of the political genesis of such efforts and how they affect populations across generations and provide opportunities for identifying needed political and community-based interventions. Further, a systems persecptive can build on existing research that examines how immigration and health policy interact to create new and unexpected inequalities for Latinx immigrants (Kline, 2018).

In addition to continuing to use existing theoretical models to understand the impact of immigration enforcement on health, future work must move beyond frameworks that focus *only* on individual health behaviors or the role of culture and focus theoretical attention on broader social, economic, and political forces (Castañeda et al., 2015). By examining the many ways in which these structures affect health, researchers can better acknowledge the social factors and forces that operate to either include or exclude individuals and communities from adequate health care as well as from resources that foster well-being. This requires concerted effort to understand the consequences of immigration as a social determinant of health itself; that is, how being an immigrant limits behavioral choices and can have a direct impact on the effects of other social positioning, such as race/ethnicity, gender, or socioeconomic status, because it places individuals in ambiguous and often hostile relationships with the state and its institutions. Accordingly, future work on immigration enforcement and health can build upon existing understandings of immigration as a social determinant and continue to theorize the relationship between undocumented immigrants, state institutions, and health.

Successful Research and Interventions

As an emerging field of research in a dynamic and shifting policy environment, there is not yet a robust amount of scholarship on successful research interventions designed to alleviate negative health-related consequences of immigration enforcement. Nevertheless, there are policy initiatives and activist responses that may mitigate some of the effects. For example, the city of San Francisco's policy climate that supports undocumented immigrants' efforts to obtain health care by adopting sanctuary city policies, providing a city identification card to all residents regardless of immigration status, and funding a health insurance program for children (Marrow, 2012) represents a direction other major cities could consider adopting. Such policies are not a panacea, however, as local providers and health care institutions face barriers in providing certain types of care that require the involvement of state and federally funded organizations. Accordingly, future research could longitudinally examine how citywide policy interventions affect overall health service utilization rates in immigrant families and suggest implementation strategies for other municipalities and for scaling up interventionsto a county or state level. Similarly, in 2016, California became the first state to request permission to allow undocumented immigrants to purchase health insurance through its state health exchange, which would offer them the same affordable options available to other residents for the first time. This effort required federal approval, however, as it sought to modify a statute of the ACA, which stalled the success of the proposal. Despite this setback, states could still devise their own programs to improve undocumented immigrants' well-being that are not linked to the ACA and would not require petitioning the federal government.

In addition to policies enacted at local levels, some activist organizations have developed programs aimed at bringing awareness to immigration enforcement policies that affect the Latinx population. Through its "Know Your Rights" campaigns, the American Civil Liberties Union (ACLU) has created educational tools that provide strategies for responding to officers when pulled over in places compliant with the Real ID law and where state enforcement efforts have been enacted (American Civil Liberties Union, 2016). Similarly, local immigrant rights organizations have continued to protest and organize in their home states to reverse immigration enforcement laws, drawing attention to their numerous negative consequences, including those that directly affect health (Kline, 2019). In Georgia and Washington, for example, immigrant rights organizations have mobilized to create areas where communality members warn each other about the presence of ICE officers, dubbing them "ICE-Free Zones."

Research and Intervention Needs and Priorities

The results of research on immigration enforcement suggest the importance of interventions on both policy and individual levels. First and foremost, following recommendations from the American Public Health Association's policy statements on Secure Communities, anti-immigration statutes, anti-immigrant racism, and border-crossing deaths (American Public Health Association, 2012), we assert the most urgent intervention needed is to end these harsh immigration policies and practices. Collectively, these and other immigrant-policing efforts contribute to health inequalities and deepen existing health disparities among immigrants living in the USA and their families, countering health equity goals.

Additional intervention recommendations include increasing rights-based training among immigrants living in hostile immigration policy climates, and enacting state-level laws that expand driver's licenses to undocumented immigrants (Rhodes et al., 2015). Moreover, given the family-related impacts of immigration enforcement, family-oriented interventions such as advocating for preserving parent–child relationships when undocumented immigrants are identified for deportation must become priorities for social service and law enforcement workers (Allen et al., 2015). There are still several intervention needs and research priorities around this topic, including expanding theoretical models to address how immigration-enforcement policies can shape numerous social dynamics in families, workplaces, community organizations, and government institutions, and as a system itself. For example, immigration-enforcement efforts can raise tensions within families, especially those with multiple immigration statuses present, resulting in persistent worries about family separation, frequent conversations about deportation and police apprehension, and heightened anxiety about keeping family units together (Valdez et al., 2013).

Future research on immigration enforcement and Latinx health should also be attentive to concerns related to gender and power and use theoretical frameworks focusing on these issues. Pressing areas include the impacts of immigration enforcement on lesbian, gay, bisexual, transgender, and queer (LGBTQ+) populations; relationships between immigration enforcement and violence linked to sex and gender; and the unique, health-related challenges undocumented and queer (UndocQueer) immigrants face in enforcement contexts. Accordingly, one of the most important theoretical approaches currently absent from immigration enforcement and health literature is the perspective of intersectionality.[1] As Viruell-Fuentes, Miranda, and Abdulrahim (2012) have argued, an intersectional approach to immigrant health must be attentive to racialization processes and policies that directly affect immigrants' health. Furthermore, an Institute of Medicine report (Graham et al., 2011) highlighted a critical need for LGBTQ+ research that includes racial diversity, and we advance these calls by directing attention to immigration status as an identity that intersects with other forms of vulnerability, such as sexual orientation and race, to shape experiences and opportunities. Adopting an intersectional research agenda can help guide future work on immigration enforcement policy and health. For example, one of the authors of this chapter (Kline) is currently examining the interplay of racial and sexual minority status and different citizenship and immigration configurations represented in the response to the Pulse nightclub shooting in Orlando, Florida (Kline & Cuevas, 2018). Moreover, future research and intervention priorities surrounding gender and power should consider women's health needs that are separate from prenatal care and children's health needs.

Lastly, echoing the importance of systems approaches in examining immigration enforcement, future researchers should understand immigration enforcement not just as a single variable among many but rather as part of a system of multiple components that affect Latinx health in the USA. Existing paradigms to advance this idea include considering immigration as a social determinant of health (Castañeda et al., 2015) and immigration status as a form of structural vulnerability (Quesada, Hart, & Bourgois, 2011). Similarly, understanding immigration enforcement, or law enforcement practices generally, as a health determinant can contribute to multilevel interventions among numerous minority groups that experience various forms of health inequality and tenuous relationships with enforcement authorities. The examination of the effects of enforcement policies must go beyond undocumented persons themselves and also capture the effects on US-citizen family members, especially children (Castañeda & Melo, 2014; Vargas & Ybarra, 2017), and on those in liminal legal statuses such as DACA, temporary protected status, or asylum seekers. Only after a full understanding of these disparities will we be able to identify the mechanisms affecting ill health and design appropriate interventions.

---

[1] Intersectionality considers how multiple forms of identity and social vulnerability interact to produce qualitatively unique life experiences for individuals. See: Crenshaw, K. (1989). Demarginalizing the intersection of race and sex: A Black feminist critique of antidiscrimination doctrine, feminist theory and antiracist politics. *U. Chi. Legal F.*, 139, and Crenshaw, K. (1991). Mapping the margins: Intersectionality, identity politics, and violence against women of color. *Stanford Law Review*, 1241–1299.

References

Aguilasocho, E. I., Rodwin, D., & Ashar, S. M. (2012). *Misplaced priorities: The failure of Secure Communities in Los Angeles County*. Irvine, CA: University of California.

Alexander, W. L., & Fernandez, M. (2014). Immigration policing and medical care for farmworkers: Uncertainties and anxieties in the East Coast migrant stream. *North American Dialogue, 17*(1), 13–30.

Allen, B., Cisneros, E. M., & Tellez, A. (2015). The children left behind: The impact of parental deportation on mental health. *Journal of Child and Family Studies, 24*(2), 386–392.

American Civil Liberties Union. (2016). Know your rights: What to do if you're stopped by police, immigration agents or the FBI. Accessed July 19. https://www.aclu.org/know-your-rights/what-do-if-youre-stopped-police-immigration-agents-or-fbi.

American Immigration Council. (2012). The 287(g) Program: A flawed and obsolete method of immigration enforcement. Accessed July 18. http://www.immigrationpolicy.org/just-facts/287g-program-flawed-and-obsolete-method-immigration-enforcement.

American Public Health Association. (2012). Opposing the DHS-ICE Secure Communities program. Accessed May 15. https://www.apha.org/policies-and-advocacy/public-health-policy-statements/policy-database/2014/07/18/11/24/opposing-the-dhs-ice-secure-communities-program.

Bernal, R. (2017). Five things to know about Texas' sanctuary city law. *The Hill*. Accessed May 15. http://thehill.com/latino/332463-five-things-to-know-about-texas-sanctuary-city-law.

Brabeck, K. M., Lykes, M. B., & Cristina Hunter, C. (2014). The psychosocial impact of detention and deportation on US migrant children and families. *American Journal of Orthopsychiatry, 84*(5), 496.

Brenner, M. H. (1995). Political economy and health. In B. C. Amick, S. Levine, A. R. Tarlov, & D. C. Walsh (Eds.), *Society and health* (pp. 211–246). New York, NY: Oxford University Press.

Carrasquillo, O., Carrasquillo, A. I., & Shea, S. (2000). Health insurance coverage of immigrants living in the United States: Differences by citizenship status and country of origin. *American Journal of Public Health, 90*(6), 917.

Castañeda, H. (2016). Health care along the US/Mexico border. In L. Manderson, E. Cartwright, & A. Hardon (Eds.), *The Routledge handbook of medical anthropology* (pp. 269–273). New York: Routledge.

Castañeda, H., Holmes, S. M., Madrigal, D. S., DeTrinidad Young, M.-E., Beyeler, N., & Quesada, J. (2015). Immigration as a social determinant of health. *Annual Review of Public Health, 36*(1), 1.1–1.18.

Castañeda, H., & Melo, M. A. (2014). Health care access for Latino mixed-status families barriers, strategies, and implications for reform. *American Behavioral Scientist, 58*(14), 1891–1909.

Castañeda, H., & Melo, M. A. (2019). Geographies of confinement for immigrant youth: Checkpoints and immobilities along the US/Mexico border. *Law & Policy, 41*(1), 80–102.

Chavez, M. L., Soriano, M., & Oliverez, P. (2007). Undocumented students' access to college: The American dream denied. *Latino Studies, 5*(2), 254–263.

Coleman, M. (2007). Immigration geopolitics beyond the Mexico-US border. *Antipode, 39*(1), 54–76.

Coleman, M. (2012). The "local" migration state: The site-specific devolution of immigration enforcement in the US South. *Law & Policy, 34*(2), 159–190.

Cornelius, W. A. (2001). Death at the border: Efficacy and unintended consequences of US immigration control policy. *Population and Development Review, 27*(4), 661–685. http://www.jstor.org/stable/2695182.

Dang, B. N., Giordano, T. P., & Kim, J. H. (2012). Sociocultural and structural barriers to care among undocumented Latino immigrants with HIV infection. *Journal of Immigrant and Minority Health, 14*(1), 124–131.

De León, J. (2015). *The land of open graves: Living and dying on the migrant trail*. Oakland, CA: University of California Press.

Department of Homeland Security. (2016). Real ID frequently asked questions for the public. Accessed July 18. https://www.dhs.gov/real-id-public-faqs.

Derose, K. P., Bahney, B. W., Lurie, N., & Escarce, J. J. (2009). Immigrants and health care access, quality, and cost. *Medical Care Research and Review, 66*(4), 355–408.

Doty, R. L. (2011). Bare life: Border-crossing deaths and spaces of moral alibi. *Environment and Planning D: Society and Space, 29*(4), 599–612.

Dreby, J. (2015). *Everyday illegal: When policies undermine immigrant families*. Oakland, CA: University of California Press.

Fairchild, A. L. (2004). Policies of inclusion: Immigrants, disease, dependency, and American immigration policy at the dawn and dusk of the 20th century. *American Journal of Public Health, 94*(4), 528–539.

Falcon, S. (2001). Rape as a weapon of war: Advancing human rights for women at the US-Mexico border. *Social Justice, 28*(2), 31–50.

Fishbein, M. (1979). A theory of reasoned action: Some applications and implications. *Nebraska Symposium on Motivation, 27*, 65–116.

Flynn, M., Eggerth, D. E., & Jacobson, C. J. (2015). Undocumented status as a social determinant of occupational safety and health: The workers' perspective. *American Journal of Industrial Medicine, 58*(11), 1127–1137.

Gany, F., Novo, P., Dobslaw, R., & Leng, J. (2014). Urban occupational health in the Mexican and Latino/Latina immigrant population: A literature review. *Journal of Immigrant and Minority Health, 16*(5), 846–855.

Goldman, D. P., Smith, J. P., & Sood, N. (2005). Legal status and health insurance among immigrants. *Health Affairs, 24*(6), 1640.

Graham, R., Berkowitz, B., Blum, R., Bockting, W., Bradford, J., de Vries, B., ... Kasprzyk, D. (2011). The health of lesbian, gay, bisexual, and transgender people: Building a foundation for better understanding. Washington, DC: Institute of Medicine.

Greenberg, M. R. (2006). The diffusion of public health innovations. *American Journal of Public Health, 96*(2), 209–210.

Hacker, K., Chu, J., Leung, C., Marra, R., Pirie, A., Brahimi, M., ... Marlin, R. P. (2011). The impact of immigration and customs enforcement on immigrant health: perceptions of immigrants in Everett, Massachusetts, USA. *Social Science & Medicine, 73* (4), 586–594.

Hall, M., & Greenman, E. (2015). The occupational cost of being illegal in the United States: Legal status, job hazards, and compensating differentials. *International Migration Review, 49*(2), 406–442.

Hardy, L. J., Getrich, C. M., Quezada, J. C., Guay, A., Michalowski, R. J., & Henley, E. (2012). A call for further research on the impact of state-level immigration policies on public health. *American Journal of Public Health, 102*(7), 1250–1253.

Hatzenbuehler, M. L., Prins, S. J., Flake, M., Philbin, M., Frazer, M. S., Hagen, D., et al. (2017). Immigration policies and mental health morbidity among Latinos: A state-level analysis. *Social Science and Medicine, 174*, 169–178.

Holley-Walker, D. (2011). Searching for equality: Equal protection clause challenges to bans on the admission of undocumented immigrant students to public universities. *Michigan State Law Review, 357*.

Ibarra, A. B., & Terhune, C. (2017). California withdraws bid to allow undocumented to buy unsubsidized plans. Accessed May 15. http://khn.org/news/california-withdraws-bid-to-allow-undocumented-immigrants-to-buy-unsubsidized-obamacare-plans/.

Johnson, J. C. (2014). Memorandum: Secure Communities. November 20.

Kline, N. (2017). Pathogenic policy: Immigrant policing, fear, and parallel medical systems in the US South. *Medical Anthropology, 36*(4), 396–410.

Kline, N. (2019). *Pathogenic Policing: Immigration Enforcement and Health in the US South*. Rutgers University Press.

Kline, N. (2018). Life, death, and dialysis: Medical repatriation and liminal life among undocumented kidney failure patients in the United States. *PoLAR: Political and Legal Anthropology Review, 41*(2), 216–230.

Kline, N., & Cuevas, C. (2018). Resisting identity erasure after pulse: Intersectional LGBTQ+ Latinx Activism in Orlando, FL. *Chiricú Journal: Latina/o Literatures, Arts, and Cultures, 2*(2), 68–71.

Kullgren, J. T. (2003). Restrictions on undocumented immigrants' access to health services: The public health implications of welfare reform. *American Journal of Public Health, 93*(10), 1630.

LeBrón, A. M. W., Lopez, W. D., Cowan, K., Novak, N. L., Temrowski, O., Ibarra-Frayre, M., et al. (2018). Restrictive ID policies: Implications for health equity. *Journal of Immigrant and Minority Health, 20*(2), 255–260.

Leischow, S. J., & Milstein, B. (2006). Systems thinking and modeling for public health practice. *American Journal of Public Health, 96*(3), 403–405.

Lopez, W. D., Kruger, D. J., Delva, J., Llanes, M., Ledón, C., Waller, A., … Harner, M. (2017). Health implications of an immigration raid: Findings from a Latino community in the midwestern United States. *Journal of Immigrant and Minority Health, 19*(3), 702–708.

Luke, D. A., & Stamatakis, K. S. (2012). Systems science methods in public health: Dynamics, networks, and agents. *Annual Review of Public Health, 33*, 357.

Marrow, H. B. (2012). Deserving to a point: Unauthorized immigrants in San Francisco's universal access healthcare model. *Social Science and Medicine, 74*(6), 846–854.

Menjívar, C. (2006). Liminal legality: Salvadoran and Guatemalan immigrants' lives in the United States. *American Journal of Sociology, 111*(4), 999–1037.

Miles, T. J., & Cox, A. B. (2014). Does immigration enforcement reduce crime? Evidence from Secure Communities. *Journal of Law and Economics, 57*(4), 937–973.

Miranda, P. Y., Yao, N., Snipes, S. A., BeLue, R., Lengerich, E., & Hillemeier, M. M. (2017). Citizenship, length of stay, and screening for breast, cervical, and colorectal cancer in women, 2000–2010. *Cancer Causes and Control, 28*(6), 589–598.

Mueller, C. W., & Bartlett, B. J. (2017). US immigration policy regimes and physical disability trajectories among Mexico–US immigrants. *Journals of Gerontology: Series B*, gbx026.

National Conference of State Legislatures. (2016). States offering driver's licenses to immigrants. Accessed May 15. http://www.ncsl.org/research/immigration/states-offering-driver-s-licenses-to-immigrants.aspx.

Nevins, J. (2007). Dying for a cup of coffee? Migrant deaths in the US-Mexico border region in a neoliberal age. *Geopolitics, 12*(2), 228–247.

Ngai, M. M. (2014). *Impossible subjects*. Illegal aliens and the making of modern American–updated edition. Princeton, NJ: Princeton University Press.

Novak, N. L., Geronimus, A. T., & Martinez-Cardoso, A. M. (2017). Change in birth outcomes among infants born to Latina mothers after a major immigration raid. *International Journal of Epidemiology, 46*(3), 839–849.

Núñez, G., & Heyman, J. (2007). Entrapment processes and immigrant communities in a time of heightened border vigilance. *Human Organization, 66*(4), 354–365.

Ortega, A. N., Fang, H., Perez, V. H., Rizzo, J. A., Carter-Pokras, O., Wallace, S. P., et al. (2007). Health care access, use of services, and experiences among undocumented Mexicans and other Latinos. *Archives of Internal Medicine, 167*(21), 2354.

Pham, H. (2005). The constitutional right not to cooperate-local sovereignty and the federal immigration power. *University of Cincinnati Law Review, 74*, 1373.

Pham, H., & Van, P. H. (2010). Economic impact of local immigration regulation: An empirical analysis. *Immigration & Nationality Law Review, 31*, 687.

Philbin, M. M., Flake, M., Hatzenbuehler, M. L., & Hirsch, J. S. (2018). State-level immigration and immigrant-focused policies as drivers of Latino health disparities in the United States. *Social Science and Medicine, 199*, 29–38.

Quesada, J., Hart, L. K., & Bourgois, P. (2011). Structural vulnerability and health: Latino migrant laborers in the United States. *Medical Anthropology, 30*(4), 339–362.

Rhodes, S. D., Mann, L., Simán, F. M., Song, E., Alonzo, J., Downs, M., et al. (2015). The impact of local immigration enforcement policies on the health of immigrant hispanics/latinos in the United States. *American Journal of Public Health, 105*(2), 329–337.

Rodriguez, C. M. (2008). The significance of the local in immigration regulation. *Michigan Law Review,* NYU Law School, Public Law Research Paper No. 08-22. https://ssrn.com/abstract=1006091.

Ross, J., Felsen, U. R., Cunningham, C. O., Patel, V. V., & Hanna, D. B. (2017). Outcomes along the HIV care continuum among undocumented immigrants in clinical care. *AIDS Research and Human Retroviruses, 33*(10), 1038–1044.

Siddiqi, A., Zuberi, D., & Nguyen, Q. C. (2009). The role of health insurance in explaining immigrant versus non-immigrant disparities in access to health care: Comparing the United States to Canada. *Social Science and Medicine, 69,* 1452–1459.

Slack, J., & Whiteford, S. (2011). Violence and migration on the Arizona-Sonora border. *Human Organization, 70*(1), 11–21.

Stanton, R. (2017). Washtenaw County plans to financially assist undocumented immigrants. Accessed May 4. http://www.mlive.com/news/ann-arbor/index.ssf/2017/05/washtenaw_county_to_financiall.html.

Stokols, D. (1992). Establishing and maintaining healthy environments: Toward a social ecology of health promotion. *American Psychologist, 47*(1), 6.

Stuesse, A., & Coleman, M. (2014). Automobility, immobility, altermobility: Surviving and resisting the intensification of immigrant policing. *City & Society, 26*(1), 105–126.

Suárez-Orozco, C., Todorova, I. L., & Louie, J. (2002). Making up for lost time: The experience of separation and reunification among immigrant families. *Family Process, 41*(4), 625–643.

Suárez-Orozco, C., Yoshikawa, H., Teranishi, R., & Suárez-Orozco, M. (2011). Growing up in the shadows: The developmental implications of unauthorized status. *Harvard Educational Review, 81*(3), 438–473.

Taylor, J. (2017). Attorney general orders crackdown on 'sanctuary cities,' threatens holding funds. National Public Radio. Accessed May 5. http://www.npr.org/2017/03/27/521680263/attorney-general-orders-crackdown-on-sanctuary-cities-threatens-holding-funds.

Thompson, G., & Cohen, S. (2014). More deportations follow minor crimes, records show. *The New York Times.* Accessed July 18, 2016.

Trevino, J. A. (1998). Border violence against illegal immigrants and the need to change to border patrol's current complaint review process. *Immigration & Nationality Law Review, 19,* 481.

Valdez, C. R., Padilla, B., & Valentine, J. L. (2013). Consequences of Arizona's immigration policy on social capital among Mexican mothers with unauthorized immigration status. *Hispanic Journal of Behavioral Sciences, 35*(3), 303–322.

Vargas, E. D., & Ybarra, V. D. (2017). U.S. citizen children of undocumented parents: The link between state immigration policy and the health of Latino children. *Journal of Immigrant and Minority Health, 19*(4), 913–920.

Villazor, R. C. (2010). Sanctuary cities and local citizenship. *Fordham Urban Law Journal, 37*(2), 573.

Viruell-Fuentes, E. A., Miranda, P. Y., & Abdulrahim, S. (2012). More than culture: Structural racism, intersectionality theory, and immigrant health. *Social Science and Medicine, 75*(12), 2099–2106.

Wallace, S. P., Torres, J., Sadegh-Nobari, T., & Pourat, N. (2013). *Undocumented and Uninsured: Barriers to affordable care for immigrant population.* Los Angeles, CA: UCLA Center for Health Policy Research.

Ward, L. S. (2010). Farmworkers at risk: The costs of family separation. *Journal of Immigrant and Minority Health, 12*(5), 672–677.

Warren, R. (2016). US undocumented population drops below 11 million in 2014, with continued declines in the Mexican undocumented population. *Journal on Migration and Human Security, 4*(1), 1.

White, K., Yeager, V. A., Menachemi, N., & Scarinci, I. C. (2014). Impact of Alabama's immigration law on access to health care among Latina immigrants and children: Implications for national reform. *American Journal of Public Health, 104*(3), 397–405.

Zayas, L. H., & Bradlee, M. H. (2014). Exiling children, creating orphans: When immigration policies hurt citizens. *Social Work, 59*(2), 167–175.

Chapter 13
Three Ecologies of the Urban Environment and the Health of Latinx Communities

Francisco Lara-Valencia and Hilda García-Pérez

Abstract In the USA, the Latinx population has been identified as a minority group subject to disproportionate exposure to unhealthy environments. Given that a vast majority of Latinx persons live in highly segregated neighborhoods in metropolitan areas, an understanding of how urban environments affect Latinx persons' health opportunities is vital for reducing health disparities. In this chapter, we explore some dimensions of the urban environment and explain its relevance to Latinx communities' health. We provide an overview of the social composition and spatial distribution of the Latinx population. Then, we present a conceptual model describing a general pathway of how the social, built, and natural ecologies of the urban environment influence Latinx communities' health. We illustrate empirically how these ecologies interact at the neighborhood level to affect Latinx persons' physical activity. We conclude with a list of actionable policy alternatives that can address urban health problems in Latinx neighborhoods.

Keywords Latinx populations · Residential segregation · Environment–health nexus · Urban environments · Physical activity

The burgeoning body of research on the social determinants of health has increased the attention to the significant disparities in morbidity and mortality across multiple subpopulations and their association with complex contextual variables. Although hardly a novel perspective, this approach emphasizes the need to restore the broken link between epidemiology and social urban analysis amidst the growing evidence that health outcomes are influenced by the interaction and intersection of biologic, societal, and environmental factors (Angotti & Sze, 2009; Corburn, 2007; Lawrence, 2004). At first, studies embracing a socio-ecological view of health examined primarily income, education, support networks, and other factors that are related to the social life of a person and can be ascribed to individual subjects. Later, researchers gradually started to focus their attention more on factors that are not specific to indi-

---

F. Lara-Valencia (✉)
School of Transborder Studies, Arizona State University, Tempe, AZ, USA
e-mail: Francisco.Lara@asu.edu; fcolara@asu.edu

H. García-Pérez
Department of Population Studies, El Colegio de la Frontera Norte, Nogales, Sonora, México

© Springer Nature Switzerland AG 2020
A. D. Martínez and S. D. Rhodes (eds.), *New and Emerging Issues in Latinx Health*, https://doi.org/10.1007/978-3-030-24043-1_13

viduals and affect large groups because they share common living and working spaces (Evans, Whitehead, & Diderichsen, 2001; Woolf & Aron, 2013). Ultimately, this shift in focus led to the recognition that morbidity and mortality foreshadow patterns that are directly correlated with observable variations in the density of community-level factors and therefore predicate a gradient of exposure of groups and individuals to their effects (Galea, & Vlahov, Freudenberg, 2005; Galea & Vlahov, 2005).

In urban settings, this gradient exists because the distribution of social and physical environments that are conducive to good health is not evenly dispersed across social groups and spaces, resulting in clustering of disease and other situations that affect the ability of people to reach their potential in life. Because certain social groups, particularly racial and ethnic minorities, are consistently more exposed than others to the detrimental or beneficial effects of certain environments, it has become increasingly clear that health disparities have an inequity component that can be addressed only through interventions at the community level (Angotti & Sze, 2009; Woolf & Aron, 2013).

In the context of the USA, the Latinx population has been identified as a minority group subject to a disproportionate exposure to unhealthy environments. For instance, in a statewide study using pollutant concentration estimates for California, researchers found that cancer risk from exposure to ambient air toxins was higher among Latinx persons compared with members in other racial/ethnic groups. This association persisted even after controlling for other variables that predict localized ambient pollution burdens, such as land use, household income, population density, and home ownership (Pastor, Morello-Frosch, & Sadd, 2005). These findings were independently validated by survey results indicating that the Latinx population is the most likely racial/ethnic group in this state to consider regional air pollution a serious problem (45%), followed by the [non-Hispanic] black (black) (36%), [non-Hispanic] white (white) (29%), and Asian (24%) populations (Public Polity Institute of California, 2007).

The Latinx population is also disproportionately affected by overweight and obesity. According to data from the National Health and Nutrition Examination Survey (NHANES) 2011–2014, 42.5% of Latinx adults are obese. Obesity especially targets poor Latinx women and children. Approximately 45.7% of adult Latinx women are obese, as well as 21.9% of Latinx youth (Ogden, Carroll, Fryar, & Flegal, 2015). The effect of overweight and obesity is significant, as 18% of Mexican-origin Latinx adults have diabetes compared with 9.6% of non-Latinx white adults (National Center for Health Statistics, 2017). The findings of a number of studies agree that, aside from biological factors, obesity in Latinx communities reflects the limited availability of affordable, healthy food in racial/ethnic minority neighborhoods, along with urban conditions that discourage physical activity (Abercrombie et al., 2008; Lopez & Hynes, 2009; Sister, Wolch, & Wilson, 2010; Wolch, Wilson, & Fehrenbach, 2005; Zenk, Schulz, Odoms-Young, & Lockett, 2009). Thus, in addition to income and education, inadequate access to a healthy living environment is the feature of the urban places that are key to explain the prevalence of chronic diseases in Latinx communities.

Given that a vast majority of Latinx persons live in metropolitan areas, with most of them living in highly segregated neighborhoods, an understanding of whether and how urban environments affect Latinx persons' health opportunities is vital for reducing disparities in health (Logan, 2011). In this chapter, we explore some dimensions of the urban environment and explain its relevance to the health of Latinx communities. We first provide an outlook of the Latinx population, with an emphasis on its social composition and spatial distribution. We then present a conceptual model describing a general pathway of how the social, built, and natural ecologies of the urban environment influence the health of Latinx communities. Then, drawing on research we conducted in the Phoenix Metropolitan Area, we illustrate how these ecologies intersect and interact at the neighborhood level, affecting the active lifestyle opportunities of Latinx persons. We conclude with a list of actionable policy alternatives that potentially can address urban health problems in Latinx neighborhoods.

The Latinx Population and the City

"Latinx" is a generic term used to designate a diverse and changing segment of the US population that shares a strong connection with the cultures and societies of Latin America and the Spanish-speaking Caribbean. In 2015, with a population of 54.2 million, Latinx persons constituted 17.1% of the total US population and were the largest racial/ethnic minority in the nation (U.S. Census, 2015). The Mexican-origin population makes up the largest Latino subgroup (63.8%), followed by Puerto Rican (9.5%) and Cuban (3.7%) populations. Starting in the early 1980s, a surge in the number of migrants from Central and South America increased the contribution of persons from Salvador, Guatemala, Colombia, and other countries in the total Latinx population. Concurrently, the US Latinx population, while still highly concentrated in a few states, has diversified its geographic footprint, with individuals in recent years finding new places to settle beyond traditional Latinx gateways such as Los Angeles, Houston, or Chicago. The dispersal of Latinx in the USA has coincided with the rise of immigration from Mexico and Central America since the 1980s, with a significant number of newly arrived immigrants settling increasingly in smaller metropolitan and non-metropolitan areas in the South and the Midwest (Carr, Lichter, & Kafala, 2013; Stepler & Lopez, 2016; Tienda & Fuentes, 2014). Combined with the higher fertility of immigrant families already settled in the USA, changes in migration patterns during the latter quarter of the twentieth century contributed to an even a greater diversity of the Latinx population in terms of national origin, birthplace, legal status, and settlement patterns (Tienda & Fuentes, 2014).

Despite these changes, one thing that has remained unaffected is the fact that the Latinx population is basically an urban one. In 2015, 93.5% of Latinx resided in a metropolitan area, compared with 85.4% of the US general population. In 2018, 10 metropolitan areas alone housed almost one in two Latinx persons, with Los Angeles, New York, Miami, Houston, and Chicago at the top of the list of Latinx metro areas. The primary reason Latinx persons concentrate in cities is the work opportunities urban places provide, but also the accessibility to affordable housing, education, health services, and other resources that can be afforded only by high population density (Tienda & Fuentes, 2014). In fact, three specific trends indicate that the spatial distribution of the Latinx population is pointing toward a sustained growth of the Latinx urban imprint.

First, regardless of their size, most metropolitan areas in the USA have experienced an expansion in the Latinx population in the last 20 years, with so-called new-destination metropolitan areas such as Atlanta and New Orleans registering the highest growth pace and traditional Latinx metropolitan areas such as Los Angeles and New York with the largest absolute increase (Suro & Singer, 2002; Tienda & Fuentes, 2014). This trend is likely to continue even after the slowdown of immigration from Latin America, as most of the Latinx persons in these places are US-born citizens (Stepler & Lopez, 2016). Second, Latinx persons have increased their presence in suburban areas, joining a national trend in which black and Asian persons are also participating. Since 1980, the growth of the suburban Latinx population outpaced the growth of Latinx persons residing in central cities, and now, more than 54% of Latinx individuals reside in the suburbs (Onésimo Sandoval & Jennings, 2012; Suro & Singer, 2002). Third, the escalation of anti-immigrant policies and sentiments in recent years has been associated with a reduction of mobility and rising levels of residential segregation affecting Latinx communities (Amuedo-Dorantes, Puttitanun, & Martinez-Donate, 2013; Tienda & Fuentes, 2014; Varsanyi, 2010). These trends are likely to reinforce the persisting concentration of Latinx persons in cities and further the salience of hypersegregated barrios in many metropolitan areas.

Nexus Between the Urban Environment and Community Health

Within the past two decades, there has been a rapid proliferation of research on the nexus between the urban environment and health within the social epidemiologic literature (Northridge, Sclar, & Biswas, 2003). Fitzpatrick and LaGory (2011) suggest that the interest in understanding the role of environmental factors on health outcomes arises from the recognition that individual and household-level factors have limited explanatory power in isolation from the environmental context that shapes and supports human living (Fitzpatrick & LaGory, 2011). Additional impetus for this interest comes from the repeated observation that many health outcomes correlate with differences across geographic areas in the density and dispersal of influential environmental factors. In fact, the findings of some reviews suggest that both individual and environmental factors seem to be part of a reinforcing cycle that creates and reproduces health disparities across social, racial, and ethnic groups (D'Amato et al., 2015; Woolf & Aron, 2013).

Although offering critical information for new insights regarding the impact of environmental factors on health, this research has also drawn some criticism for being too narrowly focused on isolating singular environmental influences on health. For example, while determining the role of the number and dispersion of grocery stores in urban neighborhoods could be important for understanding the food choices of inner-city residents, it is clearly incorrect to assume that simply bringing new supermarkets to a neighborhood will change unhealthy eating habits or solve food insecurity of residents (Angotti & Sze, 2009). Stuck in tenacious and pervasive poverty, quotidian food practices among a majority of Latinx families are under constant siege. Feeding family members is an act in which food choices are shaped primarily by severe budgetary constraints, work-schedule pressures, precarious employment, scant household savings, and an increasingly restricted safety net. In addition, the spatial distribution of grocery stores in cities and its limiting effect on the food choices available to residents of inner-city neighborhoods is an expression of the combined effect of three interrelated forces that operate at different temporal and spatial scales: residential segregation, economic restructuring, and reorganization in the retail food industry (Zenk et al., 2009). Therefore, although the food landscape plays an important role in the reproduction of unhealthy nutrition practices, any attempt to explain them will be incomplete if the structural factors that concentrate poverty in Latinx neighborhoods and regulate availability and accessibility to food in a market-driven economy are not taken into account.

Hence, understanding the influence of urban environments on health, but particularly explaining disparities in health among different subpopulations and neighborhoods requires a conceptual framework that can explicate cities as social systems embedded in larger milieus (Northridge et al., 2003). Comprehensive conceptions of the influence of the urban environment in producing health disparities must encompass the social fabric and institutions that generate and reproduce the spatial isolation and marginalization of racial/ethnic minority groups and maintain the privilege of the majority, and the physical systems—built and natural—that provide material support to the functionality of dominant social structures (Fitzpatrick & LaGory, 2011; Galea et al., 2005; Galea & Vlahov, 2005).

Following from this perspective, the health of urban populations is a function of multiple factors, spawn from the social, built, and natural urban environments (see Fig. 13.1). This framework assumes that these three ecologies of the urban environment are embedded in an all-encompassing and evolving milieu that is driven by shifting societal values, population dynamics, global climate change, technologic innovation, and politics and governance. These larger forces are not deterministic, but their influence over cities is apparent on the impact of national policies and climate change or migration, to mention some of the structural forces that condition the ability of cities to secure prosperity and sustainability in an increasingly interconnected and competitive society.

The framework also borrows from social epidemiology the notion that the urban environment operates its influence over health outcomes through a pathway that includes distal and proximate factors (Klitzman, Matte, & Kass, 2006; Markevych et al., 2017). For example, urban sprawl and strict zoning, two distal factors linked to the built environment, result in high car dependency and substantial vehicular emissions, which in turn, lead to poor air quality, a proximal factor for respiratory diseases

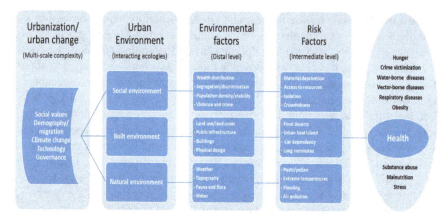

Fig. 13.1 Urban environment–health nexus. *Source* Adapted from Galea et al. (2005) and from Klitzman et al. (2006)

such as asthma. Clearly, the concentration of airborne pollutants in a particular area is influenced by topography and atmospheric conditions, so built environmental factors often interact with natural factors in influencing the respiratory health of populations exposed to poor air quality. The point here is that this framework also admits that the elements of the urban environment are not independent of each other and their influence on health outcomes does not necessarily follow a linear pathway. The three ecologies of the urban environment and their influence on health are described briefly.

Social Environment The social urban environment refers to the group of values, norms, and institutions that shape individual and collective behaviors, with implications for public health. Many cities, for example, have passed laws that tax the sale of sugary drinks with the intention of discouraging their consumption and reducing the incidence of obesity and associated health problems (Colchero, Popkin, Rivera, & Ng, 2016; Levell, O'Connell, & Smith, 2016). Another example is the investment that a community makes to support after-school programs providing recreational and educational opportunities to children in racial/ethnic minority neighborhoods. These two examples illustrate elements in the social environment that reflect a deliberate, proactive community action seeking to steer human behavior in a certain and desirable direction. Some other elements of the social environment with influence on health are less explicit in their intentionality, but they are equally tangible. This is the case of social values and norms that sort individuals into societal categories and expose them to a variety of contexts on the basis of race, ethnicity, gender, income, and other traits.

Residential segregation is perhaps the most concrete expression of how social norms that categorize people on a variety of scales results in fragmented communities and creates spaces that isolate individuals within socially and physically homogenous spaces (Acevedo-Garcia, Lochner, Osypuk, & Subramanian, 2003; Logan, 2011; Schulz, Williams, Israel, & Lempert, 2002). Both concentration and isolation patterns seem to facilitate the reproduction of unhealthy behaviors associated with cardiovascular diseases and communicable diseases, such as tuberculosis, as well as limiting the access to primary health care, two conditions that contribute to the Latinx-white health gap (Anderson & Fullerton, 2014; Kramer & Hogue, 2009; Li, Wen, & Henry, 2017). These patterns also expose Latinx persons to disproportionate levels of urban violence, which is positively correlated with sedentarism and higher obesity rates (Forsyth et al., 2015; Lin et al., 2016). It is important to acknowledge that the social environment can be experienced at multiple scales, often simultaneously, including household, neighborhood, city, region, and even global scales. Embedded within an increasingly interconnected network of spaces, contemporary social environments are open structures subject to the influence of people, ideas, information, and values that are multisourced and in constant flux (Galea et al., 2005).

Built Environment The built environment encompasses all the systems created by humans to shelter, connect, and support all forms of human activity in cities and their hinterland (Morello-Frosch & Jesdale, 2006; Northridge et al., 2003). By definition, cities are spaces that concentrate the highest density of such systems, as expressed in the concentration of housing, office buildings, parks, plazas, malls, streets, and other infrastructure networks that characterize urban places. As noted by Schulz and Northridge (2004), the built environment influences health through a range of pathways. Structures such as houses and office buildings, for example, are known to function as vessels of unhealthy indoor environments because their lack of maintenance, construction materials, technologies, and sanitary conditions promote the accumulation of mold, lead, or pests that increase the incidence of respiratory, neurologic, and infectious diseases. The spatial arrangement of workplaces, stores, housing, and other urban facilities resulting from strict zoning regulations can also have an impact on health by limiting the accessibility of jobs, consumption, and affordable housing, and by limiting the modes of transportation available to city residents (Sallis et al., 2016). The findings of some studies suggest that the atmosphere created by the form, accessibility, and aesthetic character of neighborhoods and other urban spaces influence children and adolescents' level of engagement in physical activity (Christian et al., 2015; Timperio, Crawford, Ball, & Salmon, 2017; Timperio, Crawford, Telford, & Salmon, 2004).

Natural Environment The natural environment refers to external tangible elements and processes that are produced by energy exchanges that occur continuously in nature and create ecologies in which the human body exists and which can influence its behavior and development. This environment includes landforms, soil types, vegetation, fauna, and climate. Although it was a reasonable assumption to think about the natural environment as a constant factor in models explaining urban health, the increasing unpredictability and variability of the global climate and the cauda of devastation and death caused by hurricanes and drought in cities across the world are making this supposition clearly untenable (Northridge et al., 2003). All of these factors are important to health because they can be both a resource and a hazard, depending on the ability of a society to maintain the delicate balance between human needs and nature's needs. The natural environment can affect health through physical exposure, such as extreme variations in temperatures. Between 2006 and 2010, an average of 2,000 weather-related deaths occurred in the USA, of which most can be attributed to exposure to excessive natural cold or excessive natural heat (Berko, Ingram, Saha, & Parker, 2014). Extreme heat affects human health through heat stress and can exacerbate underlying medical conditions that lead to increased morbidity. Basu and Ostro (2008) estimated that, with each 10 °F increase in ambient temperature, there is a 2.6% increase in cardiovascular mortality, with the most significant risk associated with ischemic heart disease. Similarly, a growing body of the literature has documented that the rise in the prevalence of asthma and allergies is associated with increased air pollution in urbanized areas (Baldacci et al., 2015; D'Amato, Liccardi, D'Amato, & Cazzola, 2001). Research has identified specific physiological mechanisms by which air pollutants may promote airway sensitizing that may elevate the allergenicity of pollen and other airborne irritants present in urban areas (D'Amato, 2002; D'Amato et al., 2001, 2015). The impact of weather-related and ambience pollution on health also varies significantly across socioeconomic groups, racial/ethnic groups, regions, and neighborhoods (Morello-Frosch & Jesdale, 2006; Pastor et al., 2005).

Latinx Health and Urban Living

In this section, we use the framework described to explore the importance of the urban environment for the engagement of Latinx persons in active lifestyles. An active lifestyle, including regular leisure-time physical activity, can help individuals control weight, reduce the risk of cardiovascular disease, type 2 diabetes, metabolic syndrome, and some cancers; strengthen bones and muscles; and improve mental health and mood (Crespo, 2000; Powell & Blair, 1994; U.S. Surgeon General, 1999). As suggested by the results of a number of studies, Latinx persons do not engage in sufficient physical activity and may not be getting all the physiological and psychological health benefits associated with an active lifestyle, particularly leisure-time physical activity (Casper & Harrolle, 2013; Crespo, 2000; Cronan, Shinew, Schneider, Stanis, & Chavez, 2008; Lindsay, Sussner, Greaney, & Peterson, 2009). Research findings have indicated that the urban environment disproportionately affects the ability of Latinx persons to engage in an active lifestyle. First, Latinx persons are more likely to live in neighborhoods perceived as dangerous or unwelcoming, a circumstance that may discourage residents from engaging in outdoor activities, thus increasing the chance of sedentarism and isolation. Second, fragmented and homogenous spaces in metropolitan areas limit mobility and increase car dependency, reinforcing the propensity of Latinx persons toward sedentary lifestyles. Third, lack of greenery and expansive, hard surface buildup in Latinx neighborhoods upset natural processes, increasing air pollution and thermal discomfort, thus discouraging residents' outdoor activity.

In particular, neighborhood parks have long been advocated as an essential ingredient for active urban living for all ethnic/racial groups (Loukaitou-Sideris, 1995; Jones,

Brainard, Bateman, & Lovett, 2009; Wolch et al., 2005). Particularly, in increasingly multiethnic and socially fragmented urban contexts, public parks are potentially a key resource for leisure, solace, sense of community, and quality of life (Byrne & Wolch, 2009; Wolch, Byrne, & Newell, 2014). Accordingly, the results of a considerable number of studies suggest that urban parks contribute to healthier lifestyles by providing city residents with outdoor recreational opportunities, including green areas, open space, playgrounds, sport fields, and other amenities that encourage participation in different forms of physical activity. Proximity and density of parks have received great attention in these studies because people living closer to parks are more likely to exercise regularly—leading to weight loss, increased energy, and better health in general (Cohen, McKenzie, Sehgal, Williamson, Golinelli, & Lurie, 2007; Giles-Corti, Broomhall, Knuiman, Collins, Douglas, Ng, Lange, &Donovan, 2005; Kaczynski & Henderson, 2007; Nagel, Carlson, Bosworth, &Michael, 2008). Moreover, some researchers report that individuals living close to a park are more likely to report better self-perceived health than individuals who do not (Maas, Verheij, Groenewegen, De Vries, & Spreeuwenberg, 2006). The availability of parks has also been linked to mental and psychological well-being, as parks can create opportunities for social interaction, which in turn reduces isolation and increases life satisfaction, particularly among vulnerable populations (Kaźmierczak, 2013; Wood, Hooper, Foster, & Bull, 2017). Overall, research findings indicate a positive link between parks and people's health and well-being (Maas, Verheij, Spreeuwenberg, & Groenewegen, 2008; Bedimo-Rung, Mowen, & Cohen, 2005; Chiesura, 2004).

Spatial equity research—the body of knowledge that systematically studies the geographic distribution of environmental burdens and amenities as a function of sociopolitical factors and processes (Jones et al., 2009; Sister et al., 2010; Talen, 1997)—has documented an unequal supply of public parks with regard to both race and ethnicity and socioeconomic status in many US cities. For example, in a study conducted in Los Angeles, white neighborhoods had 31.8 acres of park space for every 1,000 people, compared with 1.7 acres in black neighborhoods, and 0.6 acres in Latinx neighborhoods (Pincetl, Wolch, Wilson, & Longcore, 2003). Other studies also provide evidence that Latinx neighborhoods are likely to contain considerably fewer parks than non-Latinx neighborhoods, thereby reducing opportunities for an active lifestyle and recreation (Garcia, 2014; García, Gee, & Jones, 2016; Johnson Gaither, 2011; Kozlowski, 2008). Furthermore, the findings of other research indicate that parks in predominantly minority neighborhoods have fewer amenities and offer a less-than-pleasant experience for park goers than do parks located in predominantly non-minority neighborhoods in the suburbs (Bruton & Floyd, 2014; Jenkins et al., 2015; Sister et al., 2010; Suminski et al., 2012; Vaughan et al., 2013).

With the aim of illustrating in direct ways the nexus between the urban environment and health, we studied how residents of Latinx neighborhoods interact with their immediate living space for leisure-time physical activity. Using the greater Phoenix Metropolitan Area as a case study (Fig. 13.2), we explored the meaning and significance of neighborhood urban environments from Latinx women seeking an active lifestyle for themselves and their families. We evaluated three aspects.

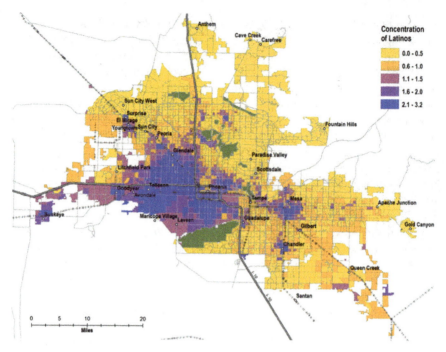

Fig. 13.2 Concentration of Latinx populations in the Phoenix Metropolitan Area in 2010. *Source* Lara-Valencia, & Garcia-Perez, (2018)

- What the women say about the importance of maintaining an active lifestyle.
- The women's perceptions of what makes public open space, especially parks, a resource for active living.
- Strategies the women use to overcome barriers resulting from the concrete social, built, and natural ecologies of Latinx neighborhoods in the Phoenix Metropolitan Area.

Exploring the way residents of Latinx neighborhoods relate to public parks from these three angles allows us to examine how the various aspects of urban environment discussed above interact and intersect in the context of a metropolitan area in rapid demographic and cultural transformation.

Before we present some findings, we noted that the analysis presented here is part of a comparative multicity project on women's perceptions of neighborhood resources and hazards for leisure-time physical activity. Here, we report the interviews with 12 Latinx women living in the Phoenix Metropolitan Area in 2017. The participants' ages ranged from 27 to 48 years old, with a median of 35.7 years (Table 13.1). The length of residence in the area ranged from 1 to 34 years (median, 18.6 years). The majority of the participants were married or living as married (83%), had at least 1 year of high school education (83%), and were primarily immigrants from Mexico (83%). Most of the interviews were conducted in Spanish (92%) in a park during the spring months.

Challenges of Being Active

Generally speaking, Latinx women understand and value the benefits of being physically active. Almost all mentioned that they try to exercise regularly and also try to facilitate the participation of their children in sports and other forms of physical activity. Women cited benefits like keeping their weight in check, complying with medical recommendations, feeling well, or simply relaxing after a long day of work. Regardless of the source of their motivation, most of the women mentioned their home or neighborhood as a primary place for physical exercise.

On the very enthusiastic end of the spectrum was Patricia,[1] a Mexican immigrant in her forties who is a mother of three. Patricia moved to the Phoenix suburb of Glendale 24 years ago and, like most of the participants, has had to balance work and family demands, while finding some personal time to exercise, which frequently ends up being a location in the neighborhood. As she told us during the interview:

> [I exercise] with the objective of feeling well, because lately I have been depressed, exhausted, and with exercise I feel more motivated. I have been to the gym, and nothing! Lately, I have been going to the neighborhood park early in the morning.

Through the interview, Patricia explained that exercise time for her is not only residual, but also has to complement her family's needs in terms of recreation and exercise. In Patricia's case, complementarity means that exercise time and place for her and her family have to overlap in order for her to stay physically active. As she explained:

> Since my children do sports, I take advantage of their practice periods to do some exercise like jogging or running, or simply walking.

Similarly, Marina, an American woman of Central American decedent who is in her early thirties and runs a home-base daycare to support her four children, explained that despite doing a lot of physical work in her job, such as bending, lifting, and cleaning, she still exercises in the neighborhood.

> Yes, sometimes I go for a walk to the neighborhood park and sometimes I go to the homes of my friends to exercise in [a] group.

For all women, motherhood and entry to the workforce are of the utmost significance in terms of their ability to be physically active. Bertha, an immigrant from Mexico and mother of two daughters, explains her level of activity before and after she becomes a mother.

---

[1] All individuals' names in this chapter are pseudonyms.

Table 13.1 Sociodemographic characteristics of Latinx women interviewed

Park and city	Pseudonym	Age (years)	Marital status	Highest level of education	No. of children	Employed outside the home	Birth country	No. of years of residency in the area
Kiwanis (Tempe)	Zaida[a]	34	Married	High school	4	Yes	United States	34
Kiwanis (Tempe)	Bertha	32	Married	High school	2	Yes	México	19
Sherwood (Mesa)	Cecilia	28	Married	High school	3	Yes	México	7
Sherwood (Mesa)	Marina[b]	32	Divorced	High school	4	Yes	United States	32
San Marcos (Chandler)	Delia	45	Married	Middle school	4	No	México	9
San Marcos (Chandler)	Ana	41	Single	College	0	Yes	México	29
San Marcos (Chandler)	Lupita	33	Married	Elementary school	3	No	México	12
Cesar Chávez (Phoenix)	Diana	31	Married	High school	1	No	México	15
Cesar Chávez (Phoenix)	Vilma	32	Married	High school	3	No	México	1
Cesar Chavez (Phoenix)	Alicia	27	Living as married	High school	2	No	México	18
Veterans (Tolleson)	Teresa	48	Living as married	High school	1	No	México	17
Veterans (Tolleson)	Patricia	43	Living as married	High school	3	No	México	24

[a]Zaida is an indigenous Mexican-American woman. She is part of the Yaqui community that lived in the town of Guadalupe, AZ
[b]Marina is a US-born woman of Central American descent
Source Neighborhood Environment and Leisure-Time Physical Activity Among Adult Women. Arizona State University. Obesity Solutions; ASU-Mayo Clinic, 2017

...before, when I was 18 or 19... I had a job and I was able to go to the mountain to hike and all those things. But now I can't do that, I have my daughters... I am a mom and also have a job. It is quite difficult...I have less time.

Overall, the circumstances of these Latinx women highlight the unquestionable relevance of the neighborhood environment for active living in the Phoenix Metropolitan Area. As suggested by the interviewees, being physically active could be challenging even for women who are knowledgeable and inclined to engage in physical exercise. For the women in these interviews, close-to-home facilities like neighborhood parks provide physical activity opportunities that are not only affordable but also essential, given the unyielding time constrains many of them face in their double role as mothers and employees. Other elements of the neighborhood's built environment, such as sidewalks and tree canopies along streets, if properly maintained and planned, may also help women to navigate the pressures of daily life that act as barrier for active living. In fact, given prevailing theories on the positive impacts of walkable neighborhoods with access to parks for promoting physical activity, it would be easy to assume that improving walkability and accessibility to parks will be an appropriate intervention to pursue in Latinx neighborhoods of the Phoenix Metropolitan Area. However, even though such actions are steps in the right direction, transforming neighborhoods in spaces that encourage and sustain an active living requires more than simple physical interventions.

Neighborhood Parks as Assets for Active Living

A look at Latinx women's experiences and perceptions regarding neighborhood parks reveals much about the significance of the urban environment for physical activity of Latinx women in the Phoenix Metropolitan Area. Through their own activity and that of their families, women are able to interact with the various elements of their neighborhood's urban environment that affect their ability to use parks, streets, and other local open spaces for exercise or play. As conveyed by the interviews, the study participants have a significantly nuanced understanding of parks as a resource, and through their narratives they are able to unpack and weight each of the ecologies that shape the potential of Latinx neighborhoods for an active lifestyle.

All the women acknowledged the existence of a park in their neighborhood. However, many of them told us that the parks and their surroundings are not safe, and as a result, were not a good place for them or their families to exercise or play. Consider, for example, the following observation by Zaida, a Yaqui indigenous woman in her thirties—an observation that was similar to that in a number of other interviews.

I wouldn't go to walk [especially at night]. Some of the streets in my neighborhood are dark, there is too much traffic, and drivers don't pay attention to speed limits....

Male-dominated environments were commonly mentioned as ongoing problems in some of the neighborhoods. Women described how this situation affected their ability to use nearby parks or simply going out for a walk.

> You don't feel safe on the street or the park; I live near a trailer park and sometimes they (adult males) are out there simply sitting outside their homes... Some of them seem to be fixing their cars or their homes, but sometimes they just look at you and you don't feel comfortable. I prefer to go to another park or a gym, so I can feel comfortable. (Patricia)

Crime and substance abuse in the neighborhood were often described as factors that inhibited the women from visiting local parks. They considered the presence of homeless individuals, discarded drug paraphernalia, and broken bottles as indications of risk of violence they chose to avoid. Mothers did not want their children exposed to people using drugs or being victims of violence, so they preferred to stay indoors or go to other places in the metropolitan area. Another common concern among the women was the presence of unleashed dogs in the street and parks of their neighborhood. Two women described their experience with this kind of incivility in the following manner:

> Sometimes people come [to the park] with their dogs and they are unleashed... The last time I was here, about two weeks ago, they had a Pitbull here and did not have a leash...It was unleashed! (Marina)

> No, I don't like to walk on the street...I always see unleashed dogs and I am afraid of them. I don't like my neighborhood for walking! (Bertha)

The women were asked about what amenities and features of the parks in their neighborhood they liked the most or were a concern. Their responses indicated that a variety of facilities, size, and design are important factors influencing the value of neighborhoods for physical activity and recreation. Most of the women agreed that the Phoenix Metropolitan Area has an adequate number of parks, but said that parks in Latinx neighborhoods need to adapt to the needs of the residents. For instance, most parks in Latinx neighborhoods have the same layout and amenities, including soccer fields and basketball courts, but lack walking paths or large free-play areas where young children can play safely. Diana, a 31-year-old Mexican immigrant, criticized the uniformity of parks in the area and highlighted the qualities of an ideal park.

> [Parks] are so square! They only have basketball courts, tennis courts, soccer fields... we need a little bit more of variety, not only basketball and soccer. Yes, almost everywhere is the same! I like a park with trees and walking paths that are not straight, where you can go up and down.

Later in the interview, Diana described how much she enjoys being in a park where trees are abundant to shade the path while she walks, and where the design of the path would allow her to reach her daily fitness goals easier. She mentioned that these features are not present in the park near her home. That park is small, it has few trees, and after ten turns around its perimeter, exercising becomes monotonous and boring.

Some of the interviewed women noted that parks in their neighborhood are so small that visitors of different age groups compete for space and equipment. High visitation of small park areas produces saturation, which in turn, reduces the attractiveness of Latinx neighborhoods parks, especially for mothers with small children. As explained during the interviews, overpopulated playgrounds, particularly by teenagers who do not have dedicated spaces, are ground for tension, unwanted physical contact, and accidents affecting mostly young children. The following account by Bertha, a Mexican woman in her thirties, was repeated by many women in the study.

> [The park] near to my house, I don't like it, I don't like it! It is hard, the environment... too much people! Too much people saying obscenities and kids fighting... and my two daughters see things....

The women were attracted to parks with open space, greenery, and tree canopy. Some expressed their dissatisfaction with the lack of replacement of trees fallen during the monsoon season, which makes parks less green and, in consequence, less appealing. They also showed preference for parks with large open spaces where their children could play freely and safely. Consider for example, the following observation by Cecilia, a Mexican woman in her late twenties with three children.

> This park has a lot of open views. Right now, for example, I am here seated with my toddler and I can see where my two-year old boy is playing. I can see him! ...there is a high visibility and there is a lot of grass. I like it because the playground's equipment is not too high or dangerous.

The hot summers of the Arizona desert constrain outdoor activities to a narrow window of time encompassing early mornings and early evenings. As noted earlier, even though the women see parks as an important recreational asset, many are not able to use them because the parks frequently lack proper lighting during the so-called good hours for exercise. These good hours of exercise also often coincide with homeless and young people loitering or engaging in activities deemed unacceptable by some of the women. As described by Vilma, a 32-year-old Mexican immigrant who moved to Phoenix one year ago:

> I don't know if I should go [to the park], it does not look safe ...there are many [homeless] men that are doing other things... they are not going to exercise or play.

In general, the women's descriptions of their interactions with neighborhood parks are influenced by a variety of factors, including prominently perceived safety in and around the site, but also by the opportunities for physical activity resulting from its design, equipment, and greenery. One highlight of the descriptions is that individual women are most likely to relate to parks as bundles of amenities and services embedded in the neighborhood and linked to the three ecologies of the urban environment: social, built, and natural. This so-called bundling is a reflection of how close these three ecologies are intertwined. For example, the perceived safety of a park is directly affected by its design, which includes physical characteristics such as poor visibility of play areas, limited lighting, isolation, poor maintenance, and surrounding land uses, among others. Through appropriate design, parks planners could balance the negative impacts of a social environment that is perceived as threatening by women in Latinx neighborhoods. Another example of the interaction between ecologies is how good lighting could augment the night time usability of parks during the hot summer days of Arizona, which can also be mitigated by tree canopies and water bodies that are known to reduce ambient temperatures through shading and evapotranspiration.

Not All Parks Are Created Equal

The findings of a significant proportion of the research examining the nexus between the urban environment and health suggest profound disparities across racial/ethnic groups in the distribution of environmental factors, such as access to green space or walkable neighborhoods (García et al., 2016; Stodolska, 2015). Most of these studies tend to focus on quantitative dimensions of accessibility to those factors, such as distance to the nearest neighborhood park or the number of street intersections within the neighborhood. Although these types of studies contribute to essential analyses to understand the impact of environmental factors on active-living opportunities across social groups, they often overlook the subjective and perceived quality of those factors. Interestingly, studies in this field have also failed to produce conclusive findings on the magnitude and pervasiveness of these disparities and their cause.

In contrast, the Latinx women in this study are unequivocally convinced that urban environments, but especially parks, are not equal across neighborhoods. Among other things, we learned that women are very sensitive to conditions and features of parks. The women made it clear that parks' social, physical, and natural characteristics are as important as proximity to their homes. In fact, many of the interviewed women traveled to different neighborhoods to use a park that offered the amenities and conditions they considered desirable: choice of recreational activity, large park space, safety, and cleanliness.

For example, Bertha traveled 20 min three times a week to gain access to an open space that provides the recreational opportunities that she and her family need. One of the most frequent referred motivations for this type of recreational commuting is that the destination park is "prettier," it has "a little bit more light" at sunset, "has better mountain views," and people in the park are simply "exercising or playing." Clearly, the inequitable distribution of active-living environmental factors like safety, cleanliness, greenness, and well-designed neighborhood parks has not been overlooked by these Latinx women in this area.

We already mentioned many of the conditions of urban environments in Latinx neighborhoods that forced these women to avoid engagement with the outdoors or push them to other recreational destinations in the metro area. One factor that deserves special mention is the rigidity of open-space design that homogenizes use and produces parks that seem predisposed against diversity and change. Women in Latinx neighborhoods in the Metropolitan Phoenix Area perceived parks as male-oriented spaces that failed to accommodate the needs of diverse user groups and especially exclude women with caregiving responsibilities. Exclusion is particularly severe for women who face economic, social, or physical constraints that prevent them from traveling to other neighborhoods where urban environments offer more and better recreational opportunities and amenities.

Unpacking the Urban Environment–Health Nexus

Most city residents get their leisure-time physical activity in their neighborhood, and close-to-home open public spaces are frequently the most likely places to engage in physical activity (Casper & Harrolle, 2013). Therefore, urban environments in Latinx neighborhoods play a crucial role in facilitating or preventing active living and their associated health benefits. The environments do this by providing opportunities for children, adolescents, adults, and older adults to engage with the place they live during their leisure time and utilitarian physical activities.

Although proximity to open space, such as neighborhood parks, is important in determining whether residents in Latinx neighborhoods will engage in active living, we have argued and provided evidence that focusing on only one of the ecologies of the urban environment is not enough. As indicated earlier, a host of socio-environmental factors act as constraints that impede the translation of the availability of open space into active lifestyles among Latinx persons. To start with, demanding occupations and family responsibilities limit the availability for Latinx individuals to engage in leisure-time physical activity. Indeed, for some of the women interviewed in the study in the Phoenix Metropolitan Area, freeing time for exercise was a challenging proposition, considering the amount of physical effort that they and other income earners in their family exerted during a regular workday. Nonetheless, the perceived health benefits of an active lifestyle motivate many of these Latinx women to pursue leisure-time physical activity, which forces them to negotiate a variety of obstacles in their neighborhoods. These obstacles include streets that are unsafe for pedestrians, isolated parks where residents feel threatened by crime and incivilities, play areas that fail to accommodate the activity needs of different groups, or poorly designed spaces that are unlikely to bring pleasure or result in frequent visits. As we learned from the women interviewed, the parks in the area vary in quality, and existing differences in their recreational and amenity value justify traveling to get to parks where the desirable mix of social, built, and natural environmental elements is available.

The fact that engagement in active living is a multifactorial and multiscalar outcome is widely recognized, but research using this approach in the study of the Latinx urban environments is hard to find. There are several reasons for this. First, it is difficult to avoid the tendency in this type of research to fragment urban realities into pieces that are both appealing to academic audiences and can be easily processed by a well-established disciplinary apparatus. As explained by Corburn (2007), professionalization, technocratization, and bureaucratization are factors underlying the difficulty of bringing together the realms of public health and urban planning. Second, urban and public health researchers have hesitated to abandon the safety of established methodologic approaches based on mere quantification and need to embrace new methodologic approaches mixing quantitative tools (e.g., surveys, geospatial mapping) with visual ethnographies, focus groups, and other qualitative methodologies. Therefore, approaches that unbundle the multifactorial and multiscalar processes that link neighborhood urban environments and residents' active lifestyles still need to be adopted. Third, prevailing conceptions of the influence of the urban environment on health are not only narrow and restrictive but also fail to accept the larger sociospatial processes, such as segregation and racial discrimination, that produce environmental inequities affecting Latinx persons and persons in other urban minority groups.

Conclusions and Recommendations for Future Research

This chapter represents an initial effort to map the complex relationship between neighborhood urban environments and the health of Latinx communities. The intention has been to highlight the point that the conditions that influence the level of physical activity of Latinx persons are complex and suggest a need for comprehensive approaches, recognizing that lifestyles leading to better health are the net effect of interacting and overlapping social, built, and natural neighborhood ecologies. Besides the obvious conceptual and analytic implications of this, there is also a need for all-inclusive strategies, including policies and programs to bring about changes in each of these ecologies if the goal is to actively pursue a healthier Latinx population. Overall, such changes should have as a priority the removal of barriers to physical activity and the conversion of neighborhoods into safe, accessible, and attractive places for all Latinx individuals. The transformation of Latinx neighborhoods into active-living spaces requires the application of old and new ideas, many of which were suggested in the accounts of the Latinx women we talked to in the Phoenix Metropolitan Area.

First, a good place to start is to see Latinx neighborhoods as disarticulated spatial systems that need to be reconnected by linking streets, school yards, parks, and other public facilities in a network for active human mobility. Many cities in the USA, and around the world, are using this approach to promote walking, cycling, running, and mobility because of their beneficial effect on public health and sense of community (Sallis et al., 2016). The creation of these types of networks is an intervention that is likely to contribute to the reduction of obesity and the incidence of non-communicable diseases among residents of Latinx neighborhoods. Furthermore, such networks provide a way to expand the amount of available public open space while augmenting near-to-home opportunities for recreation and exercise by improving the accessibility of parks and creating trails connecting parks and other public spaces within the neighborhood. Having additional walking venues closer to residences may encourage individuals to increase their level of physical activity, particularly for residents with demanding work schedules or transportation constraints.

Second, perceived safety is as a factor that will affect the beneficial impact of the creation of such network. It is imperative then, that signs of disorder in the neighborhood, such as vandalism, trash, unleashed dogs, uncontrolled traffic, and loitering be eliminated. Many of these things require effective actions to control crime, improve street and park lighting, and eliminate so-called hideouts for engaging in undesirable behaviors. As Stodolska (2015) suggested, it is also important to obtain current information about perceived safety issues, not only from residents using neighborhood parks, but also from nonusers, as they may be affected the most by existing safety issues.

Third, equally important are efforts to redesign public open space, including local streets and parks, in order to accommodate a diverse demand for active-living opportunities from women, men, children, and older adults living in Latinx neighborhoods. It is obvious that if residents of Latinx neighborhoods are to derive the greatest health benefit of public parks, diverse types of park amenities and services must be provided. The creation of active environments supportive of a diverse demand should focus on designing neighborhood parks that are safe and attractive especially to Latinx women, as they tend to be less physically active than women who identify with other US ethnic/racial groups and who (as are other women) are particularly sensitive to conditions that affect their perception of parks as a hazard or a resource and have significant influence in the level of activity of other family members.

Fourth, cities should organize regular events to encourage neighborhood residents to engage in physical activity. Examples include walking, yoga, dance groups, and other organized activities that appeal to Latinx residents and meet the needs of a diverse group of users. Indeed, opportunities for both moderate and vigorous activities are needed, particularly for women and older adults—two groups clearly excluded by park facilities that are often biased toward men and youth (Cohen et al., 2016). In particular, many Latinx women will be encouraged to participate if such efforts, as suggested by Stodolska (2015), include such things as childcare services and activities for the entire family.

Lastly, in agreement with many other scholars, we want to emphasize that the creation of active, supportive urban environments should be a regular function not only for urban planning departments but also for public health departments in cities and towns in metropolitan areas (Christian et al., 2015; Corburn, 2007; Northridge et al., 2003; Sallis et al., 2016). Urban planners and public health professionals should set a priority to reconnect their practices and priorities with the needs of minority populations who are particularly affected by inadequate and outdated planning, designs, and maintenance of streets, parks, public transportation, and other environmental elements that could trigger the activation of residents in Latinx neighborhoods.

References

Abercrombie, L. C., Sallis, J. F., Conway, T. L., Frank, L. D., Saelens, B. E., & Chapman, J. E. (2008). Income and racial disparities in access to public parks and private recreation facilities. *American Journal of Preventive Medicine, 34,* 9–15.

Acevedo-Garcia, D., Lochner, K. A., Osypuk, T. L., & Subramanian, S. V. (2003). Future directions in residential segregation and health research: A multilevel approach. *American Journal of Public Health, 93,* 215–221.

Amuedo-Dorantes, C., Puttitanun, T., & Martinez-Donate, A. P. (2013). How do tougher immigration measures affect unauthorized immigrants? *Demography, 50,* 1067–1091.

Anderson, K., & Fullerton, A. (2014). Residential segregation, health, and health care: Answering the Latino question. *Race and Social Problems, 6,* 262–279.

Angotti, T., & Sze, J. (2009). Environmental justice practice: implications for interdisciplinary urban public health. In N. Freudenberg, S. Klitzman, & S. Saegert (Eds.), *Urban health and society: Interdisciplinary approaches to research and practice* (pp. 19–42). San Francisco: Jossey-Bass.

Baldacci, S., Maio, S., Cerrai, S., Sarno, G., Baiz, N., Simoni, M., et al. (2015). Allergy and asthma: Effects of the exposure to particulate matter and biological allergens. *Respiratory Medicine, 109,* 1089–1104.

Basu, R., & Ostro, B. D. (2008). A multicounty analysis identifying the populations vulnerable to mortality associated with high ambient temperature in California. *American Journal of Epidemiology, 168,* 632–637.

Bedimo-Rung, A. L., Mowen, A. J., & Cohen, D. A. (2005). The Significance of Parks to Physical Activity and Public Health: A Conceptual Model. *American Journal of Preventive Medicine ,28*(2):159–168.

Berko, J., Ingram, D. D., Saha, S., & Parker, J. D. (2014). Deaths attributed to heat, cold, and other weather events in the United States, 2006–2010. In *National health statistical reports* (p. 15). Hyattsville, MD: National Center for Health Statistics.

Bruton, C. M., & Floyd, M. F. (2014). Disparities in built and natural features of urban parks: Comparisons by neighborhood level race/ethnicity and income. *Journal of Urban Health, 91,* 894–907.

Byrne, J., & Wolch, J. (2009). Nature, race, and parks: past research and future directions for geographic research. *Progress in Human Geography , 33* (6), 743–765.

Carr, P., Lichter, D., & Kafala, M. (2013). Can immigration save small-town America? In *Research and policy brief series,* issue 53. Ithaca, NY: Community and Regional Development Institute. https://cardi.cals.cornell.edu/sites/cardi.cals.cornell.edu/files/shared/documents/ResearchPolicyBriefs/Policy-Brief-April13.pdf.

Casper, J. M., & Harrolle, M. G. (2013). Perceptions of constraints to leisure time physical activity among Latinos in Wake County, North Carolina. *American Journal of Health Promotion, 27,* 139–142.

Cohen, D., McKenzie, T., Sehgal, A., Williamson, S., Golinelli, D., & Lurie, N. (2007). Contribution of public parks to physical activity. *American Journal of Public Health ,97.*

Chiesura, A. (2004). The role of urban parks for the sustainable city. *Landscape and Urban Planning, 68*(1), 129–138.

Christian, H., Zubrick, S. R., Foster, S., Giles-Corti, B., Bull, F., Wood, L., et al. (2015). The influence of the neighborhood physical environment on early child health and development: A review and call for research. *Health & Place, 33,* 25–36.

Cohen, D. A., Han, B., Nagel, C. J., Harnik, P., McKenzie, T. L., Evenson, K. R., et al. (2016). The First National Study of Neighborhood Parks. *American Journal of Preventive Medicine, 51,* 419–426.

Colchero, M. A., Popkin, B. M., Rivera, J. A., & Ng, S. W. (2016). Beverage purchases from stores in Mexico under the excise tax on sugar sweetened beverages: Observational study. *BMJ, 352.*

Corburn, J. (2007). Reconnecting with our roots. *Urban Affairs Review, 42,* 688–713.

Crespo, C. J. (2000). Encouraging physical activity in minorities: Eliminating disparities by 2010. *Physician & Sportsmedicine, 28,* 36–51.

Cronan, M. K., Shinew, K. J., Schneider, I., Stanis, S. A. W., & Chavez, D. (2008). Physical activity patterns and preferences among Latinos in different types of public parks. *Journal of Physical Activity and Health, 5,* 894–908.

D'Amato, G. (2002). Environmental urban factors (air pollution and allergens) and the rising trends in allergic respiratory diseases. *Allergy, 57*(Suppl 72), 30–33.

D'Amato, G., Holgate, S. T., Pawankar, R., Ledford, D. K., Cecchi, L., Al-Ahmad, M. … Annesi-Maesano, I. (2015). Meteorological conditions, climate change, new emerging factors, and asthma and related allergic disorders. A statement of the World Allergy Organization. *World Allergy Organization Journal, 8,* 25.

D'Amato, G., Liccardi, G., D'Amato, M., & Cazzola, M. (2001). The role of outdoor air pollution and climatic changes on the rising trends in respiratory allergy. *Respiratory Medicine, 95,* 606–611.

Evans, T., Whitehead, M., & Diderichsen, F. (2001). The social basis of disparities in health. In T. Evans, M. Whitehead, F. Diderichsen, A. Bhuiya, & M. Wirth (Eds.), *Challenging inequities in health: From ethics to action* (pp. 13–23). New York: Oxford University Press.

Fitzpatrick, K., & LaGory, M. (2011). *Unhealthy cities: Poverty, race, and place in America.* London: Routledge.

Forsyth, A., Wall, M., Choo, T., Larson, N., Van Riper, D., & Neumark-Sztainer, D. (2015). Perceived and police-reported neighborhood crime: Linkages to adolescent activity behaviors and weight status. *Journal of Adolescent Health, 57,* 222–228.

Galea, S., Freudenberg, N., & Vlahov, D. (2005). Cities and population health. *Social Science & Medicine, 60*(5), 1017–1033.

Garcia, J. (2014). *Does living in Latino neighborhoods affect risk for obesity? Findings from a study of social capital and parks availability in Los Angeles neighborhoods* (Unpublished dissertation). Los Angeles, CA: University of California.

García, J. J., Gee, G. C., & Jones, M. (2016). A critical race theory analysis of public park features in Latino immigrant neighborhoods. *Du Bois Review: Social Science Research on Race, 13,* 397–411.

Giles-Corti, B., Broomhall, M. H., Knuiman, M., Collins, C., Douglas, K., Ng, K., Lange, A., & Donovan, R. J. (2005). Increasing walking: How important is distance to, atractivenness and size of public open space?. *America Journal of Preventive Medicine, 28*(2):169–176.

Jenkins, G., Yuen, H., Rose, E., Maher, A., Gregory, K., & Cotton, M. (2015). Disparities in quality of park play spaces between two cities with diverse income and race/ethnicity composition: A pilot study. *International Journal of Environmental Research and Public Health, 12,* 8009.

Johnson Gaither, C. (2011). Latino park access: Examining environmental equity in a "New Destination" county in the South. *Journal of Park and Recreation Administration, 29*(4), 37–52.

Jones, A. P., Brainard, J., Bateman, I. J., & Lovett, A. A. (2009). Equity of access to public parks in Birmingham, England. *Environmental Research Journal, 3,* 237–256.

Kaczynski, A. T., & Henderson, K. A. (2007). Environmental correlates of physical activity: A review of evidence about parks and recreation. *Leisure Sciences, 29.*

Kaźmierczak, A. (2013). The contribution of local parks to neighbourhood social ties. *Landscape and Urban Planning, 109,* 31–44.

Klitzman, S., Matte, T., & Kass, D. (2006). The urban physical environment and its effects on health. In N. Freudenberg, S. Galea, & D. Vlahov (Eds.), *Cities and the health of the public* (pp. 61–84). Nashville, TN: Vanderbilt University Press.

Kozlowski, J. C. (2008). Equity in Latino neighborhood parks. *Parks and Recreation, 43,* 26–28.

Kramer, M. R., & Hogue, C. R. (2009). Is segregation bad for your health? *Epidemiologic Reviews, 31,* 178–194.

Lara-Valencia, F., & Garcia-Perez, H. (2018). Disparities in the provision of public parks in neighbourhoods with varied Latino composition in the Phoenix Metropolitan Area. *Local Environment, 23*(12), 1107–1120.

Lawrence, R. J. (2004). Housing and health: From interdisciplinary principles to transdisciplinary research and practice. *Futures, 36,* 487–502.

Levell, P., O'Connell, M., & Smith, K. (2016). Sugary drinks tax: Response from the Institute for Fiscal Studies. *The Lancet, 387,* 1907–1908.

Li, K., Wen, M., & Henry, K. A. (2017). Ethnic density, immigrant enclaves, and Latino health risks: A propensity score matching approach. *Social Science and Medicine, 189,* 44–52.

Lin, A. R., Menjívar, C., Ettekal, A. V., Simpkins, S. D., Gaskin, E. R., & Pesch, A. (2016). "They will post a law about playing soccer" and other ethnic/racial microaggressions in organized activities experienced by Mexican-origin families. *Journal of Adolescent Research, 31,* 557–581.

Lindsay, A. C., Sussner, K. M., Greaney, M. L., & Peterson, K. E. (2009). Influence of social context on eating, physical activity, and sedentary behaviors of Latina mothers and their preschool-age children. *Health Education & Behavior, 36,* 81–96.

Logan, J. R. (2011). Separate and unequal: The neighborhood gap for blacks, Hispanics and Asians in metropolitan America. *Project US2010.* https://s4.ad.brown.edu/Projects/Diversity/Data/Report/report0727.pdf.

Lopez, R. P., & Hynes, H. P. (2009). Obesity, physical activity and the urban environment: Public health research needs. In H. P. Hynes & R. P. Lopez (Eds.), *Urban health: Readings in social, built, and physical environments of U.S. cities* (pp. 169–181). Sudbury, MA: Jones and Bartlett.

Loukaitou-Sideris, A. (1995). Urban Form and Social Context: Cultural Differentiation in the Uses of Urban Parks. *Journal of Planning Education and Research 14*(2), 89–102.

Markevych, I., Schoierer, J., Hartig, T., Chudnovsky, A., Hystad, P., Dzhambov, A. M. … Fuertes, E. (2017). Exploring pathways linking greenspace to health: Theoretical and methodological guidance. *Environmental Research, 158,* 301–317.

Maas, J., Verheij, R., Groenewegen, P., De Vries, S., & Spreeuwenberg, P. (2006). Green space, urbanity, and health: How strong is the relation?. *Journal of Epidemiol and Community Health, 60*(7), 587–592.

Maas, J., Verheij, R., Spreeuwenberg, P., & Groenewegen, P. (2008). Physical activity as a possible mechanism behind the relationship between green space and health: A multilevel analysis. *BMC Public Health, 8*

Morello-Frosch, R., & Jesdale, B. M. (2006). Separate and unequal: Residential segregation and estimated cancer risks associated with ambient air toxics in U.S. metropolitan areas. *Environmental Health Perspectives, 114,* 386–393.

Nagel, C. L., Carlson N. E., Bosworth, M., & Michael, Y. L. (2008). The Relation between Neighborhood Built Environment and Walking Activity among Older Adults. *American Journal of Epidemiology, 168*(4), 461–468.

National Center for Health Statistics. (2017). *Health, United States, 2016: With chartbook on long-term trends in health.* Hyattsville, MD: National Center for Health Statistics.

Northridge, M. E., Sclar, E. D., & Biswas, P. (2003). Sorting out the connections between the built environment and health: A conceptual framework for navigating pathways and planning healthy cities. *Journal of Urban Health: Bulletin of the New York Academy of Medicine, 80,* 556–568.

Ogden, C. L., Carroll, M. D., Fryar, C. D., & Flegal, K. M. (2015). Prevalence of obesity among adults and youth: United States, 2011–2014. In *NCHS data brief* (p. 8). Hyattsville, MD: National Center for Health Statistics.

Onésimo Sandoval, J. S., & Jennings, J. (2012). Barrios and hyper barrios: How Latino neighborhoods changed the urban built environment. *Journal of Urbanism: International Research on Placemaking and Urban Sustainability, 5,* 111–138.

Pastor, M., Morello-Frosch, R., & Sadd, J. L. (2005). The air is always cleaner on the other side: Race, space, and ambient air toxics exposures in California. *Journal of Urban Affairs, 27,* 127–148.

Pincetl, S., Wolch, J., Wilson, J., & Longcore, T. (2003). *Toward a sustainable Los Angeles: A "nature's services" approach.* Los Angeles, CA: Center for Sustainable Cities, University of Southern California.

Powell, K. E., & Blair, S. N. (1994). The public health burdens of sedentary living habits: Theoretical but realistic estimates. *Medicine and Science in Sports and Exercise, 26,* 851–856.

Public Polity Institute of California. (2007). Latino attitudes and the environment. In *Just the facts*: San Francisco: Public Polity Institute of California. http://www.ppic.org/content/pubs/jtf/JTF_LatinoAttitudesEnvironmentJTF.pdf.

Sallis, J. F., Bull, F., Burdett, R., Frank, L. D., Griffiths, P., Giles-Corti, B., et al. (2016). Use of science to guide city planning policy and practice: How to achieve healthy and sustainable future cities. *Lancet, 388,* 2936–2947.

Schulz, A., & Northridge, M. E. (2004). Social determinants of health: Implications for environmental health promotion. *Health Education & Behavior, 31,* 455–471.

Schulz, A. J., Williams, D. R., Israel, B. A., & Lempert, L. B. (2002). Racial and spatial relations as fundamental determinants of health in Detroit. *Milbank Quarterly, 80,* 677–707.

Sister, C., Wolch, J., & Wilson, J. (2010). Got green? Addressing environmental justice in park provision. *GeoJournal, 75,* 229–248.

Stepler, R., & Lopez, M. H. (2016). *U.S. Latino population growth and dispersion has slowed since onset of the Great Recession* (p. 53). Washington, DC: Pew Research Center. http://www.pewhispanic.org/2016/09/08/latino-population-growth-and-dispersion-has-slowed-since-the-onset-of-the-great-recession/.

Stodolska, M. (2015). Recreation for all: Providing leisure and recreation services in multi-ethnic communities. *World Leisure Journal, 57,* 89–103.

Suminski, R. R., Connolly, E. K., May, L. E., Wasserman, J., Olvera, N., & Lee, R. E. (2012). Park quality in racial/ethnic minority neighborhoods. *Environmental Justice, 5,* 271–278.

Suro, R., & Singer, A. (2002). *Latino growth in metropolitan America: Changing patterns, new locations*. Washington, DC: The Brookings Institution, Center on Urban and Metropolitan Policy, and Pew Hispanic Center.

Talen, E. (1997). The social equity of urban service distribution an exploration of park access in Pueblo, Colorado, and Macon, Georgia. *Urban Geography, 18,* 521–541.

Tienda, M., & Fuentes, N. (2014). Hispanics in metropolitan America: New realities and old debates. *Annual Review of Sociology, 40,* 499.

Timperio, A., Crawford, D., Ball, K., & Salmon, J. (2017). Typologies of neighbourhood environments and children's physical activity, sedentary time and television viewing. *Health & Place, 43,* 121–127.

Timperio, A., Crawford, D., Telford, A., & Salmon, J. (2004). Perceptions about the local neighborhood and walking and cycling among children. *Preventive Medicine, 38,* 39–47.

U.S. Census. (2015). *2011–2015 American Community Survey 5-year estimates*. U.S. Census Bureau: Washington, DC.

U.S. Surgeon General. (1999). *Physical activity and health: A report of the Surgeon General*. Atlanta. GA: Centers for Disease Control and Prevention.

Varsanyi, M. (2010). *Taking local control: Immigration policy activism in U.S. cities and states*. Redwood City, CA: Stanford University Press.

Vaughan, K. B., Kaczynski, A. T., Wilhelm Stanis, S. A., Besenyi, G. M., Bergstrom, R., & Heinrich, K. M. (2013). Exploring the distribution of park availability, features, and quality across Kansas City, Missouri by income and race/ethnicity: An environmental justice investigation. *Annals of Behavioral Medicine, 45*(Suppl 1), S28–S38.

Wolch, J., Wilson, J. P., & Fehrenbach, J. (2005). Parks and park funding in Los Angeles: An equity-mapping analysis. *Urban Geography, 26,* 4–35.

Wolch, J., Byrne, J., & Newell, J. (2014). Urban green space, public health, and environmental justice: The challenge of making cities 'just green enough'. *Landscape and Urban Planning, 125,* 234–244.

Wood, L., Hooper, P., Foster, S., & Bull, F. (2017). Public green spaces and positive mental health—Investigating the relationship between access, quantity and types of parks and mental wellbeing. *Health & Place, 48,* 63–71.

Woolf, S. H., & Aron, L. (2013). *U.S. health in international perspective: Shorter lives, poorer health*. Washington, DC: The National Academies Press.

Zenk, S. N., Schulz, A. J., Odoms-Young, A. M., & Lockett, M. (2009). Interdisciplinary, participatory research on urban food environments and dietary behavior. In N. Freudenberg, S. Klitzman, & S. Saegert (Eds.), *Urban health and society: Interdisciplinary approaches to research and practice* (pp. 45–61). San Francico: Jossey-Bass.

Chapter 14
Racial/Ethnic Discrimination, Intersectionality, and Latina/o Health

Alana M. W. LeBrón and Edna A. Viruell-Fuentes

Abstract In this chapter, we summarize the existing literature on self-reported experiences of racial/ethnic discrimination and health status among Latina/o persons in the USA, explore the implications for Latina/o/x health, and identify future directions of research in this critical area. We reviewed 25 peer-reviewed articles that quantitatively examined the association between self-reported discrimination and mental or physical health, published between 2000 and 2016. The reviewed studies were primarily cross-sectional and few compared Latina/o subgroups. We encourage researchers to examine the health impacts of racial/ethnic discrimination on Latina/o health through intersectionality theory to assess discrimination across multiple intersecting social statuses. We also recommend that researchers examine the longitudinal health consequences of structural forms of racism such as carceral policies, educational policies, environmental quality, immigration enforcement, residential segregation, and health care access and quality across spatial contexts.

Keywords Discrimination · Immigration policies · Intersectionality theory · Latinx health · Racism

Anti-immigrant and anti-Latina/o/x ideologies and policy proposals advanced following the 2016 election of Donald J. Trump as President of the USA illustrate the persistent and dynamic context of racialization of Latina/o/x persons in the twenty-first century. In the month following the election, the country experienced a sharp increase in hate incidents in public and private spaces, 29% of which were anti-immigrant in nature and 14% of which were classified as anti-Latina/o/x (Southern Poverty Law Center, 2016). Hate incidents represent one important aspect of racism in

---

A. M. W. LeBrón (✉)
Department of Population Health and Disease Prevention and Department of Chicano/Latino Studies, University of California, Irvine,
CA, USA
e-mail: alebron@uci.edu

Department of Chicano/Latino Studies, University of California, Irvine, CA, USA

E. A. Viruell-Fuentes
Department of Latina/Latino Studies, University of Illinois, Urbana-Champaign,
IL, USA

© Springer Nature Switzerland AG 2020
A. D. Martínez and S. D. Rhodes (eds.), *New and Emerging Issues in Latinx Health*, https://doi.org/10.1007/978-3-030-24043-1_14

the USA, joining other forms of personally mediated racism and institutional racism as components of structural racism. In 2016, 52% of Latina/o/x persons reported regular or occasional experiences of discrimination linked with their racialized status (Krogstad & Lopez, 2016). These reports varied by nativity, age, and educational attainment, indicating the intersectional nature of racism (Krogstad & Lopez, 2016). These processes have important implications for health inequities[1] and for health patterns among Latina/o/x persons.

As a structural determinant of health, racism operates through institutions and policies that shape access to health-promoting resources, such as housing; community social and economic resources; exposure to physical environments; educational and employment opportunities; and the opportunity to reside in the USA (Jones, 2000; Viruell-Fuentes, Miranda, & Abdulrahim, 2012; Williams & Mohammed, 2013). Racism also structures and is reinforced by ideologies and representations that reify policies that negatively shape the opportunities of communities targeted with racism and emboldens personally mediated racism (Jones, 2000; Viruell-Fuentes et al., 2012; Williams & Mohammed, 2013). Racism thus not only shapes access to resources that are fundamental to promoting health, but also serves as a profound and persistent life stressor that has cumulative effects on health and well-being (Lewis, Cogburn, & Williams, 2015; Williams & Mohammed, 2013).

Variations in health patterns among Latina/o/x persons discussed in other chapters in this volume necessitate an examination of the contributions of racism to these patterns. While an increasingly prominent line of inquiry has established linkages between racism and physical and mental health for non-Latina/o Black persons (henceforth, *Black persons*), the literature regarding the health implications of racism for Latina/o persons, and variations in these associations by social statuses, is still emerging. The primary goal of this chapter is to summarize and synthesize the existing literature on self-reported experiences of racial/ethnic discrimination and health status among Latina/o persons in the USA, discuss implications for the health of Latina/o/x populations, and identify future directions for research in this critical area.

The literature on racism and health reviewed in this chapter is based on responses by Latina/o persons' to validated surveys that assess experiences of discrimination that individuals attributed to their racial/ethnic status, as well as general experiences of discrimination that individuals did not restrict to their racial/ethnic status. It is difficult to separate multiple, intersecting social statuses when examining the experiences with racism among Latina/o persons (Viruell-Fuentes et al., 2012). Accordingly, we conceptualize measures of both racial/ethnic discrimination and general discrimination as capturing experiences with racism. Additionally, we conceptualize other measures (e.g., subscales of the Hispanic Stress Inventory and indicators of fear of deportation) as assessing a subset of experiences with and vigilance toward racism (Cavazos-Rehg, Zayas, & Spitznagel, 2007; Cervantes, Fisher, Padilla, & Napper, 2016; Cervantes, Padilla, & Salgado de Snyder, 1991). While there is a body

---

[1] We define health inequities as differences in health that are systematic, preventable, unjust, and actionable (Whitehead, 1991).

of literature that addresses acculturative stress among Latina/o persons (Abraído-Lanza, Armbrister, Flórez, & Aguirre, 2006; Abraído-Lanza, Chao, & Flórez, 2005; Abraído-Lanza, Echeverría, & Flórez, 2016), which, as noted, sometimes includes subscales related to discrimination, our review is focused on the literature that explicitly sought to address the links between discrimination and health, conceptually and empirically.

Racialization Processes and Racial Categories

Race/ethnicity are socially constructed categories that capture the historical and contemporary consequences of differential access to social, political, and economic opportunities (Almaguer, 2009; Omi & Winant, 2015). Throughout the latter part of the 20th century and the beginning of the 21st century, the term *Latina/o* (as opposed to Hispanic) has been used to foreground the histories of colonization of, and contemporary foreign policy towards, some Latin American countries or territories by the US, all of which have contributed to the presence and position of Latinas/os within the US racial/ethnic structure.

As an intrinsic component of racialization processes, racial/ethnic categories are created, contested, inhabited, transformmed, and eventually destroyed (Omi & Winant, 2015). Currently, social movements are elevating intersectional and queer analyses and strategies to understand and address racialization processes. Accordingly, there is a growing discussion of strategies to incorproate a range of gender and queer identities when referring to persons of Latin American origin or descent. One such strategy involves moving away from the term *Latino* (intending to encompass women and men, though linguistically a masculine term) and towards labels that include cis-women (e.g., *Latina*), cis-men (e.g., *Latino*), and persons who do not identify along gender binaries (e.g., *Latin@* or *Latinx*).

Consistent with racialization processes, these discussions, practices, and responses are ongoing and dynamic. For example, as in this edited volume, the term *Latinx* is increasingly being used to refer to persons of Latin American origin or descent. Affected community members and members of dominant social structures have responded to this movement in a range of ways, including but not limited to: embracing the term Latinx to refer broadly to people of Latin American origin or descent; recognizing queer identities by specifically referring to queer persons or populations as Latinx; and/or resisting practices that refer to cis-Latinas and cis-Latinos as Latinx.

Our review encompasses literature on racial/ethnic discrimination and the health of people in Latin American descent or origin published between 2000 and 2016, at which time, the literature largely lacked an intersectional and queer analytic lens. We use the term *Latina/o* when referring to findings from specific studies to reflect the state of this literature. When discussing health patterns at the population level, we include queer identities by using the term *Latina/o/x*. Recognizing great heterogeneity within the Latina/o/x population, we refer to specific country or territory of origin or descent whenever possible. We return to these issues in our conclusion, wherein we call for scholarship that advances intersectional and queer lenses to the study of racial/ethnic discrimination and health among individuals and communities of Latin American origin and descent in the United States.

Racism Trickles Down to Matters of Health

Racism is a dynamic social process through which racial/ethnic meanings and differences are constructed and reconstructed across historical moments and social contexts, with deleterious consequences for those targeted with racism (Almaguer, 2009; Omi & Winant, 2015; Schwalbe et al., 2000). Ascribed racial/ethnic meanings produce and are used to justify social, economic, and political inequities that are patterned by race/ethnicity and profoundly shape access to health-promoting resources and institutions (Jones, 2000). Often unfolding in the form of ideologies, institutional practices or policies, and interpersonal processes, racism serves to limit access to health-promoting resources according to an individual's or group's ascribed, (de)valued status and produce race-related stressors (Almaguer, 2009; Jones, 2000; Omi & Winant, 2015; Schwalbe et al., 2000). Processes of racism also invoke other social statuses, such as gender, socioeconomic position, nativity, and citizenship (Viruell-Fuentes et al., 2012). These processes that shape social hierarchies and identities are fluid and relational, while also obdurate, and interact over time and within particular contexts (Collins, 1990, 2012; Crenshaw, 1989; Ford & Airhihenbuwa, 2010; Hankivsky, 2012).

Consistent with processes of racism that ascribe social labels and statuses, the US Office of Management and Budget (OMB), designated Latina/o/x persons as a "Hispanic" social group[2] (OMB, 1997) and as the only recognized "ethnic" group in the USA, regardless of country or territory of origin or descent. Latina/o/x persons have a longstanding and complex history with racism in the USA (Acuña, 2011; Almaguer, 2009). However, partly due to the above-mentioned state-driven processes of labeling Latina/o/x persons as an ethnic group, rather than a racial group, the development of scholarship focused on the health implications of racism for Latina/o/x persons is still emerging. That is, studies that center on ethnicity motivate attention to cultural distinctions across groups and on attributions of health differentials to cultural processes. In contrast, studies that highlight "race" seek to attend to how the multiple dimensions of racism, such as the role of institutional and interpersonal racism, shape health and well-being. Consequently, while Latina/o/x persons as a group, and subgroups within this heterogeneous population, have experienced historical and contemporary racism, the great majority of the Latina/o health liter-

---

[2]Some individuals and communities with social, historical, and/or birth ties to Latin American countries or colonized territories identify with the term *Latina/o/x* as a strategy to resist government-driven racial/ethnic labels and embrace their political status and history as a social bloc, rather than identify with their colonizer (i.e. Spain) (Alcoff, 2005; Hayes-Bautista & Chapa, 1987).

ature has focused on culture and acculturation to explain health outcomes among Latina/o persons (Hunt, Schneider, & Comer, 2004; Viruell-Fuentes, 2007; Viruell-Fuentes et al., 2012).

Structural racism, including ideologies, policies, and institutional and interpersonal practices, often finds expression in day-to-day experiences (Viruell-Fuentes et al., 2012),[3] some of which are captured in existing quantitative measures of self-reported discrimination[4] (Krieger, Smith, Naishadham, Hartman, & Barbeau, 2005; Williams & Mohammed, 2009, 2013). While some of the literature involving quantitative measures of discrimination characterizes these reports of discrimination as "perceived discrimination," we conceptualize these reports as "self-reported discrimination." As Krieger and colleagues (2005) explain, "While self-reported experiences must be perceived, not all perceived experiences are necessarily reported, depending on individuals' willingness or ability to report them" (p. 1578). Additionally, nomenclature of "perceived discrimination" may erroneously be interpreted as the experience not having occurred or as not being discriminatory, and risks minimizing the structural conditions that give rise to experiences of discrimination. Furthermore, referring to quantitative measures of discrimination as "self-reported discrimination" acknowledges that the process of interpreting discriminatory experiences is shaped by exposure to contextually specific racialization processes and thus identifying and articulating experiences of discrimination within that context.

What follows is a review of the literature examining the social patterning of discrimination and associations between discrimination and health for Latina/o persons. We begin by describing the most common quantitative measures of discrimination, then summarize the literature regarding the patterning of discrimination among Latina/o persons, and synthesize the literature examining associations between discrimination and health. We conclude with an analysis of this literature and provide recommendations for future research.

Measuring Racial/Ethnic Discrimination

Racial/ethnic discrimination is conceptualized as capturing exposure to processes that restrict access to resources such as quality education, employment, housing, health care, goods, and services, and the opportunity to remain in the USA and/or outside of carceral institutions on the basis of race/ethnicity (Almaguer, 2009; Nagel, 1994; Omi & Winant, 2015; Schwalbe et al., 2000). In addition to capturing exposure to the production of inequalities through restricted access to institutional, material, and social resources and opportunities, several measures of discrimination capture exposure to psychosocial stressors associated with these processes (Lewis et al., 2015; Williams & Mohammed, 2013).

---

[3]For a discussion of the health implications of internalized racism and stereotype threat, please see (Williams & Mohammed, 2013).
[4]Throughout this chapter, we refer to self-reported discrimination as *discrimination*.

Several widely available quantitative scales capture micro- and macro-level aspects of experiences of discrimination (Bastos, Celeste, Faerstein, & Barros, 2010; Lewis et al., 2015; Paradies et al., 2015; Pascoe & Richman, 2009; Williams & Mohammed, 2013). One of the most common scales applied in the literature on discrimination and health among Latina/o persons that we reviewed is the Everyday Unfair Treatment Scale (Williams, Yu, Jackson, & Anderson, 1997), which assesses exposure to day-to-day indignities (e.g., being treated with less courtesy or respect) and inferior service or treatment (e.g., receiving poorer service than others, people act as if they are afraid of you) (Williams et al., 1997). The experiences captured in the Everyday Unfair Treatment Scale are conceptualized as being rooted in systems of oppression, but are not necessarily linked with a particular institutional source or setting. Studies involving the Everyday Unfair Treatment Scale often query about experiences of unfair treatment or discrimination generally, then ask the respondent to attribute their experience(s) to a range of social statuses (e.g., gender, age, socioeconomic position, where they live, language use, nativity, race, ethnicity, sexual orientation, and ability). Some studies restricted survey questions or analyses to experiences of discrimination that respondents specifically attributed to their racial/ethnic identity or national origin or descent. Other studies considered experiences of discrimination regardless of attribution, and yet other studies evaluated the health implications of discrimination that respondents attributed to multiple social statuses or identities.

Other scales used in the articles we reviewed, albeit far less frequently than the Everyday Unfair Treatment Scale, include: the Experiences of Discrimination Scale (Krieger, 1990; Krieger et al., 2005), the Reactions to Race module (Purnell et al., 2012), the Perceived Racism Scale for Latinos (Collado-Proctor, 1999), the Perceived Ethnic Discrimination Questionnaire (Brondolo et al., 2005), and subscales of acculturation scales (e.g., Acculturation Stress Subscale of the Social, Attitudinal, Familial, and Environmental Scale) (Mena, Padilla, & Maldonado, 1987). This range of scales used to assess Latina/o persons' experiences with discrimination reflects the multiple life domains in which different forms of discrimination may unfold.

Overall, these measures attempt to capture processes that are involved in the construction and maintenance of inequalities that are associated with and reinforce systems of racial oppression. Although some of these scales were developed based on an understanding of the racialized experiences of Black persons in the USA in the 1990s, these measures have proven useful in our understanding of the links between discrimination and health among Latina/o persons.

Social Patterning of Self-reported Discrimination

Consistent with intersectionality theory (Collins, 1990, 2015; Crenshaw, 1991), Latina/o among persons the prevalence of self-reported discrimination varies by several social statuses and identities, with some patterns varying according to the specific characteristics of the sample and the measure used to assess discrimination. A consistent finding across studies is that younger Latina/o persons report more frequent experiences of discrimination than their older counterparts (Finch, Kolody, & Vega, 2000; LeBrón et al., 2014, 2017; Pérez, Fortuna, & Alegría, 2008) after accounting for socioeconomic position, gender, nativity, and/or indicators of length of US residence or citizenship status. This finding of more frequent reports of discrimination among younger Latina/o persons suggests that social factors associated with age may pattern experiences of discrimination and/or the likelihood of reporting them. Younger Latina/o/x persons may encounter more frequent discrimination than older adults, perhaps attributed to stigma associated with both their racial/ethnic identity and age, or to structural patterns of their day-to-day lives (e.g., employment or caregiving responsibilities).

Gender may also shape the patterning of self-reported discrimination, although evidence is mixed. Finch and colleagues (2000) found that Mexican American and Mexican immigrant men in California were more likely than women to report discrimination attributed to their racial/ethnic subgroup, after accounting for nativity, social and economic characteristics, and geographic context. Similarly, Pérez and colleagues (2008) found that in a national sample, Latino men were more likely than Latina women to report discrimination, controlling for nativity, Latina/o identity, age, and socioeconomic position. In contrast, LeBrón and colleagues (2014, 2017) found no gender differences in the reported frequency of discrimination for Latina/o adults with diabetes in Detroit, MI, after accounting for nativity and social and economic status. One possible explanation for these different patterns may have to do not only with the specific scales used to measure discrimination, but also with the geographic context in which these studies took place. That is, these differing findings suggest that there may be differences in the patterning of discrimination linked with contextual characteristics of communities that have had longstanding and large Latina/o/x populations, relative to community contexts with smaller Latina/o/x populations, and new destination communities where the Latina/o/x population has experienced recent growth. Studies that examine gender differences in discrimination across geographic contexts and alongside other social statuses (e.g., age, nativity, and socioeconomic position) are needed to better understand how gender shapes experiences and/or reporting of discrimination.

The social patterning of discrimination by educational attainment is also mixed. For a nationally representative sample of Latina/o adults (Pérez et al., 2008) and a study of Latina/o adults from a Midwestern city (LeBrón et al., 2014), Latina/o persons with more than a high school education or at least a high school education, respectively, reported more frequent discrimination than their counterparts with lower educational attainment. In contrast, Finch and colleagues (2000) reported that among Mexican American and Mexican immigrant adults in California, the patterning of reported discrimination by educational attainment was more nuanced: Adults with 7–11 years of education reported more frequent discrimination attributed to their racial/ethnic subgroup than adults with lower educational attainment, and no difference in these patterns for adults with a high school education or higher. Further complicating these patterns, LeBrón and colleagues (2017) found that for Latina/o adults in Detroit, MI, the patterning of educational attainment with racial/ethnic discrimination varied by the specific type of discriminatory experiences: Greater educational attainment was associated with more frequent reports of poorer service and being treated as if the participant was not smart due to their racial/ethnic subgroup. In contrast, educational attainment was not associated with experiences of being treated with less respect, treated unfairly, or threatened or harassed due to their racial/ethnic subgroup. The authors posited that the context of discrimination in which race/ethnicity *and* educational attainment may be salient—such as educational settings, workplaces, or settings in which one's intelligence or knowledge may be invoked—may have shaped the salience of educational attainment in these dimensions of racial/ethnic discrimination.

Together, these patterns suggest the importance of including more nuanced measures of educational attainment in considerations of the social patterning of discrimination for Latina/o/x persons. These differences across studies may be shaped by the aggregation of Latina/o subgroups in the former studies; differences in the social, political, and economic contexts across study locations (e.g., national sample, Midwest, California); and/or differences across measures (i.e., general discrimination vs. discrimination attributed to specific racial/ethnic group and/or to the specific type of experiences of discrimination).

Another important dimension of the experience and reporting of discrimination is immigrant generation or nativity and, for immigrants,[5] length of US residence or age at migration. Pérez and colleagues (2008) report that while they found no difference in reports of discrimination by immigrant generation, Latina/o adults who arrived to the continental USA between ages 7 and 24 (as opposed to their age at the time of the survey) were less likely to report discrimination than those who arrived to the continental USA at a younger age. LeBrón and colleagues (2014) found that US-born Latina/o persons and Latinx Latina/o immigrants who resided in the USA for a longer period reported more frequent discrimination than immigrants with a shorter time period in the USA. In addition, another study of Latina/o adults in Detroit, MI, found that US-born Latina/o persons reported more frequent racial/ethnic discrimination than their immigrant counterparts, though the strength of these associations was non-linear and contingent upon length of US residence for Latina/o immigrants and the specific dimension of discrimination assessed (LeBrón et al., 2017). The authors posited that the immigration policy context upon entry to the USA might shape these non-linear associations of length of US residence with racial/ethnic discrimination for immigrant Latina/o persons relative to US-born Latina/o persons. That is, non-linear associations of length of US residence with reports of discrimination may reflect length of exposure to racialization processes in the USA as well as cohort effects of immigration policies or contexts of reception when Latina/o immigrants migrated to the USA given that immigration policies and sentiments toward Latina/o persons vary according to the sociopolitical context (Chavez, 2013; Viruell-Fuentes et al., 2012).

---

[5]Our use of the term "immigrant" refers to individuals and communities born outside of the United States who have or may be perceived to settle in the United States, or who migrated to the USA with the intent of settling. Due to their birthright citizenship, we refer to Puerto Ricans as "migrants" when referencing to studies involving Puerto Ricans who were born in Puerto Rico and resided in the continental USA at the time of the study.

Taken together, the association of immigrant generation and, for (im)migrants, length of US residence or age at migration, with self-reported discrimination may reflect the implications of coming of age in the USA for exposure to racialization processes and/or ways of understanding the US racial/ethnic structure that may be learned over time or through experiences with US institutions (Viruell-Fuentes, 2007). Additionally, these patterns may reflect cohort effects of immigration policies or other social and economic policies that may shape Latina/o persons' experiences and reporting of discrimination (LeBrón et al., 2017). Indeed, Finch et al. (2000) found that patterns of discrimination that respondents linked with their racial/ethnic subgroup vary by a complex interplay of nativity, citizenship status, and language use.

Measures of discrimination have been developed with the goal of capturing multilevel, dynamic systems of racial oppression (Krieger et al., 2005; Williams et al., 1997). Accordingly, patterns of discrimination may vary across policy contexts, including national, state, and local policies and the extent to which such policies are inclusionary or exclusionary toward Latina/o/x populations. As indicated in this review of the literature, it is difficult to capture self-reported experiences with structural forms of racism that limit a person's due process, cause material deprivation, restrict access to other health-promoting resources, and which serve as profound stressors. Studies that take historical, national, state, and local sociopolitical contexts into account in the study of racial/ethnic discrimination begin to address this challenge.

For example, given the historical construction of Latina/o persons as perpetual foreigners (Chavez, 2013), an emerging body of literature has considered the role of increasingly restrictive immigration policies in processes that racialize Latina/o persons. Almeida, Biello, Pedraza, Wintner, & Viruell-Fuentes (2016) report that for a national sample of Latina/o adults, those residing in states with more anti-immigrant policies implemented between 2005 and 2011 reported greater discrimination than their counterparts in states with fewer anti-immigrant policies passed over the same period. Patterns of discrimination linked with the state immigration policy context varied by country or territory of origin and immigrant generation. The positive association of anti-immigrant policies and discrimination was strongest for third-generation Latina/o persons relative to first- and second-generation Latina/o persons and for Latina/o persons of Mexican, Cuban, or any other country of origin compared to Puerto Ricans. These findings suggest that state-level anti-immigrant policies that have unfolded in the early twenty-first century heightened the context of discrimination for Latina/o persons, with adverse effects that extend beyond immigrants to US-born Latina/o persons, and with particularly acute effects for Latina/o persons with ties to Mexico and other Latin American countries.

Together, these variations in discrimination across several social statuses suggest important differences within the Latina/o/x population. The social patterning of discrimination discussed above may reflect differences in interpretation or readiness to characterize encounters with racism, internalized racism and other aspects of Latina/o/x racialized status. Attending to differences in the reported frequency of discrimination is important because such differences may contribute to differential effects of discrimination on health, or to differential estimations of the health implications of self-reported discrimination.

Self-reported Discrimination and Health

We identified and reviewed 25 peer-reviewed articles that quantitatively examined the association between self-reported discrimination and mental or physical health. Studies included in this review were published between 2000 and 2016 and included at least 30 Latina/o adults (aged 18 and older), in order to make inferences of the reported associations to the Latina/o/x population. For the purposes of this review, we excluded studies where health care discrimination was the only measure of discrimination. The majority of the identified studies were national in scope and/or from cities or metropolitan areas in the Southwestern or Northeastern USA, with a handful of studies conducted with samples from the Midwest. Though this literature varies in the specific scales used to assess the frequency of self-reported discrimination or discrimination-related stress, the most common scale utilized in these studies was the Everyday Unfair Treatment scale (Williams et al., 1997). In the sections that follow, we characterize the literature evaluating associations between discrimination and health for Latina/o persons and consider mechanisms by which discrimination may shape the health of Latina/o/x persons.

Self-reported Discrimination and Mental Health

Twelve out of the 25 studies we reviewed examined associations of discrimination and indicators of mental well-being for Latina/o persons. This literature suggests a consistent and robust association of discrimination with adverse mental health outcomes. Discrimination, in general, was positively associated with psychological distress for a national sample of Latina/o persons (Molina, Alegría, & Mahalingam, 2013); symptoms of post-traumatic stress disorder for a multiracial sample of pregnant women in Michigan (Seng, Lopez, Sperlich, Hamama, & Reed Meldrum, 2012); psychotic experiences for a national multiracial sample, including Latina women (Oh, Yang, Anglin, & DeVylder, 2014); anxiety and depressive disorders for a national sample of Latina/o immigrants (Leong, Park, & Kalibatseva, 2013); number of poor mental health days for Latina/o persons in New York City (Stuber, Galea, Ahern, Blaney, & Fuller, 2003); and diabetes-related distress and depressive symptoms for Latina/o persons with diabetes in Detroit, MI (LeBron et al., 2014).

Other studies have examined the mental health implications of discrimination that Latina/o persons attribute to their specific racial/ethnic subgroup. Discrimination that respondents linked with their racial/ethnic subgroup was positively associated with depressive symptoms for Mexican Americans and Mexican immigrants in California (Finch et al., 2000; Flores et al., 2008); psychological distress for a sample of

Latina/o persons (predominantly Cubans and Puerto Ricans) in Florida (Moradi & Risco, 2006) and in a sample of Mexican and Central American immigrant day laborers in a southwestern city (Negi, 2013); poorer mental health status for a multiracial sample in New Hampshire (Gee, Ryan, Laflamme, & Holt, 2006); and elevated symptoms of depression and anxiety for a multiracial sample of men who have sex with men in Los Angeles, CA (Choi, Paul, Ayala, Boylan, & Gregorich, 2013).

The strength of the association of self-reported discrimination with mental well-being may be shaped by multiple intersecting identities. Two studies identified in this literature review (Choi et al., 2013; Seng et al., 2012) suggest that discrimination that respondents attributed to multiple marginalized identities may be more strongly associated with poor mental health. Similarly, the mental health implications of discrimination may be stronger for Latina women relative to Latino men. Finch and colleagues (2000) reported that the positive association of discrimination attributed to racial/ethnic subgroup with depressive symptoms was stronger for Mexican women than Mexican men. Likewise, Molina and colleagues (2013) reported stronger associations of discrimination with psychological distress for Mexican women relative to Cuban and Puerto Rican men. The authors conjecture that these differential impacts of discrimination on mental health by gender and Latina/o subgroup may be linked with Mexican women's management of multiple chronic stressors, some of which were encompassed within the measure of discrimination. Additionally, the authors note that Puerto Rican men in this sample reported high levels of discrimination, while Cuban men in this sample reported low levels of discrimination. Though the authors do not disentangle these associations for Mexican women relative to Mexican men, this study illustrates the need to consider the role of multiple social statuses in shaping experiences with discrimination and its health impacts. This literature suggests complex dynamics between experiences of discrimination, discrimination attributed to racial/ethnic subgroup, gender, and mental well-being. To better understand these complexities, research is needed that considers the ways in which racialized experiences are gendered (and vice versa) and their implications for health outcomes.

The mental health implications of experiences of discrimination may be compounded by or operate through stress responses to discrimination. Indeed, Gee et al. (2006) reported that greater discomfort with discrimination linked with racial/ethnic subgroup was associated with worse psychological well-being for a multiracial sample that included Mexican Americans, Latina/o adults of other countries of origin or descent, and Black adults in New Hampshire.

Self-reported Racial/Ethnic Discrimination and Self-reported General or Physical Health

As with indicators of mental well-being, several studies suggest a consistent association of discrimination more generally and discrimination attributed to racial/ethnic subgroup with: adverse self-rated general health (Flores et al., 2008); poor self-rated physical health (Finch, Hummer, Kol, & Vega, 2001; Molina et al., 2013; Ryan, Gee, & Laflamme, 2006); higher number of days of poor general health (Otiniano & Gee, 2012); higher number of days with activity limitations (Otiniano & Gee, 2012); lower quality of life (Seng et al., 2012); and higher number of self-reported indicators of acute physical symptoms (Flores et al., 2008; Lee & Ferraro, 2009; Pilver, Desai, Kasl, & Levy, 2011). Each of these studies included Latina/o persons and controlled for several social and economic characteristics. However, for a multiracial sample, Stuber and colleagues (2003) did not find support for the hypothesis of an association of discrimination attributed to racial/ethnic subgroup or discrimination more generally with days of poor physical health.

Though this association of discrimination with self-reported general or physical health was robust across eight of the nine identified studies, only a handful of studies examined potential variations in the association of discrimination and self-rated health for Latina/o persons by gender. Flores and colleagues (2008) reported that the inverse association of discrimination with self-rated general health was stronger for Mexican-origin men than women. In more specific tests of intersectionality, Seng and colleagues (2012) found that for a multiracial sample of pregnant women, discrimination, and a greater number of marginalized identities that respondents attributed to their experiences of discrimination, were associated with worse quality of life. Pilver and colleagues (2011) report that the intensity and attribution of experiences of discrimination shape the association of discrimination and health for a non-stratified multiracial national sample. Discrimination on the basis of gender and racial/ethnic subgroup was more strongly associated with premenstrual dysphoric disorder, and there was a stronger association of more subtle forms of reported discrimination with premenstrual dysphoric disorder than blatant forms of discrimination.

In terms of variations in self-rated health by social statuses or identities related to migration (i.e., nativity, length of US residence), Finch, Hummer, Kol, and Vega, (2001) found no differences in these associations for a sample of Mexican American or Mexican immigrant adults. With regard to differences in self-reported health by Latina/o subgroup, in a more specific examination of the association of discrimination with physical health symptoms, frequency of discrimination was positively associated with acute physical symptoms (e.g., headaches, chest or heart pains, upset stomach, hot or cold spells, feeling week, and back pain) for Puerto Rican and Mexican American adults in Chicago, IL (Lee & Ferraro, 2009). These studies, as a whole, highlight the need to examine patterns by Latina/o/x subgroup and other social experiences, such as citizenship, nativity, and length of US residence.

Self-reported Discrimination and Anthropometrically or Clinically Assessed Indicators of Health

Discrimination may also shape health by adversely affecting clinically and anthropometrically assessed indicators of physical health, although evidence of these associations, based on nine studies identified in this review, is mixed. The majority of identified studies examining how discrimination becomes embodied are based on multiracial samples that include Latina/o persons. Racially stratified models suggest no cross-sectional association of discrimination with blood pressure for a national sample of middle-aged Latina women (Brown, Matthews, Bromberger, & Chang, 2006), blood pressure for unionized Latina/o workers in the greater Boston area (Krieger et al., 2008); nor overweight, obesity, and waist circumference for Latina/o adults in Chicago, IL (Hunte & Williams, 2009).

Some studies involving aggregated multiracial groups suggest that discrimination is associated with cardiovascular and metabolic risk. Ryan and colleagues (2006) reported a U-shaped association of racial/ethnic discrimination with systolic blood pressure, but not diastolic blood pressure for US-born and immigrant Black and Latina/o immigrants in New Hampshire. That is, adults reporting the lowest and the highest levels of racial/ethnic discrimination had higher systolic blood pressure than adults reporting some experiences of discrimination. These associations did not differ for Black adults relative to Latina/o adults.

The patterning of discrimination with indicators of cardiovascular risk also varies jointly by age and indicator of health. For example, Moody and colleagues (2016) reported that racial/ethnic discrimination was more strongly associated with elevated diastolic blood pressure for middle- and older-aged Black and Latina/o adults compared to younger adults, and discrimination was positively associated with nocturnal systolic blood pressure, regardless of age.

The association of discrimination with health may also vary by gender and indicator of cardiovascular health. McClure, Martinez et al. (2010) and McClure, Snodgrass et al. (2010) report that among a sample of predominantly Mexican immigrant farmworkers in Oregon, racial/ethnic discrimination-related stress predicted elevated systolic blood pressure (SBP) among men but not women, controlling for age and length of US residence. Additionally, racial/ethnic discrimination-related stress was more strongly associated with elevated systolic blood pressure for men of lower socioeconomic position relative to men of higher socioeconomic position (assessed by indicators of educational attainment, personal income, and household income).

It is possible that the implications of discrimination for cardiovascular or metabolic health may manifest over a longer period of time. We identified only one study that included Latina/o persons that examined the longitudinal association of discrimination with a clinical indicator of health (Kwarteng et al., 2016). Kwarteng et al. (2016) found that baseline frequency of discrimination was positively associated with increases in central adiposity over a six-year period for an aggregated sample of Latina/o Black, and non-Latina/o white adults (white adults) in Detroit, MI.

In cross-sectional studies, discrimination may be more visible for indicators of health that may be more responsive to racialized stressors in the short term, such as immune function. Indeed, Bogart, Landrine, Galvan, Wagner, & Klein (2013) found that among HIV-positive Latino men who have sex with men, discrimination across multiple domains was associated with greater severity of anti-retroviral medication side effects and more AIDS symptoms. Similarly, McClure, Martinez et al. (2010) report that for a sample of predominantly Mexican-origin farm workers in Oregon, racial/ethnic discrimination-related stress predicted elevated levels of Epstein-Barr virus antibodies (an indicator of immune function) among men, but not women. Further, this association was stronger for men of higher socioeconomic position compared to men of lower socioeconomic position. If the health implications of discrimination are visible for immune responses in the short term, it is possible that the immune response triggered by discriminatory experiences may be a bellwether for subsequent responses to stressors that affect other physical health outcomes (e.g., metabolic and cardiovascular risk) later in the life course. Together this literature suggests that the associations of discrimination with anthropometric indicators of health status are mixed, with some findings varying by age, gender, and by the intensity and timing of experiences of discrimination relative to the assessment of health status.

Mechanisms by Which Discrimination Shapes Health and Health Inequities for Latinx Persons

The self-reported discrimination measures described above and the conceptual frameworks that guide the body of literature reviewed here point to multiple mechanisms through which discrimination affects health. Indeed, the studies reviewed above rely on several theoretical frameworks that seek to tease out the social, psychological, and physiological mechanisms through which discrimination affects health. Several studies characterize discrimination as a vulnerability for adverse health outcomes that operates through biopsychosocial and stress processes. For instance, "the biopsychosocial model" approaches health with the understanding that biological, psychological, and social factors comprise a complex system that influences health (Engel, 1977). In a more specific extension of the biopsychosocial model, "the stress process framework" posits that marginalized social statuses increase exposure to stressors and that stress processes catalyzed by responses to stressors may accumulate to adversely affect health (Lazarus & Folkman, 1984; Pearlin, Menaghan, Lieberman, & Mullan, 1981). It follows from this framework that discrimination is a stressor—the exposure to which (including the form, frequency, and intensity of the exposure) and its health consequences are shaped by social statuses, such as race/ethnicity.

Building upon stress process theories (Lazarus & Folkman, 1984), some of the studies we reviewed are informed by the Minority Stress Model (Meyer, 1995, 2003). This model posits that racial/ethnic "minorities" experience stressors outlined in stress process frameworks, as well as stressors that are unique to "minorities" due to racist structures and processes. As such, the Latina/o/x population—a racialized group—are exposed to stressors related to their ascribed racialized status. This model also proposes that communities disproportionately burdened by racism may develop individual and collective strategies to cope with and overcome these stressors. In sum, this model suggests that discrimination-related stressors heighten vulnerability for adverse health outcomes for Latina/o/x persons and that variations in these associations within the heterogeneous Latina/o/x population, as well as access to psychosocial and institutional resources to buffer or disrupt the effects of discrimination, may contribute to complex associations between discrimination and health.

With regard to the measurement of discrimination, some measures capture experiences that may alter opportunities for social and economic opportunity and advancement—that is, fundamental determinants of health (House, Kessler, & Herzog, 1990; Link & Phelan, 1995; Phelan, Link, & Tehranifar, 2010)—while others assess day-to-day barriers and indignities experienced by stigmatized racial/ethnic populations.

The experiences of discrimination captured in these measures point to the physiopsychosocial stress pathways through which discrimination may affect health, outlined by the conceptual frameworks discussed above. Notably, the findings from emerging literature reviewed above suggest that the health implications of reported discrimination may be visible more immediately for mental well-being, self-reported health, and immune function. As such, this literature suggests that discrimination may shape mental health, self-reported health, and immune function through physiopsychosocial stress pathways. That is, the psychological distress brought about by experience(s) of discrimination, effortful coping with discrimination, and/or other stressors catalyzed by restricted access to resources and/or threats to an affirming identity (Geronimus, 2000; James, 1993) not only directly impact mental well-being and assessments of one's health, but also physiological processes related to immune function.

The evidence base analyzed in this chapter also suggests that discrimination is inimical for the cardiovascular and metabolic health of Latina/o persons. In particular, the mixed literature regarding the association of self-reported discrimination with cardiovascular and metabolic risk suggests that the health implications of discrimination may cumulate over time to manifest in poor cardiovascular and metabolic risk later in the life course. Further work, however, is needed to better understand the cumulative effects of discrimination over the life course.

The measures of discrimination used in the reviewed studies capture reported experiences of discrimination assessed at the individual level and may not necessarily capture mechanisms through which more structural forms of discrimination affect health. Additionally, these measures do not assess contemporary forms of racialization that have escalated in recent years, such as escalations in racializing hate speech and hate crimes that have been perpetrated in primary education settings, college campuses, neighborhoods, religious institutions, and in social media and political rhetoric. Additionally, an emerging literature links increasingly restrictive immigration policies, a component of structural racism, with reduced access to health-promoting resources and declines in health for Latina/o persons (Gee & Ford, 2011; Kline, 2016; LeBrón, Schulz, & Mentz, 2018; Lopez et al., 2016; Novak, Geronimus, & Martinez-Cardoso, 2017; Pedraza, Cruz Nichols, & LeBrón, 2017; Rhodes et al., 2015). Anti-immigrant ideologies, policies, and practices and their expression at multiple levels represent structural-level mechanisms that affect health—all of which require further theorizing and empirical assessment.

Methodological Issues, Limitations, and Future Considerations

The literature reviewed here should be considered within the context of several limitations, all of which point to important areas of future research. First, the self-reported measures of discrimination used in the studies we reviewed capture more visible forms of racism, including discrimination initiated by persons or by individuals at the interface of institutions. These measures do not fully capture structurally embedded forms of racism, such as race-based residential segregation, racial ideologies, immigration policies and practices, racial profiling, carceral policies and practices, environmental quality, educational opportunity patterned by residential segregation or state education policies, and healthcare access and quality, among others. Studies examining the health implications of these structural forms of racism are important to consider as they provide critical insights into the health consequences and legacies of institutional systems of racism such as restricted access to housing that shapes the persistence of race-based residential segregation; exposure to environmental risk factors; and educational quality (Schulz et al., 2017; McConnell, 2012). It would also be important to examine the health consequences of community and family separation, or the threat thereof, through policing of Latina/o/x communities and restrictive immigration policies that have heightened immigration-related detentions and deportations affecting Latina/o/x communities (Cox & Miles, 2013; Golash-Boza & Hondagneu-Sotelo, 2013; McConnell, 2013; Rios, 2011).

Relatedly, findings reported here indicate further need to theorize and consistently examine the health implications of discrimination across social contexts, such as traditional gateway communities with longstanding and sizable Latina/o/x populations, new destination communities characterized by recent and substantial growth of the Latina/o/x population, and communities with a smaller, though well-established Latina/o/x population. For example, in an examination of Southern new destination regions with sizable and well-established white and Black communities, Marrow (2011, 2009) finds that Latina/o persons manage complex racial structures and racialization processes in the midst of increasingly restrictive immigration policies that have emerged in response to the growth of the Latina/o immigrant population. Addressing how racialized practices and expressions of structural racism unfold in different spatial contexts would enhance our understanding of the variations in the association between discrimination and health by geographic context found in our review.

Second, the cross-sectional nature of the majority of the above-mentioned studies has important implications. As with all cross-sectional designs, the associations between discrimination and health reported herein, while strongly suggestive, do not demonstrate causality. In addition, such designs may contribute to an underestimation of the magnitude of the effect of discrimination on certain physical health indicators. That is, it is possible that discrimination may contribute to more immediate effects on mental health, self-rated health, and immune function, while taking longer to become expressed in physical health, such as cardiovascular and metabolic risk. Several studies we reviewed used scales that queried about experiences of discrimination in the past year or over the life course, and as such, it is possible that these studies capture some of the cumulative effects of discrimination on health. Nevertheless, studies are needed that enable us to better understand the effects of discrimination on conditions that take longer to manifest, as well as its overall cumulative effects on health.

Third, this relatively small emerging literature demonstrating an association of reported discrimination and health was most consistent for self-reported indicators of mental and physical health. While self-rated health is a robust measure of morbidity and mortality (Idler & Benyamini, 1997; Latham & Peek, 2013; Schnittker & Bacak, 2014), use of self-reported measures of both the independent (i.e., self-reported discrimination) and the outcome variables (i.e., mental health, self-reported general, or physical health) is subject to same-source bias (Mitchell, 1985; Podsakoff & Organ, 1986; Thorndike, 1920). In addition, when assessing self-reported health among Latina/o/x persons, attention to the language of interview is necessary to avoid methodological biases due translation (Viruell-Fuentes, Morenoff, Williams, & House, 2011). Furthermore, self-reported measures of discrimination are subject to a number of processes, including naming and reporting discrimination (Viruell-Fuentes, 2007). These reporting processes may overshadow the reporting of forms of racism that may be less visible on a day-to-day basis or which individuals may be less prepared to name.

Fourth, while some studies identified in this review advance an intersectional analysis of the social patterning of discrimination and implications for health, the characteristics of the samples used in the studies we reviewed impede the development of a more robust intersectional assessment of the association of discrimination and Latina/o/x health. Several studies, for instance, included multiracial samples, and many of these multiracial samples included a relatively and numerically small sub-sample of Latina/o/x persons. The ability to extend an intersectional analysis to these studies was often precluded by the relatively small size of the Latina/o sample and/or the aggregation of Latina/o participants with other racial groups. Therefore, an analysis of how gender and gender identities, citizenship status, class, sexuality, and other social statuses may intersect with race/ethnicity are not systematically addressed in the discrimination and Latina/o health literature, as of yet.

In addition, the majority of studies we reviewed included a sizable proportion of Mexican American or Mexican immigrant adults, reflecting the largest Latina/o/x subgroup in the USA (Stepler & Brown, 2016). Due to small sample sizes of Latina/o persons representing other Latin American countries or territories, several studies aggregated Latina/o persons into a pan-ethnic category, preventing a comparison of the social patterning of discrimination across groups and contributing to the homogenization of the Latina/o population.

Fifth, while some studies examined the health implications of discrimination that participants attributed to race/ethnicity, national origin, or gender, none of the studies we reviewed examined the health implications of language as a racializing marker. This omission in the literature may contribute to a limited understanding of the processes by which racism operates to shape access to resources, opportunities for advancement, and exposure to psychosocial stressors. In the case of Latina/o health research, language is typically subsumed under the concept of acculturation; the limitations of which have been highlighted by multiple scholars (Hunt et al., 2004; Viruell-Fuentes, 2007; Viruell-Fuentes et al., 2012). Future research that places language within a racialization framework is needed to gain a fuller picture of the multiple ways in which racism operates to impact the health of Latina/o/x persons. Relatedly, because the goal of our review was to assess and characterize our understanding of the racism and health literature, we focused our review on studies that explicitly and directly used discrimination as a guiding conceptual framework. As such, we did not review possible related literature, such as the health effects of acculturative stress.

Sixth, for the purposes of this chapter, we interpreted general discrimination measures as markers of racial/ethnic discrimination, although these are holistic measures of discrimination and may not be (exclusively) capturing racial/ethnic discrimination. It is possible that reports of "discrimination" that are not restricted to race/ethnicity might be often understood as racial/ethnic discrimination by racialized groups. Nevertheless, future research that explicitly assesses experiences of discrimination across multiple intersecting social statuses is necessary.

Additionally, it is possible that some reports of discrimination captured in the literature reviewed above may pertain to experiences of discrimination perpetrated by within-group members. However, the majority of studies reviewed did not include survey items that explicitly asked about the social status(es) of the perpetrator(s) of discrimination, such as the perpetrator's institutional role (e.g., institutional agent or bureaucrat), the perpetrator's peer group membership (e.g., neighbor, student, patient), nor the perceived race/ethnicity of the perpetrator. Because within-group discrimination is an expression of larger structural racism (Jones, 2000; Viruell-Fuentes, 2011); from a population-health perspective, we argue that these questions are only useful to the extent to which they elucidate mechanisms to shift institutional and cultural environments to eliminate, reduce, or disrupt structural racism.

Recommendations for Future Research

Studies are warranted that evaluate racism as a structural determinant of health, considering the ways in which racism toward Latina/o/x persons is (re)produced in the twenty-first century. This includes, for example, examining the health implications of housing, educational, employment, environmental, immigration, and social welfare policies and practices that shape day-to-day life opportunities, for individuals and communities. In addition, a further theorizing and empirical examination of how experiences of racialization unfold across spatial contexts would help shed light on the findings from the emerging literature reviewed in this chapter. While we did not examine emerging research on anti-immigrant environments and health (see Kline & Castañeda, Chap. 12), it is important to underscore that immigration policies are part and parcel of the country's long history of racialized nativism, and as such merit careful attention.

Additionally, studies are needed that assess the health implications of vigilance toward racism and spillover effects of racism toward important peers, communities, or a particular population. Future research is necessary that follows Latina/o/x persons over time and assesses exposure to the multiple ways in which racism unfolds, considering variation in and frequency and intensity of exposures, as well as pathways to health and health inequities over the life course.

In addition, more research is needed on the kinds of social institutions and resources that buffer the effects of racism on health. The health impacts of psychosocial or institutional buffers may vary according to the form of racism and/or health indicator. It is possible that some social buffers may temporarily promote mental health, but have longer-term consequences for other somatic symptoms. Future research is warranted that explores psychosocial and institutional resources on which Latina/o/x persons may draw to protect against the adverse health implications of racism.

Theoretically, a fuller application of intersectionality theory (Collins, 1990, 2015; Crenshaw, 1991) in examining the links between discrimination and health among Latina/o/x persons is critical. In other words, studies that examine the intersections between racism and other forms of marginalization, such as gender, class, citizenship status, sexual orientation, among others, would greatly enhance our understanding of the patterns outlined herein. Indeed, advancing the study of the health implications of racialization processes as they relate to peoples' multiple identities necessitates a queer analytic approach (Anzaldúa, 2009).

In addition, research regarding the association of discrimination and Latina/o/x health would be strengthened by considering population-based theories about the implications of racism for health inequities. For instance, Chae, Nuru-Jeter, Lincoln, and Francis (2011) advance a socio-psychobiological framework for studying how enduring and contemporary systems of racial oppression become embodied and produce racial differences in health. The socio-psychobiological framework builds on previous frameworks to posit that racism (rather than race) shapes health through the psychological, behavioral, and biological embodiment of social inequalities. Studies that examine the health implications of discrimination for Latina/o/x persons informed by such theories and frameworks would situate this area of inquiry within the racialized sociopolitical context in which Latina/o/x persons navigate. In addition, studies that consider cumulative effects of discrimination on health over the life course, and in relation to other stigmatized social locations are also necessary.

Relatedly, given the limitations of quantitative discrimination measures described above, qualitative studies that examine experiences of racism as they intersect with multiple identities and statuses are needed to better understand the mechanisms by which racism shapes health. For example, some qualitative studies indicate a possible underreporting of discrimination among Latina/o persons, a pattern that is shaped by exposure to and understanding of the US racial structure (Tovar & Feliciano, 2009; Viruell-Fuentes, 2007). Additionally, an emerging qualitative literature focused on the health implications of restrictive immigration policies for Latina/o communities is beginning to implicate structures in these processes (LeBrón, Schulz, Gamboa, Reyes, Viruell-Fuentes, & Israel, 2018; Garcia, 2017; Kline, 2016), and contributes to strengthening our understanding of the dynamic nature of experiences with structural racism and variation across social statuses.

Further, structural and intersectional inquiries of the health impacts of racism for Latina/o/x persons through systems affecting housing, policing, education, occupational settings, and health care are necessary. Furthermore, the literature reviewed above calls for future health research that considers various dimensions of exposure to discrimination including age of exposure and length of exposure over the life course, particularly given that, for immigrants, exposure may vary depending on their age of arrival in the USA. Moreover, few studies included in this review consider the health implications language as a racializing marker (Viruell-Fuentes, 2011). Future studies, that evaluate the health implications of discrimination based on language use, and the intersection of language-based discrimination with racial/ethnic discrimination, are warranted.

Conclusions

This chapter provides a review of the emerging literature that evaluates the health implications of discrimination for Latina/o persons in the early twenty-first century. By characterizing the breadth and depth of this literature, as well as variations in findings across studies, often according to measure of discrimination, health indicator, sample, or social statuses, this chapter sheds light on the health implications of racial/ethnic discrimination. This chapter also offers future directions for research regarding discrimination and Latina/o/x health. Novel aspects of this chapter include disentangling the literature according to measure of discrimination (e.g., general or race/ethnicity-specific), and its attention to these patterns within the heterogeneous Latina/o population.

Given the historical and current contexts of racism in the country, it remains of critical importance to consider the health and health equity implications of racism against Latina/o/x persons. Strategies to dismantle racism, and the inequalities that are symptomatic of these processes, are of critical importance for promoting the social and economic well-being and health of Latina/o/x persons, the fastest growing racial/ethnic group in the USA. As we advance scholarship, policies, and practices to dismantle racism, we encourage scholars and practitioners to carefully consider the social statuses and identities that racial labels make visible and those which they obscure. The use of intersectional labels, such as Latinx, needs to be accompanied by an analytical stance that contributes to eliminating all forms of oppression.

Acknowledgements We thank Brenda Gisela García for her assistance with preparing this chapter.

References

Abraído-Lanza, A. F., Armbrister, A. N., Flórez, K. R., & Aguirre, A. N. (2006). Toward a theory-driven model of acculturation in public health research. *American Journal of Public Health, 96*(8), 1342–1346.

Abraído-Lanza, A. F., Chao, M. T., & Flórez, K. R. (2005). Do healthy behaviors decline with greater acculturation? Implications for the Latino mortality paradox. *Social Science and Medicine, 61*(6), 1243–1255.

Abraído-Lanza, A. F., Echeverría, S. E., & Flórez, K. R. (2016). Latino immigrants, acculturation, and health: Promising new directions in research. *Annual Review of Public Health, 37*(1), 219–236.

Acuña, R. F. (2011). *Occupied America: A history of Chicanos*. Boston: Longman.

Alcoff, L. M. (2005). Latino vs. Hispanic: The politics of ethnic names. *Philosophy & Social Criticism, 31*(4), 395–407.

Almaguer, T. (2009). *Racial fault lines: The historical origins of white supremacy in California*. Berkeley: University of California Press.

Almeida, J., Biello, K. B., Pedraza, F., Wintner, S., & Viruell-Fuentes, E. (2016). The association between anti-immigrant policies and perceived discrimination among Latinos in the U.S.: A multilevel analysis. *SSM—Population Health, 2,* 897–903.

Anzaldúa, G. (2009). To(o) Queer the writer – Loca, escritor, y chicana. In *The Gloria Anzaldúa Reader* (pp. 163–175). Duke University Press.

Bastos, J. L., Celeste, R. K., Faerstein, E., & Barros, A. J. D. (2010). Racial discrimination and health: A systematic review of scales with a focus on their psychometric properties. *Social Science and Medicine, 70*(7), 1091–1099.

Bogart, L. M., Landrine, H., Galvan, F. H., Wagner, G. J., & Klein, D. J. (2013). Perceived discrimination and physical health among HIV-positive black and latino men who have sex with men. *AIDS and Behavior, 17*(4), 1431–1441.

Brondolo, E., Kelly, K. P., Coakley, V., Gordon, T., Thompson, S., Levy, E., ... Contrada, R. J. (2005). The perceived ethnic discrimination questionnaire: Development and preliminary validation of a community version 1. *Journal of Applied Social Psychology, 35*(2), 335–365.

Brown, C., Matthews, K. A., Bromberger, J. T., & Chang, Y. (2006). The relation between perceived unfair treatment and blood pressure in a racially/ethnically diverse sample of women. *American Journal of Epidemiology, 164*(3), 257–262.

Cavazos-Rehg, P. A., Zayas, L. H., & Spitznagel, E. L. (2007). Legal status, emotional well-being and subjective health status of Latino immigrants. *Journal of the National Medical Association, 99*(10), 1126–1131.

Cervantes, R. C., Fisher, D. G., Padilla, A. M., & Napper, L. E. (2016). The hispanic stress inventory version 2: Improving the assessment of acculturation stress. *Psychological Assessment, 28*(5), 509–522.

Cervantes, R. C., Padilla, A. M., & Salgado de Snyder, N. (1991). The hispanic stress inventory: A culturally relevant approach to psychosocial assessment. *Psychological Assessment, 3*(3), 438–447.

Chae, D. H., Nuru-Jeter, A. M., Lincoln, K. D., & Francis, D. D. (2011). Conceptualizing racial disparities in health: Advancement of a socio-psychobiological approach. *Du Bois Review, 8*(1), 63–77.

Chavez, L. (2013). *The Latino threat: Constructing immigrants, citizens, and the nation*. Stanford: Stanford University Press.

Choi, K. H., Paul, J., Ayala, G., Boylan, R., & Gregorich, S. E. (2013). Experiences of discrimination and their impact on the mental health among African American, Asian and Pacific Islander, and Latino men who have sex with men. *American Journal of Public Health, 103*(5), 868–874.

Collado-Proctor, S. (1999). The perceived racism scale for Latina/os: A multidimensional assessment of the experience of racism among latina/os. *Dissertation Abstracts International: Section B: The Sciences and Engineering*.

Collins, P. H. (1990). *Black feminist thought: Knowledge, consciousness, and the policitcs of empowerment*. Boston: Unwin Hyman.

Collins, P. H. (2015). Intersectionality's definitional dilemmas. *Annual Review of Sociology, 41*(1), 1–20.

Connell, R. (2012). Gender, health and theory: Conceptualizing the issue, in local and world perspective. *Social Science and Medicine, 74*(11), 1675–1683.

Cox, A. B., & Miles, T. J. (2013). Policing immigration. *University of Chicago Law Review, 80*(1), 87–136.

Crenshaw, K. (1989). Demarginalizing the intersection of race and sex: A black feminist critique of antidiscrimination doctrine, feminist theory and antiracist policies. *The University of Chicago Legal Forum, 1989*(1), 139–167.

Crenshaw, K. (1991). Mapping the margins: Intersectionality, identity politics, and violence against women of color. *Stanford Law Review, 43*(6), 1241.

Engel, G. L. (1977). The need for a new medical model: a challenge for biomedicine. *Science, 196*(4286), 129–136.

Finch, B. K., Hummer, R. A., Kola, B., & Vega, W. A. (2001). The role of discrimination and acculturative stress in the physical health of Mexican-origin adults. *Hispanic Journal of Behavioral Sciences, 23*(4), 399–429.

Finch, B., Kolody, B., & Vega, W. (2000). Perceived discrimination and depression among Mexican-origin adults in California. *Journal of Health and Social Behavior, 41*(3), 295–313.

Flores, E., Tschann, J. M., Dimas, J. M., Bachen, E. A., Pasch, L. A., & de Groat, C. L. (2008). Perceived discrimination, perceived stress, and mental and physical health among Mexican-origin adults. *Hispanic Journal of Behavioral Sciences, 30*(4), 401–424.

Ford, C. L., & Airhihenbuwa, C. O. (2010). The public health critical race methodology: Praxis for antiracism research. *Social Science and Medicine, 71*(8), 1390–1398.

Garcia, S. J. (2017). Racializing "illegality": An intersectional approach to understanding how Mexican-origin women navigate an anti-immigrant climate. *Sociology of Race and Ethnicity, 3*(4), 474–490.

Gee, G. C., & Ford, C. L. (2011). Structural racism and health inequities. *Du Bois Review Social Science Research on Race, 8*(01), 115-132. https://doi.org/10.1017/S1742058X11000130.

Gee, G. C., Ryan, A., Laflamme, D. J., & Holt, J. (2006). Self reported discrimination and mental health status among African descendants, Mexican Americans, and other Latinos in the New Hampshire REACH 2010 Initiative: The added dimension of immigration. *American Journal of Public Health, 96*(10), 1821–1828.

Geronimus, A. T. (2000). To mitigate, resist, or undo: Addressing structural influences on the health of urban populations. *American Journal of Public Health, 90*(6), 867.

Golash-Boza, T., & Hondagneu-Sotelo, P. (2013). Latino immigrant men and the deportation crisis: A gendered racial removal program. *Latino Studies, 11*(2013), 271–292.

Hankivsky, O. (2012). Women's health, men's health, and gender and health: Implications of intersectionality. *Social Science and Medicine, 74*(11), 1712–1720.

Hayes-Bautista, D. E., & Chapa, J. (1987). Latino terminology: Conceptual bases for standardized terminology. *American Journal of Public Health, 77*(1), 61–68.

House, J. S., Kessler, R. C., & Herzog, A. R. (1990). Age, socioeconomic status, and health. *The Milbank Quarterly, 68*(3), 383–411.

Hunt, L. M., Schneider, S., & Comer, B. (2004). Should "acculturation" be a variable in health research? A critical review of research on US Hispanics? *Social Science and Medicine, 59*(5), 973–986.

Hunte, H. E. R., & Williams, D. R. (2009). The association between perceived discrimination and obesity in a population-based multiracial and multiethnic adult sample. *American Journal of Public Health, 99*(7), 1285–1292.

Idler, E. L., & Benyamini, Y. (1997). Self-rated health and mortality: A review of twenty-seven community studies. *Journal of Health and Social Behavior, 38*(1), 21–37.

James, S. A. (1993). Racial and ethnic differences in infant mortality and low birth weight. A psychosocial critique. *Annals of Epidemiology, 3*(2), 130–136.

Jones, C. P. (2000). Levels of racism: A theoretic framework and a gardener's tale. *American Journal of Public Health, 90*(8), 1212.

Kline, N. (2016). Pathogenic policy: Immigrant policing, fear, and parallel medical systems in the U.S. south. *Medical Anthropology, 36*(4), 396–410.

Krieger, N. (1990). Racial and gender discrimination: Risk factors for high blood pressure? *Social Science and Medicine, 30*(12), 1273–1281.

Krieger, N., Chen, J. T., Waterman, P. D., Hartman, C., Stoddard, A. M., Quinn, M. M., … Barbeau, E. M. (2008). The inverse hazard law: Blood pressure, sexual harassment, racial discrimination, workplace abuse and occupational exposures in US low-income black, white and Latino workers. *Social Science and Medicine, 67*(12), 1970–1981.

Krieger, N., Smith, K., Naishadham, D., Hartman, C., & Barbeau, E. M. (2005). Experiences of discrimination: Validity and reliability of a self-report measure for population health research on racism and health. *Social Science and Medicine, 61*(7), 1576–1596.

Krogstad, J. M., & Lopez, G. (2016). *Roughly half of Hispanics have experienced discrimination*. Washington, D.C. Retrieved from http://www.pewresearch.org/fact-tank/2016/06/29/roughly-half-of-hispanics-have-experienced-discrimination/.

Kwarteng, J. L., Schulz, A. J., Mentz, G. B., Israel, B. A., Shanks, T. R., & Perkins, D. W. (2016). Neighbourhood poverty, perceived discrimination and central adiposity in the U.S.A: Independent associations in a repeated measures analysis. *Journal of Biosocial Science, 48*(6), 709–722.

Latham, K., & Peek, C. W. (2013). Self-rated health and morbidity onset among late midlife U.S. adults. *Journals of Gerontology—Series B Psychological Sciences and Social Sciences, 68*(1), 107–116.

Lazarus, R. S., & Folkman, S. (1984). *Stress, appraisal, and coping*. New York: Springer.

LeBrón, A. M. W., Schulz, A. J., & Mentz, G. B., et al. (2018). Impact of change over time in self-reported discrimination on blood pressure: Implications for inequities in cardiovascular risk for a multi-racial urban community. *Ethnicity & Health*. https://doi.org/10.1080/13557858.2018.1425378.

LeBrón, A. M. W., Schulz, A. J., Gamboa, C., Reyes, A., Viruell-Fuentes, E. A., Israel, B. A. (2018). "They are Clipping Our Wings": Health implications of restrictive immigrant policies for Mexican-origin women in a northern border community. *Race and Social Problems, 2018*, 1–19. https://doi.org/10.1007/s12552-018-9238-0.

LeBrón, A. M. W., Spencer, M., Kieffer, E., Sinco, B., Piatt, G., & Palmisano, G. (2017). Correlates of interpersonal ethnoracial discrimination among Latino adults with diabetes: Findings from the REACH Detroit study. *Journal of Ethnic & Cultural Diversity in Social Work, 26*(1–2), 48–67.

LeBron, A. M. W., Valerio, M. A., Kieffer, E., Sinco, B., Rosland, A.-M., Hawkins, J., … Spencer, M. (2014). Everyday discrimination, diabetes-related distress, and depressive symptoms among African Americans and Latinos with diabetes. *Journal of Immigrant and Minority Health, 16*(6), 1208–1216.

Lee, M. A., & Ferraro, K. F. (2009). Perceived discrimination and health among Puerto Rican and Mexican Americans: Buffering effect of the lazo matrimonial? *Social Science and Medicine, 68*(11), 1966–1974.

Leong, F., Park, Y. S., & Kalibatseva, Z. (2013). Disentangling immigrant status in mental health: Psychological protective and risk factors among Latino and Asian American immigrants. *American Journal of Orthopsychiatry, 83*(2, Part 3), 361–371.

Lewis, T. T., Cogburn, C. D., & Williams, D. R. (2015). Self-reported experiences of discrimination and health: scientific advances, ongoing controversies, and emerging issues. *Annual Review of Clinical Psychology, 11,* 407–440.

Link, B. G., & Phelan, J. (1995). Social conditions as fundamental causes of disease. *Journal of Health and Social Behavior, 35*(1), 80–94.

Lopez, W. D., Kruger, D.J., Delva, J., Llanes, M., Ledon, C., Waller, A... Israel, B. (2016). Health implications of an immigration raid: Findings from a Latino community in the Midwestern United States. *Journal of Immigrant & Minority Health, 19*(3), 702–708.

Marrow, H. B. (2009). New immigrant destinations and the American colour line. *Ethnic and Racial Studies, 32*(6), 1037–1057.

Marrow, H. B. (2011). *New destination dreaming immigration, race, and legal status in the rural American South*. Stanford: Stanford University Press.

McClure, H. H., Martinez, C. R., Snodgrass, J. J., Eddy, J. M., Jiménez, R. A., Isiordia, L. E., & McDade, T. W. (2010). Discrimination-related stress, blood pressure and epstein-barr virus antibodies among Latin American immigrants in Oregon, U.S. *Journal of Biosocial Science, 42*(4), 433–61.

McClure, H. H., Snodgrass, J. J., Martinez, C. R., Eddy, J. M., Jiménez, R. A, & Isiordia, L. E. (2010). Discrimination, psychosocial stress, and health among Latin American immigrants in Oregon. *American Journal of Human Biology, 22*(3), 421–423.

McConnell, E. D. (2012). House poor in Los Angeles: Examining patterns of housing-induced poverty by race, nativity, and legal status. *Housing Policy Debate, 22*(4), 605–631.

McConnell, E. D. (2013). Who has housing affordability problems? Disparities in housing cost burden by race, nativity, and legal status in Los Angeles. *Race and Social Problems, 5*(3), 173–190.

Mena, F. J., Padilla, A. M., & Maldonado, M. (1987). Acculturative stress and specific coping strategies among immigrant and later generation college students. *Hispanic Journal of Behavioral Sciences, 9*(2), 207–225.

Meyer, I. H. (1995). Minority stress and mental health in gay men. *Journal of Health and Social Behavior, 36*(1), 38–56.

Meyer, I. H. (2003). Prejudice, social stress, and mental health in lesbian, gay, and bisexual populations: Conceptual issues and research evidence. *Psychological Bulletin, 129*(5), 674–697.

Mitchell, T. R. (1985). An evaluation of the validity of correlational research conducted in organizations. *Academy of Management Review, 10*(2), 192–205.

Molina, K. M., Alegría, M., & Mahalingam, R. (2013). A multiple-group path analysis of the role of everyday discrimination on self-rated physical health among Latina/os in the USA. *Annals of Behavioral Medicine, 45*(1), 33–43.

Moradi, B., & Risco, C. (2006). Perceived discrimination experiences and mental health of Latina/o american persons. *Journal of Counseling Psychology, 53*(4), 411–421.

Moody, B. D. L., Waldstein, S. R., Tobin, J. N., Cassells, A., Schwartz, J. C., & Brondolo, E. (2016). Lifetime racial/ethnic discrimination and ambulatory blood pressure: The moderating effect of age. *Health Psychology, 35*(4), 333–342.

Nagel, J. (1994). Constructing ethnicity: Creating and recreating ethnic identity and culture. *Social Problems, 41*(1), 152–176.

Negi, N. J. (2013). Battling discrimination and social isolation: Psychological distress among Latino day laborers. *American Journal of Community Psychology, 51*(1–2), 164–174.

Novak, N. L., Geronimus, A. T., & Martinez-Cardoso, A. M. (2017). Change in birth outcomes among infants born to Latina mothers after a major immigration raid. *International Journal of Epidemiology, 46*(3), 839–849.

Oh, H., Yang, L. H., Anglin, D. M., & DeVylder, J. E. (2014). Perceived discrimination and psychotic experiences across multiple ethnic groups in the United States. *Schizophrenia Research, 157*(1–3), 259–265.

Omi, M., & Winant, H. (2015). *Racial formation in the United States* (3rd ed.). New York: Routledge.

Otiniano, A. D., & Gee, G. C. (2012). Self-reported discrimination and health-related quality of life among Whites, Blacks, Mexicans and Central Americans. *Journal of Immigrant and Minority Health, 14*(2), 189–197.

Paradies, Y., Ben, J., Denson, N., Elias, A., Priest, N., Pieterse, A., ... Gee, G. (2015). Racism as a determinant of health: A systematic review and meta-analysis. *PLoS ONE, 10*(9), e0138511.

Pascoe, E. A., & Richman, L. S. (2009). Perceived discrimination and health: A meta-analytic review. *Psychological Bulletin, 135*(4), 531–554.

Pearlin, L. I., Menaghan, E. G., Lieberman, M. A., & Mullan, J. T. (1981). The stress process. *Journal of Health and Social Behavior, 22*(4), 337–356.

Pedraza, F., Cruz Nichols, V., & LeBrón, A. M. W. (2017). Cautious citizenship: The deterring effect of immigration issue salience on health care use and bureaucratic interactions among Latino U.S. citizens. *Journal of Health Politics, Policy and the Law, 42*(5), 925–960.

Pérez, D. J., Fortuna, L., & Alegría, M. (2008). Prevalence and correlates of everyday discrimination among U.S. latinos. *Journal of Community Psychology, 36*(4), 421–433.

Phelan, J. C., Link, B. G., & Tehranifar, P. (2010). Social conditions as fundamental causes of health inequalities: theory, evidence, and policy implications. *Journal of Health and Social Behavior, 51*, Suppl(Spring), S28–S40.

Pilver, C. E., Desai, R., Kasl, S., & Levy, B. R. (2011). Lifetime discrimination associated with greater likelihood of premenstrual dysphoric disorder. *Journal of Women's Health (2002), 20*(6), 923–931.

Podsakoff, P. M., & Organ, D. W. (1986). Self-reports in organizational research: problems and prospects. *Journal of Management, 12*(4), 531–544.

Purnell, J. Q., Peppone, L. J., Alcaraz, K., McQueen, A., Guido, J. J., Carroll, J. K., ... Morrow, G. R. (2012). Perceived discrimination, psychological distress, and current smoking status: Results from the behavioral risk factor surveillance system reactions to race module, 2004–2008. *American Journal of Public Health, 102*(5), 844–851.

Rhodes, S. D., Mann, L., Simán, F. M., Song, E., Alonzo, J., Downs, M., ... Hall, M. A. (2015). The impact of local immigration enforcement policies on the health of immigrant Hispanics/Latinos in the United States. *American Journal of Public Health, 105*(2), 329–337.

Rios, V. M. (2011). *Punished: Policing the lives of Black and Latino Boys*. New York: New York University.

Ryan, A. M., Gee, G. C., & Laflamme, D. F. (2006). The association between self-reported discrimination, physical health and blood pressure: Findings from African Americans, Black immigrants, and Latino immigrants in New Hampshire. *Journal of Health Care for the Poor and Underserved, 17*(2 Suppl), 116–132.

Schnittker, J., & Bacak, V. (2014). The increasing predictive validity of self-rated health. *PLoS ONE, 9*(1), e384933.

Schulz, A. J., Mentz, G. B., Sampson, N., Ward, M., Anderson, R., De Majo, R., ... Wilkins, D. (2017). Race and the distribution of social and physical environmental risk: A case example from the Detroit Metropolitan area. *Du Bois Review, 13*(2), 285–304.

Schwalbe, M., Godwin, S., Holdern, D., Schrock, D., Thompson, S., Wolkomir, M., et al. (2000). Generic processes in the reproduction of inequality: An interactionist analysis. *Social Forces, 72*(2), 419–452.

Seng, J. S., Lopez, W. D., Sperlich, M., Hamama, L., & Reed Meldrum, C. D. (2012). Marginalized identities, discrimination burden, and mental health: Empirical exploration of an interpersonal-level approach to modeling intersectionality. *Social Science and Medicine, 75*(12), 2437–2445.

Southern Poverty Law Center. (2016). *SPLC hatewatch: Update: 1,094 bias-related incidents in the month following the election*. Montgomery. Retrieved from https://www.splcenter.org/hatewatch/2016/12/16/update-1094-bias-related-incidents-month-following-election%0D.

Stepler, R., & Brown, A. (2016). *Statistical portrait of Hispanics in the United States in 2013|Pew Research Center*. Retrieved from http://www.pewhispanic.org/2016/04/19/statistical-portrait-of-hispanics-in-the-united-states/.

Stuber, J., Galea, S., Ahern, J., Blaney, S., & Fuller, C. (2003). The association between multiple domains of discrimination and self-assessed health: A multilevel analysis of Latinos and Blacks in four low-income New York City neighborhoods. *Health Services Research, 38*(6 p 2),1735–1760.

Thorndike, E. L. (1920). A constant error in psychological ratings. *Journal of Applied Psychology, 4*, 25–29.

Tovar, J., & Feliciano, C. (2009). "Not Mexican-American, but Mexican:" Shifting ethnic self-identifications among children of Mexican immigrants. *Latino Studies, 7*(2), 197–221. https://doi.org/10.1057/lst.2009.18.

U.S. Office of Management and Budget. (1997). *Revisions to the standards for the classification of federal data on race and ethnicity*. Washington, D.C.

Viruell-Fuentes, E. A. (2007). Beyond acculturation: Immigration, discrimination, and health research among Mexicans in the United States. *Social Science and Medicine, 65*(7), 1524–1535.

Viruell-Fuentes, E. A. (2011). "It's a lot of work:" Racialization processes, racial identity formations, and their health implications. *Du Bois Review, 8*(1), 37–52.

Viruell-Fuentes, E. A., Miranda, P. Y., & Abdulrahim, S. (2012). More than culture: Structural racism, intersectionality theory, and immigrant health. *Social Science and Medicine, 75*(12), 2099–2106.

Viruell-Fuentes, E. A., Morenoff, J. D., Williams, D. R., & House, J. S. (2011). Language of interview, self-rated health, and the other Latino health puzzle. *American Journal of Public Health, 101*(7), 1306–1313.

Whitehead, M. (1991). The concepts and principles of equity and health. *Health Promotion International, 6*(3), 217–228.

Williams, D. R., & Mohammed, S. A. (2009). Discrimination and racial disparities in health: Evidence and needed research. *Journal of Behavioral Medicine, 32*(1), 20–47. https://doi.org/10.1007/s10865-008-9185-0.

Williams, D. R., & Mohammed, S. A. (2013). Racism and health: Pathways and scientific evidence. *American Behavioral Scientist, 57*(8), 1199–1216.

Williams, D. R., Yu, Y., Jackson, J. S., & Anderson, N. B. (1997). Racial differences in physical and mental health: Socio-economic status, stress and discrimination. *Journal of Health Psychology, 2*(3), 335–351.

Chapter 15
Divergent Dilemma: The Reconceptualization and Critical Use of Acculturation in Latinx Health Research

Airín D. Martínez

Abstract In this chapter, I delineate the historical and theoretical foundations of acculturation in anthropology, sociology, and psychology; identify popular measures of acculturation; and outline their critiques. After this multidisciplinary refresher, I explore how the process of acculturation can be conceptualized and investigated in relation to one health outcome commonly examined in Latinx health: obesity. My approach departs from stereotypes, acknowledges pre-immigration conditions, and captures the host context. My goal is to provide an example of how to conceptualize the process of acculturation specific to distinct health outcomes. I end by arguing that addressing the problems of acculturation in health research and creating new conceptualizations may help us resolve our divergent dilemma and produce research that provides meaningful information about Latinx health inequalities, both in the United States and abroad.

Keywords Acculturation · Assimilation · Obesity · Latinx health · Social determinants of health

The taken-for-granted definition of acculturation in Latinx health research often refers to adaptation processes occurring when individuals from one nation, primarily transnational migrants from Latin America, adopt the values, beliefs, behaviors, expectations, roles, and norms of the host culture, generally referring to that of the USA. It is often assumed that immigrants abandon traits from their ethnic background in this process. In Latinx health research, acculturation has been examined in relation to a myriad of health behaviors and outcomes such as diet (Ayala, Baquero, and Klinger, 2008; Delavari, Sønderlund, Swinburn, Mellor, & Renzaho, 2013), chronic disease risk factors (Daviglus et al., 2016; Mainous, Diaz, & Geesey, 2008; O'Brien, Alos, Bueno, & Whitaker, 2014), cancer screening (Savas, Vernon, Atkinson, & Fernandez, 2015), mental health (Koneru, de Mamani, Flynn, and Betancourt, 2007), risky sexual behaviors (Haderxhanaj, Rhodes, Romaguera, Bloom, & Leichliter, 2015), health care access and utilization (Bermúdez-Parsai, Geiger, Marsiglia, &

A. D. Martínez (✉)
School of Public Health & Health Sciences, University of Massachusetts-Amherst, Amherst, MA, USA
e-mail: admartinez@umass.edu

© Springer Nature Switzerland AG 2020
A. D. Martínez and S. D. Rhodes (eds.), *New and Emerging Issues in Latinx Health*, https://doi.org/10.1007/978-3-030-24043-1_15

Coonrod 2012), substance use (Serafini, Wendt, Ornelas, Doyle, & Donovan, 2017), and aging (Riosmena, Wong, & Palloni, 2013), among others.

A review of the research generally indicates that acculturation is related to Latinx health in three ways. First, the stress from the process of adapting to a new culture and environment has negative health effects, such as culture shock and depression. Second, assimilation to US culture harms health because Latinx individuals acquire unhealthy behaviors such as smoking (Blue & Fenelon, 2011), drinking (Bacio, Mays, & Lau, 2013) and poor diet (Mazur, Marquis, & Jensen, 2003). Third, the erosion of so-called protective Latinx values, beliefs, and behaviors can lead to chronic disease (Abraído-Lanza, Dohrenwend, Ng-Mak, & Turner, 1999; Bostean, 2013; Razum & Twardella, 2002; Scribner, 1996). Researchers often examine how adherence to English or Spanish leads to changes in health behaviors, declines in health outcomes such as chronic disease, or improvements in the reduction of infectious disease (Bohon & Conley, 2015).

Latinx persons who are more acculturated to US culture (usually self-reporting speaking English, ethnic affiliation, and living a longer time in the country) appear to have worse health, such as higher body mass index (BMI) and issues with substance use and abuse (Koneru et al., 2007). Conversely, more acculturation to US culture has also been associated with good health; for example, an increased consumption of fruits and vegetables (López & Yamashita, 2017; Otero-Sabogal, Sabogal, Perez-Stable, & Hiatt, 1995) and leisure-time physical activity (Berrigan, Dodd, Troiano, Reeve, & Ballard-Barbash, 2006; Daviglus et al., 2016). According to the findings of many systematic reviews, it is unclear whether acculturation is ultimately helpful or harmful to Latinx health (Abraído-Lanza et al. 1999; Abraído-Lanza, Echeverría, & Flórez, 2016; Ayala, Baquero & Klinger, 2008; Carter-Pokras et al., 2008; Koneru et al., 2007; Lara, Gamboa, Kahramanian, Morales, & Bautista, 2005; Palloni & Arias, 2003; 2004; Thomson & Hoffman-Goetz, 2009; Wallace, Pomery, Latimer, & Martinez, Salovey, 2010; Zambrana & Carter-Pokras, 2010). These inconclusive findings have often been attributed to researchers' use of different proxies and scales to examine acculturation.

This disjuncture about the effect of acculturation on Latinx health may also result from the failure to describe the two cultures that come into contact: Latin American or Latinx culture and US-American[1] culture. In turn, many assumptions are made about the cultural beliefs and health practices of US-born Latinx individuals and Latinx immigrants, which make the concept of acculturation and its proxies weak

---

[1] The term "US-American" implies the heterogeneous nature of what American culture represents. Many persons from Latin America consider themselves American, as they are from the American continent. However, in acculturation and health research, the term "American culture" is used as the baseline of comparison without defining which nation represents American culture, or within the context of the United States, which region the immigrants or racial/ethnic minorities are from.

2. Foodways are different from diets because it is not solely the food that is of empirical focus, but also the cultural, social, and economic practices that shape the production and consumption of food. In this case, health researchers have often omitted the meanings, rituals, cultural practices, and significance that food has for Latinx persons. The focus has been more on *what* they eat and not *how* they eat.

measures for Latinx health research. For example, Wallace and colleagues (2010) write:

> Latino cultural beliefs about the causes of illness, treatment and ways to prevent illness are significantly affected by religion, fear and fatalism... Outside forces, supernatural forces, evil spirits, punishment from God, or hexes by brujas [witches] are causes for physical disharmony. These perceptions may act as barriers to healthy lifestyle changes and must be considered in any health promotion intervention. (p. 2)

Wallace and colleagues' assumption that Latinx individuals' health beliefs and practices are largely informed by religion and superstitious beliefs suggests that these individuals are premodern—meaning that they do not practice health through biomedical approaches to the body or with the belief that biomedical technologies can improve health. By considering Latinx individuals as premodern subjects, researchers assume that US-born Latinx persons' and Latinx immigrants' health beliefs and practices are exclusively informed by cultural constructs such as *familism, fatalism, marianismo, machismo,* "indigenous" beliefs, religion, and "traditional diets." (Marsiglia and Keihne clearly define the concepts of *fatalism, familism, marianismo,* and *machismo* in Chap. 5). Furthermore, by relegating Latinx health to culture, we overlook sources of structural inequality emanating in the host context that can shape Latinx health disparities (see Abraído-Lanza et al., 2006; Carter-Pokras & Bethune, 2009; Viruell-Fuentes, 2007; Viruell-Fuentes, Miranda, & Abdulrahim, 2012; see also Chap. 14).

Despite more than 25 years of critiques and concept papers demanding the expansion and/or eradication of acculturation in health research, we still see articles, such as the one by Wallace and colleagues, with nothing short of inaccurate generalizations about Latinx persons and an incomplete conceptualization and poor operationalization of acculturation. In the face of reservations and critiques of acculturation in understanding or resolving Latinx health issues, researchers still include acculturation measures in their research; possibly, for fear of having their articles rejected or grant proposals penalized. In the area of Latinx health, reviewers for academic journals and external funding agencies expect the research to have included a measure or control for acculturation, even if the participants are not immigrants (i.e., second-generation or more), or if cultural adaptation is not central to the research question. Quite frankly, researchers face this divergent dilemma: to use or not to use acculturation in Latinx health research?

On the one hand, it is important to acknowledge the structural, cultural, and environmental changes that US-born Latinx persons and Latinx immigrants face in the USA and how these changes transform their physical health, health beliefs, and health practices. On the other hand, common acculturation measures fail to capture these macro-level changes that may shape health outcomes at the individual and aggregate level. How does the acquisition of the English language, ethnic affiliation, media language preference, and time in the USA help us understand changes in different health outcomes? The problem with acculturation is confusion over its meaning, its use in research, and more important, its significance in the social determinants of Latinx health and health disparities.

In this chapter, I attempt to delineate acculturation's historical and theoretical foundations in anthropology, sociology, and psychology and identify popular measures from sociology and psychology and their critiques. After this multidisciplinary refresher, I will discuss *how* the process of acculturation can be conceptualized and investigated in relation to two health outcomes commonly examined in Latinx health, diet and obesity, that departs from stereotypes, acknowledges pre-immigration conditions, and captures the host context. The hope is to provide an example of how to conceptualize the process of acculturation *specific* to distinct health outcomes. I end by arguing that addressing the problems of acculturation in health research and creating new conceptualizations may help us resolve our divergent dilemma and produce research that provides meaningful information about Latinx health inequalities, both in the USA and abroad.

A History of Acculturation in Anthropology, Sociology, and Psychology

Anthropologic Roots of Acculturation

The concept of acculturation has roots in anthropology and appears in ethnographic texts as early as the 1880s. During the nineteenth century, numerous anthropologists were examining nation-states and territories colonized by Western powers in order to find ways to subjugate these populations (Anderson, 2006) and because they assumed that indigenous populations and immigrants from less developed countries were culturally and biologically inferior (Rudmin, 2009).

For anthropologists, acculturation is a group-level process that occurs when two or more cultures come into contact with one another. As a result, there is mutual exposure and eventual adaptation of both the immigrant culture and that of the host society. However, we often just find analyses about the transmission of U.S. culture onto indigenous and racial/ethnic minorities in a Western context. Anthropologists Robert Redfield, Ralph Linton, and Melville J. Herskovits provided a definition and recommendations to study acculturation in 1936 on behalf of the Social Science Research Council (SSRC). They wrote, "Acculturation comprehends those phenomena which result when groups of individuals having different cultures come into continuous first-hand contact, with subsequent changes in the original cultural patterns of either or both group" (1936, p. 149).

This classic paper continues to be cited by social scientists and public health researchers alike. However, Redfield and colleagues' classic paper has been critiqued for its ambiguity, disregard for individual-level cultural change, and conceptualization of culture as a universal set of mutually exclusive group traits that remains universal across space and time (Chirkov, 2009). However, so much of what Redfield and colleagues wrote in that SSRC report is not even taken into consideration. For example, they recommend examining a selection of traits and to take into consideration the situation for acculturation: was the cultural encounter forced, as in colonialism? Or, was it a mutual, equal process? Also, why is the receiving group selecting certain traits over others? What advantages does it provide in the new, host society? (Redfield, Linton, & Herskovits, 1936).

With the postmodern turn in social theory during the twentieth century, there were critiques of this conceptualization of culture in anthropology, and instead a shift to perceive and examine culture as a *process* (Rosaldo, 1989) that is *not* exclusive to ethnic, racial, or indigenous groups (Waldram, 2009). For instance, Lupton (2012) examines medicine as a culture. However, given increased globalization and transnational processes, anthropologists are approaching the adaptation of migrant groups as part of "ethnoscapes" and having "diasporic identities."

Ethnoscapes refers to the transnational movement of ethnic groups' cultural practices not only through out-migration of people, but also through media and economic landscapes where migrants continue to consume multiple products from their home country to maintain social, political, and economic ties in their new settings (Appadurai, 1996). Diaspora "…refers to immigrant communities that distinctly attempt to maintain (real and/or imagined) connections and commitments to their homeland and recognize themselves and act as a collective community (Bhatia & Ram, 2009, p. 141, citing Tölöyan, 1996). Diasporic communities often form when the immigrants are not accepted, represented, or integrated into the host society (Bhatia and Ram, 2009) and often include members of later generations. To study these dynamic cultural processes, anthropologists continue to rely on ethnographic techniques that provide a thick, rich description.

Acculturation and Assimilation in Sociology

During the early twentieth century, unlike anthropologists who studied collectivities in foreign lands, urban sociologists at the University of Chicago tried to understand the cultural conflict and adaption of Eastern and Southern European immigrants who came to work in several sectors of manual labor and manufacturing in the USA. For example, W. I. Thomas and Florian Znanecki's (1923) *A Polish Peasant in Europe and America* is a classic sociologic text that presents the life of Polish immigrants in Chicago. Chicago School sociologists were also interested in examining the cultural conflict and adaptation of black persons migrating to northern US cities from southern states (DuBois, 1903; Park & Tristram, 1939, 1950). W. E. B. DuBois was interested in understanding how black individuals negotiated living with a *double consciousness,* as both black and American, marginalized from US society and dealing with inequalities that stemmed from racial stereotypes that they were biologically, intellectually, and culturally inferior.

As DuBois' complex discussion of black identity demonstrates, interpretive sociologists have a long history of understanding identity and culture as being dynamic, contextual, and situational. This means that the performance of one's identity will change not only throughout the life course, but also depending on the situation, who is present in that situation, and the social, historical, and political context in which one's life takes place (Clarke, 2005; Strauss, 1993; Thomas & Thomas, 1928). This is important for understanding the relationship between acculturation and health in the Latinx population because health researchers often do not inquire about the situations in which Latinx individuals feel compelled to speak a certain language, behave in a certain way, or engage in a certain healthy or risky behavior. Unfortunately, this approach is not widespread because quantitative methods dominate acculturation and health research in medical sociology, health psychology, and public health.

Robert E. Park spent much of his career writing about acculturation and assimilation of racial/ethnic minorities. For sociologists, assimilation refers to a process where a person from a racial/ethnic minority or immigrant group adopts the mainstream culture and becomes an integrated member of that culture. For Park, there was a "race relations cycle" of acculturation and assimilation that commenced with *contact* between the host (or mainstream) group and the immigrant (or minority) group, followed by *competition* between the groups in the labor and housing markets, which would eventually lead to *accommodation* of the minority group, and finally, *assimilation*. Park had a multicultural approach to the process of acculturation because he believed that assimilation would be achieved when members of the racial/ethnic groups intermarried and had children of mixed race, who shared values, norms, beliefs, and practices with mainstream, dominant culture. Then, if they were fully integrated into society, it would be too difficult to perceive physical and cultural differences between the groups. Acculturation was perceived as a process that eventually led to a positive outcome and improved the mental health of immigrants and their progeny because they no longer perceived the host culture as "alien," nor were they to be treated poorly by the mainstream society (Park and Tristram, 1950).

As idealistic as Park was about the future of race relations in the USA, he did not take into consideration that the country would continue to have immigration policies shaped by eugenics, Social Darwinism, and xenophobia. Park's comparison groups, black individuals and people from Eastern and Southern Europe, do not include the current major immigrant and refugee groups in the USA from Latin America and Asia. In addition, the economic and political context during Park's writings in the early twentieth century is distinct from that of our current twenty-first century with the economic development of Europe, technologic innovation, economic and cultural globalization, and the resurgence of xenophobic conservative immigration politics in Western countries.

After World War II, in sociology, the discussion of acculturation had receded and transformed to that of assimilation as Glazer and Moynihan (1963) and Gordon (1964) theorized about "cultural pluralism." Cultural pluralism is a condition in which multiple racial/ethnic groups maintain their racial/ethnic identity, values, and practices in the USA, as long as it is within the customs and laws of the dominant culture. The main critique of cultural pluralism is that each racial/ethnic group in the country does not have equal power in society, nor can these diverse groups compete equally for economic resources and political power in the same arenas, especially when white supremacy continues to exist. Sociologists' examination of acculturation now favors more macro-level analyses of racial conflict, inequality, and assimilation (Waters & Jiménez, 2005).

Alba and Nee's (2003) and Portes and Rumbaut's (2001) contemporary theories of assimilation critique and expand the unilinear explanations of acculturation provided by Chicago School sociologists (e.g., Park, 1928; Park & Burgess, 1925) and cultural pluralists (e.g., Glazer & Moynihan, 1963; Gordon, 1964). Portes and Rumbaut's (2001) theory includes three possible outcomes of acculturation: dissonant, consonant, and segmented assimilation. *Dissonant* assimilation results when children acculturate to American language and life faster than their immigrant parents, leading them to engage in riskier, deviant behavior (e.g., drug use and gang participation) outside of the purview and support of their parents and ethnic community. Eventually, persons experiencing dissonant assimilation can experience downward mobility because they experience discrimination but have weakened family and ethnic social supports. *Consonant* assimilation refers to the process in which the parents and children learn English and integrate American culture at the same rate, producing upward mobility and maintaining family support. Similar to consonant assimilation, *selective* acculturation refers to the process in which the parents and children learn English and integrate American culture, but also remain embedded in their ethnic culture and social networks. This process leads to biculturalism, social support, and less intergenerational conflict between parents and children. Meanwhile, Alba and Nee (2003) take a pluralist approach to acculturation in that they believe ethnic immigrants will eventually be integrated into US society. Nonetheless, like Portes and Rumbaut, Alba and Nee recognize that American mainstream culture is not monolithic, but in fact, diverse along with US history and geographically across the country.

Both Alba and Nee (2003) and Portes and Rumbaut (2001) would emphasize that when one studies acculturation, they also assess parents' human capital (e.g., pre-immigration socioeconomic status, political participation, and civic engagement), family structure (e.g., single parents), and modes of incorporation. Modes of incorporation refer to those social structural conditions that shape the ability for immigrants to adopt the host society's culture and become integrated in that society. For instance, how the legal, political, and local collectivities respond to immigrants by either providing opportunities to live in diverse neighborhoods, participate in public programs, and obtain gainful employment *or* excluding them and limiting them to inferior positions in the racial/ethnic hierarchy.

In relationship to health, the Latinx population, and immigrant health research, we do find poor health outcomes in relationship to more acculturation. In sociologic research, more acculturation often leads to improved economic mobility, but it depends on the *type of acculturation* that Latinx immigrants and their offspring experience. Waters, Tran, Kasinitz, and Mollenkopf (2010) examined the social outcomes of children of immigrants in the New York metropolitan area, representing European, Latin American, and Caribbean countries. The authors found that "neither type of acculturation (i.e., consonant, dissonant or segmented) nor the level of ethnic embeddedness [could] account for the variation in mobility patterns both across and within second generation groups" (pg. 1168). Unlike what Portes and Rumbaut warned, rarely did second-generation immigrants experience dissonant acculturation and downward social mobility. The basic message from contemporary sociologic theories of acculturation and assimilation is that immigrants and their offspring will have different acculturation trajectories, if they are racial/ethnic minorities they will face discrimination, and they will have different life outcomes depending on multiple variables, from parents' pre-immigration structural position and the modes of incorporation of the host society (Waters et al. 2010).

In addition to economic mobility, pre-immigration experiences, and modes of incorporation, health researchers rarely examine intermarriage with persons belonging to the dominant group, as a proxy for acculturation and assimilation. In fact, by the time of this writing, 27% of Hispanic newlyweds are married to persons outside their racial or ethnic group; this percentage is second only to that for Asian newlyweds (Livingston & Brown, 2017). To the best of my knowledge, no study has been conducted to determine if Latinx intermarriage is related to health outcomes.

With the surge of research examining the genesis and significance of globalization and transnationalism since the 1980s, some sociologists have moved toward "flexible acculturation" (Nederveen Pieterse, 2007). Flexible acculturation refers to how different social groups utilize transnational opportunities to achieve their economic, political, or social goals (Nederveen Pieterse, 2007). Related to modes of incorporation, flexible acculturation emphasizes that social positions are shaped by the nation-state, where governments and politicians actively shape the condition for immigrants and racial/ethnic minorities to acculturate. In this scenario, through ethnoscapes, both migrants to host societies and the natives of host societies have exposure to other national and ethnic cultures as a result of the transnational availability of media to construct "imagined communities" (Anderson, 1991). Similarly, immigrants and their children are able to maintain their language, cultural beliefs, and practices as a result of immigrant replenishment in traditional gateways (Waters & Jiménez, 2005) and hometown associations in the host country, the Internet and social media, and ease in importing products that are important for rituals and cultural maintenance. Several cultural aspects of society are shared across borders because of globalization.

As argued elsewhere (Martínez, 2010), one of the reasons people of racial/ethnic minorities, specifically the Latinx population, of second-generation or more, maintain their families' ethnic practices is not necessarily because they are *resistant* to the host culture, but because the host culture does not accept them and creates institutional forms of racism that do not support the full integration of US-born Latinx persons and Latinx immigrants into society—unlike what Park imagined. Similarly, flexible acculturation acknowledges that this process is not solely one that is isolated to migrants and their culture, but that governments and politicians actively shape the context of acculturation for migrants and people of racial/ethnic minorities (Lee, 2008). For example, in Donald J. Trump's first few weeks as President, he signed an executive order to build a militarized wall along the US–Mexican border and to increase the deportation of unauthorized immigrants, including those with minor criminal infractions (Executive Order No. 13767, 2017). Immigration policies like these are targeting Mexican-origin and Latinx communities in the USA, despite having a presence of hundreds of years in the country.

Acculturation in Psychology

Psychology commenced acculturation research much later than did anthropology and sociology (Waldram, 2009), where acculturation psychology emerged in the mid-twentieth century (Chirkov, 2009). What is often studied in psychology is acculturative stress (see Rudmin, 2003, 2009 for a review of acculturative stress research and measures). Barnett, Broom, Siegel, Voge, and Watson (1954) coined the term "acculturative stress" to describe immigrants' chronic culture shock, in which acculturation leads to psychologic, somatic, and social difficulties in adjusting. The assumption is that a racial/ethnic minority or immigrant group is more affected in acculturation. There is a supposition that the process of acculturation leads to mental pathologies when a person is adjusting to the new culture, and more important, being deprived of opportunities to reproduce one's native cultural practices in the new country. Symbolic interactionists and anthropologists would argue that immigrants would eventually experience their new surroundings as normal. As Rudmin (2009) points out, immigrants come to a point where they do not experience culture shock in their everyday life. Yet, as in early periods of anthropology and sociology, psychologists largely believe that assimilation, the final stage of acculturation, is a benefit to the mental health of immigrants to the USA and other Western developed countries. As noted in the discussion of modes of incorporation, acculturative stress may emanate from the process of becoming a marginalized person in the new society.

John Berry's fourfold theory (Berry, 1980; Berry, Evans, & Rawlinson, 1972; Berry, Phinney, Sam, & Vedder, 2006; Williams & Berry, 1991) is often used in Latinx and immigrant health research. This theory emphasizes that immigrants and racial or ethnic minorities could adjust to be in one of four states: separation, integration, marginalization, and assimilation. Separation refers to those persons who refuse to acculturate to the dominant culture and want to maintain their ethnic culture. Integration is the scenario in which the individual is bicultural and manifests both the host society's culture and that of his or her ancestors. Marginalization refers to persons who want to assimilate, but are not accepted by the host society. For Berry, assimilation is a point where immigrants lose their old ethnic identity and solely manifest that of the host society. However, Berry's model and acculturation scale have not provided a comprehensive explanation of cultural differences between groups or individuals, as the items for each state of acculturation are not mutually exclusive (Doucerain, Segalowitz, & Ryder, 2016; Rudmin, 2003). Schwartz and Zamboanga (2008), through a cluster factor analysis among a diverse multiethnic, multigenerational group of Latinx young adults, showed that more than four typologies of acculturation often emerge. In some international comparative studies, researchers found similar answers from ethnic immigrants living in a Western country, their counterparts in their home country who desired migration, and those with no interest in Western culture or migration (Kim, 1989). The next section explores these acculturation measures and their reflection, or lack thereof, of these theories.

Acculturation Measures

One of the reasons for providing a disciplinary and theoretical overview of acculturation is that most acculturation scales used in Latinx health research lack a theoretical foundation (Abraído-Lanza et al., 2006; Hunt, Schneider, & Comer, 2004; Lopez-Class, Castro, & Ramirez, 2011; Thomson and Hoffman-Goetz, 2009). The earliest acculturation measure documented for the Hispanic/Latino population was the Behavioral and Values Acculturation Scale developed by Szapocznik, Scopetta, Kurtines, and Aranalde (1978). Their study sought to test a behavioral and values acculturation between 379 Cuban-origin and white persons (13–75 years old) in Miami. Behavioral acculturation for them referred to "language use and preference, customs, habits, and lifestyle" that reflect the USA. Values acculturation was not defined. The authors found that changes in behaviors and values among Cuban-origin persons was a function of age at the time of exposure to US culture. Note, that the exposure to US culture is a separate variable from time in the USA. They also found that participants migrating at younger ages acculturated faster.

One of the interesting ways that Szapocznik and colleagues (1978) assessed behavioral changes among Cuban-origin persons was to contextualize the items in the behavior and values scale. That is, they asked participants to rank how they would respond to six scenarios, from discovering a family member's illicit drug use to the topic of abortion. However, it is unclear why certain options were considered to be more Cuban or American than others. For instance, in the gender values item, the researchers state the following.

In reference to women… three different points of view follow:

A. Women and men should be partners, she should work if she wants to, and at the same time share the duties of the household with her husband.
B. Woman should be a man's complement. While he goes to work, she should take care of the housework and the children.
C. Women should try to achieve their own goals, without following their husband's or traditional ideas to limit them.

As one can see, many of the options are not mutually exclusive of an ethnic culture, but may be informed by religious beliefs, couples' preferences in the household division of labor, economic position, and/or necessity. For instance, in Mexico, most women work outside the home out of necessity, and also, employers have sought female employees with the rise of globalization and the maquila industry (Fernández-Kelly, 2008). So, traditional gender roles are transforming in Latin America, too. Nevertheless, Szapocznik and colleagues' (1978) research presents something that is missing from contemporary acculturation and health research—*context*. The cultural scenarios in their values scale (e.g., gender norms and gender performance, beliefs around abortion, family involvement, illicit drug use, and sexuality) demonstrate that the cultural values and practice(s) that immigrants and ethnic minorities *acculturate to* differ by situation and cannot be limited to language and ethnic affiliation alone.

Since the development of Behavioral and Values Acculturation Scale, 26 acculturation measures have been used for research about Latinx health knowledge, attitudes, and behavior change between 1979 and 2006 (Wallace et al., 2010). Despite a large number of measures, six scales remain the most popular in Latinx health research, and they can be organized by measurement type: proxies, unidimensional, bidimensional, or multidimensional scales (Thomson and Hoffman-Goetz, 2009). Proxies are simply variables often culled from population-based surveys that serve as representatives of variables thought to be an attribute of acculturation. Proxies are the most frequently used acculturation measures in Latinx health research. For example, to examine the relationship between Latinx health and acculturation, researchers have often reverted to the language in which the survey was administered and the participant's nativity and time in the United States as proxies. Interestingly, in proxy-based acculturation research there has been little to no conceptualizing regarding why language, nativity, or time in the host society are so vital in the adaptation and exchange of cultural information.

Unidimensional scales are designed to examine how much Latinx persons retain or relinquish their Latin American ethnic culture for that of the USA. Two examples of very popular unidimensional scales used in public health include the Acculturation Rating Scale for Mexican Americans (ARSMA) (Cuellar, Harris, & Jasso, 1980) and Short Acculturation Scale for Hispanics (SASH) (Marin, Sabogal, Marin, Otero-Sabogal, & Perez-Stable, 1987). The ARSMA is a 60-item scale with a 5-point Likert scale that determines whether Mexican-origin persons are in one of five acculturation orientations: very Mexican, Mexican-oriented, bicultural, Anglo-oriented, or very Anglicized.

The ARSMA was piloted in a San Antonio hospital with Mexican immigrants and US-born Mexican psychiatric patients and medical trainees in the late 1970s. The measures include subscales in language preference (English or Spanish), ethnic identity and ethnic affiliation, media language preference, contact with family in Mexico, and food preference. Eight items from the ARSMA related to language use and ethnic background have been used to create an acculturation index for the first national epidemiologic study of persons of Cuban, Mexican, and Puerto Rican origin in the USA, the Hispanic Health Nutrition Examination Survey (HHANES) (1982–1983) and subsequently, the National Health Interview Survey (NHIS) (Carter-Pokras & Bethune, 2009, citing Burman, McMillan, Carter, and Haynes, 1987).

In direct response to the ARSMA, Marin and colleagues (1987) created a language acculturation scale that could be distributed to people of all Latin American nationalities. The definition of acculturation used to frame the SASH is "a process of changes in behavior and values by individuals" (Marin and Gamba, 1996, p. 184, citing Gordon, 1964). Similar to the ARSMA, the SASH assesses acculturation through behaviors such as language use and preference, media use, ethnic loyalty, and ethnic social relations (Marin and Gamba, 1996, p. 187), but it is shorter, with only 12 items versus 60, and does not ask about participants' contact with their home country. The main issue with unidimensional scales is that they assess acculturation as a linear process where people can occupy and enact only one racial/ethnic culture over another. Moreover, the Behavioral and Values Acculturation Scale, the ARSMA, and

SASH do not use longitudinal data to demonstrate that respondents' language and ethnic preferences remain the same throughout their lives. The Behavioral and Values Acculturation Scale and the ARSMA were piloted in only one Latinx subgroup in one geographic location, and there is little theory complementing the construction of these scales.

Facing critiques from many scholars that Latinx individuals never fully relinquish their ethnic culture in order to navigate both their ethnic culture and the US culture, bidimensional scales were created. Bidimensional scales are designed to capture Latinx individuals' orientation to both Latinx and non-Latinx culture, but usually people relate to one more than the other. In fact, studies have found that biculturalism is often, but not always, the most favorable acculturation orientation for young Latinx persons (Coatsworth, Maldonado-Molina, Pantin, & Szapocznik, 2005; Sullivan et al., 2007). Biculturalism may allow one to relate to people from both cultural contexts, but it may also create pressures (perceived or real) to meet the expectations of the receiving cultural context, the heritage cultural community, or both (Schwartz, Montgomery, & Briones, 2006).

An example of a bidimensional scale is the Bidimensional Acculturation Scale (BAS) by Marin and Gamba (1996), which discerns language use, language proficiency, and frequency of media consumption in Spanish or English; more English in any of these categories is considered to be less Hispanic. The 12 items in the BAS to represent these three dimensions in each domain, Hispanic, and non-Hispanic. Like the developers of the ARSMA (Cuellar, Arnold, & Maldonado, 1995; Cuellar et al., 1980), Marin and Gamba (1996) acknowledge that their scale is limited and does not measure an individual's or a group's change in values and norms. We can critique these measures individually for not being comprehensive measures or helpful for researchers to understand health outcomes for Latinx persons, but the measures were never meant to examine more complex cultural dimensions or the complexity of language. For instance, knowing and using a language is not necessarily indicative of acculturating to a specific cultural dimension such as dying and end-of-life care. Even among native-born persons in the USA, there is a great deal of variance in what end-of-life care should be and at what stage of illness for themselves or a family member. Now, language is an important variable to examine in Latinx health research because it is a vehicle for learning and engaging with an ethnic culture and with biomedical information. However, when, why, and how we use language is not being measured in these scales or with proxies. Many sociolinguists have found that, for Mexican-origin and Latinx persons, the English language can be a form of symbolic violence, in which people in racial/ethnic and immigrant minorities learn to describe themselves as inferior (Hill, 1998; 2015; Vélez-Ibáñez, 2017; Zentella, 2003). Language is an important variable, but when most acculturation scales merely examine language use and proficiency in English and Spanish, they overlook complex mechanisms for which language could be important for health outcomes. For example, interpretations of self-rated health (Viruell-Fuentes, Morenoff, Williams, & House, 2011), nutrition, and satiety (Martínez, 2015).

Multidimensional scales are designed to examine multiple dimensions of acculturation and the interaction between immigrant and dominant culture (Thomson &

Hoffman-Goetz, 2009); examples are the ARSMA-II (Cuellar et al. 1995) and the Hazuda Acculturation and Assimilation Scale (Hazuda, Stern, & Haffner, 1988; AAS). Cuellar and colleagues (1995) applied the definition of acculturation as proposed by Redfield, Linton, and Herskovits (1936) to create their ARSMA-II scale. They wanted to improve the first ARSMA scale by taking a multidimensional approach that measured changes in Mexican American persons' behavioral, cognitive, and affective changes at the macro- and micro-level. Unlike the first scale, which included the patient and health care workers of a Texas hospital, this version of the ARSMA was piloted with pre-adolescent and adolescent Mexican youth in Texas. Researchers have noted that because the scale was developed with Mexican youth, it may not be applicable to adults or persons of other Latin American nationalities. However, a simple Google Scholar search shows that the ARSMA-II has been cited over 2000 times, with multiple age groups and many Latin American nationalities. Despite the measure being designed to capture multiple dimensions of acculturation, it is still a linear index of acculturation in which people are either more Anglo-oriented, Mexican-oriented, or both.

The AAS (Hazuda, Stern, & Haffner, 1988) is informed by Gordon's (1964) seven stages of assimilation to examine acculturation and cardiovascular disease risk among Mexican-origin persons in the San Antonio Heart Study. The measure itself queries seven dimensions of acculturation: (1) language use during adulthood and childhood; (2) English proficiency in adulthood; (3) value placed on preserving Mexican culture; (4) attitudes toward family; (5) material success; (6) interaction with mainstream cultural group; and (7) interactions with non-Hispanic white persons during childhood and adulthood. The last measure is designed to capture structural assimilation, or whether Mexican-origin individuals are allowed entrance into large-scale institutions such as clubs, political parties, etc. However, the questions do not address the participants' interactions with such social clubs, politics, or other large institutions. More important, Hazuda and colleagues did not ask white participants about their interactions with Mexican participants or their efforts to integrate Mexican persons into their institutions.

Discussion of the ARSMA-II and the AAS demonstrate that even when acculturation scales are designed to be bidimensional or multidimensional, the common proxies consistently focus on ethnic affiliation and language use. Asking questions about how people identify with their ethnic identity and their language use and interactions with others often assumes that Latinx persons are not systematically segregated from predominantly white or English-speaking neighborhoods and that they are openly accepted by the mainstream society. Basically, the process of adapting to US culture is accessible to Latinx individuals as racial/ethnic minorities, and authors do not take into consideration exclusionary modes of incorporation. All of these measures minimize the conflict and power differential that Latinx persons and persons of other racial/ethnic minorities face in the United States. For example, learning a new language requires making mistakes and speaking with an accent. Yet, this can often be met with criticism or ridicule, and may be an opportunity for discrimination by others who are more proficient in the English language. We should come to the realization that the melting pot and multiculturalism theses of amalgamation do not stand because we have Latinx, Asian, and black persons of sixth generation or more who are still considered "Other."

More important, these questions assume that non-Latinx white persons do not share values with Latinx and Latin American persons. For example, do white individuals not have the desire to preserve their ethnic culture, maintain relationships with extended family, or make material sacrifices in order to help their family? Most acculturation and health research among Latinx persons in the USA takes a very hierarchical approach that positions a US.-born Latinx person or Latinx immigrant as the only one receiving and transforming his or her ethnic culture. Lastly, the acculturation scales presented here have been limited to one Latin American subgroup (except Marin & Gamba, 1996; Marin et al., 1987) and one US geographic location, and largely assess the same behaviors, such as language use, media preference, and ethnic affiliation. Language acquisition is very complex in the ways that shape cultural beliefs and behaviors, even the ways that people perceive their own foreign culture.

If no single factor can explain the health outcomes of US-born Latinx persons and Latinx immigrants (Bohon & Conley, 2015), why put so much emphasis on acculturation, a misunderstood and mismeasured variable? Although several critiques can be made on its conceptualization and operationalization (see Doucerain et al., 2016 for detailed critique), the process of acculturation does exist and may be related to health in very complex ways that have little to do with imagined "traditional" values or language and more to do with the modes of incorporation, environmental, and structural changes that US-born Latinx persons and Latinx immigrants face in the USA and Latin America.

In this section, I discussed how acculturation was historically constructed and studied in anthropology, sociology, and psychology because research on acculturation and health often adopts theories and measures from these three disciplines. The goal is to emphasize how the social sciences conceptualize acculturation and to seek revisions and recommendations for contemporary acculturation-health research. Next, I discuss how acculturation can be examined in relation to diet and obesity among US-born Latinx persons and Latinx immigrants in a way that departs from stereotypes, acknowledges pre-immigration conditions, and captures the host context. This is done with the hopes of understanding how acculturation can be related to health outcomes and expand knowledge that seeks to improve the health disparities in the Latinx population.

Theorizing Acculturation in Latinx Dietary Change and Obesity Research

The dietary practices of Latinx persons have been the fascination of health researchers since the 1970s. The Latinx diet is thought to be related to the longer life expectancy in this population. The Hispanic Paradox (Markides & Coreil, 1986) is a phrase used to describe an epidemiologic pattern in which Latinx immigrants have lower socioeconomic status and are often uninsured yet have a longer life expectancy, better birth-weight outcomes, a lower infant mortality rate, and some healthier practices than the white population in the USA. The Hispanic Paradox primarily refers to Mexican immigrants in the USA (Palloni & Arias, 2003; 2004) and has been attributed to selective migration (Abraído-Lanza et al., 1999), low acculturation, and genetics (Teruya & Bazargan-Hejazi, 2013). However, we are starting to find nuances in the paradox, with disparities across Latinx subgroups (Acevedo-Garcia, Soobader, & Berkman, 2007) and differences between birth cohorts and generational status (Balcazar, Grineski, & Collins, 2015). For example, in a systematic review of acculturation and health research on Mexican-origin persons in the USA, Carter-Pokras and colleagues (2008) found that US-born Mexican persons with English language proficiency and higher levels of education had better health outcomes than less educated US-born Mexican persons and Mexican immigrants. So, it is difficult to generalize the health advantages of Latinx immigrants if we do consider other mechanisms.

More recently, Latinx persons' diets have also been an object of study because of the increasing prevalence of obesity and chronic diseases in the USA (and Latin America); the prevalence of obesity is higher for US-born Latinx children (2–11 years old) (Kaur, Lamb, & Ogden, 2015), and Latinx adults than for black persons (Flegal, Carroll, Ogden, & Curtin, 2010). There is evidence to suggest that immigrant populations from low-to-middle income countries show major changes in obesogenic behaviors in the host society and that these changes are related to acculturation (O'Brien et al., 2014). However, the findings of much of the dietary acculturation research with Latinx persons are inconclusive regarding the effect of acculturation on eroding or improving their diets in the USA (Akresh, 2007). More important, despite hundreds of manuscripts on Latinx dietary acculturation, it is unclear which aspects of US culture shape the diets of US-born Latinx persons and Latinx immigrants and how this culture worsens or improves diets within this very diverse group. These polarizing findings may be attributed to several assumptions made about Latinx persons.

One of the outcomes that researchers attribute the Hispanic paradox and the increasing prevalence of obesity is the erosion of so-called Latinx traditional diets. Researchers often assume that these traditional diets in Latin America are healthier than general diets in the USA. We cannot generalize Latin American diets as healthy because they are extremely diverse, even within the same country. Moreover, as we see with the epidemiologic data, obesity and chronic disease are increasing in Latin America partly due to the globalization of food production and consumption (see Hawkes, Blouin, Henson, Drager, & Dubé, 2009; Martínez, 2015). As a result, pre-immigration traditional diets may not be so healthy after all.

We also do not know which behaviors or foods in the traditional diets are positive or negative, nor which dietary foodways[2] and foods are exclusive to a particular Latinx subgroup. Dietary acculturation researchers often assume that Latinx immigrants come to adopt negative Western dietary practices—often measured as the consumption of less fiber and more animal and saturated fats from fast food, processed food, and sweetened beverages—upon migration and settlement to the USA. The adoption of these negative Western dietary practices is thought to erode the protective aspect of the traditional diet (Pérez-Escamilla, 2009). Briefly, if we were to take a socioecologic approach to dietary change and weight outcomes, they are shaped by multiple levels of the social ecology. For instance, international trade policies shape the cost and availability of fresh produce, meat, and dairy products in the USA and Latin America. Federal welfare and food stamps programs determine eligibility and largely exclude unauthorized immigrants.

Diets are also shaped by local food environments such as the *availability of* and *accessibility to* grocery stores and healthy food vendors. Organizations such as schools, food pantries, and workplaces are other micro-food environments that US-born Latinx persons and Latinx immigrants engage within the United States. Social networks, like one's saturation in an ethnic enclave, shape cultural expectations and interactions with dietary practices, too. At the interpersonal level, family, spouses, and friends shape one's food preferences and behaviors. Then, at the individual level, diet and weight outcomes are shaped by biologic (e.g., hereditary, health conditions, and stress) and sociodemographic conditions (e.g., pre-immigration and current socioeconomic status, race, gender, and age). We are not capturing all the adaptations in the ecology (adjustments to new environment, food acquisition, diet and foodways, and interpersonal conditions) that influence dietary changes and subsequently, body weight.

If researchers are to assess dietary acculturation critically in a way that expands our understanding of Latinx dietary change and obesity disparities in the Latinx population, we have to (1) consider and measure Latinx persons' pre-immigration experiences, (2) create theoretically informed research that captures the complex process of dietary and foodways transformations, (3) document and compare the two or more cultures that are influencing one another, (4) conduct longitudinal studies that capture dietary changes throughout the life course, and (5) consider Latinx persons' context and modes of incorporation.

In most dietary acculturation studies, the researchers have not queried Latinx immigrants' foodways and eating rituals before migration, yet assume that diets are healthier in Latin America. Pre-migration dietary practices are important to examine in dietary acculturation research so that researchers can have a basis of comparison for the kinds of dietary changes Latinx immigrants are making in the USA. In the analysis of pre-migration experiences, one needs to examine Latinx persons' former structural positions and dietary practices. For example, immigrant families who belonged to the upper-middle class in Latin America may have eaten US fast foods often in their home countries. Then, because of the transnational discourse (ways of representing) that all the food in the USA is processed and unhealthy, they may severely limit eating fast and processed foods once in the USA (Martínez, 2015). This may be the artifact for findings that suggest that Latinx families with immigrants have healthier diets. Another pre-migration factor to consider in dietary acculturation research is people's exposure to the USA through transnational ties and the presence of transnational food and media companies in Latin America.

In many dietary acculturation studies, researchers measure Latinx individuals' proficiency in and use of English because it is assumed that competence in English is a mechanism for migrants to access and consume unhealthy US foods. However, transnational corporations such as Nestle or McDonalds have been marketing their products in Spanish and cultural contexts conducive to Latin American persons' eating practices. Many of the same products can often be found in most US grocers or ethnic markets. As I have asserted elsewhere (Martínez, 2010, 2013, 2016), migration to and settlement in the USA may not be necessary for Latinx immigrants to develop the so-called negative, Western dietary practices that researchers often use as proxies for dietary change such as macronutrients or the consumption of a handful of foods. Latinx immigrants' diets were already changing in Latin America to reflect those of the USA because of global and transnational processes in predominantly urban environments, whereby fast foods are accessible, processed foods are being integrated into quotidian cuisine, and the Latin American population has a disproportionate rate of obesity as a result. Although the Hispanic Community Health Survey/Study of Latinos database has diverse Latino subgroups and included a yes/no question about whether participants maintained food practices from their home country (Isasi et al., 2015), we still do not know what those food practices are and how they differ from their food and foodways in the USA.

In order to understand the mechanism between acculturation and diet, one needs to create theoretically informed measures that capture the complex process of dietary and foodways transformations. The common proxies for acculturation and the existing acculturation scales do not reflect the complex process of changing diets and foodways. Social practices of eating are just as important, if not more, than the actual foods eaten. For example, consuming one's daily nutrients in one sitting versus snacking throughout the day or sharing meals versus eating alone shapes the food one eats, how much one eats, and how the nutrients are metabolized. Similarly, diets are shaped not only by the foods available in one's food environments and healthy food access but by their religious and political leanings. This knowledge will help us discern what is becoming US-American in Latinx persons' diets, the way they acquire food, the food itself, or when and how they eat. Qualitative methods may be best to capture changes in ethnic foodways because they support the rich description of cultural processes (Goode, Theophano, & Curtis, 1984).

Flórez and Abraído-Lanza (2017) apply the theory of segmented assimilation to examine the likelihood of a second-generation Latinx person being in the obese BMI category. The great quality of this study is that the authors apply an underused, complex theory of acculturation. They also examine socioeconomic status more closely in which they predict that economic mobility for a second-generation individual is related to belonging to a higher BMI category. However, the authors do not include data on diet and foodways for each generation status group, leaving readers unclear about how becoming an affluent American leads to obesity. The study did not include a comparison of the data with those for white persons, or a clear description of the mechanisms explaining the relationship between segmented assimilation and obesity. We do not know if the function of economic mobility or dietary acculturation is the mechanism related to higher weights between first- and second-generation Latinx persons. We are not sure how transnational ties to family in Latin America shape obesity-related behaviors. If a person comes from an affluent or upper-middle class family in Latin America, that can also shape their eating habits. We are certainly not sure if the study sample had better modes of incorporation, such as experiencing less racism, racial segregation, or living in a city with better access to healthy foods than other cities.

In the earlier review of anthropologic, sociologic, and psychologic theories, acculturation is a multidirectional process that occurs between two or more groups. Multiple dimensions of culture, not just language use and ethnic affiliation, need to be captured in dietary acculturation research. Just as the Latinx population is a heterogeneous racial/ethnic group in which diet is shaped by food environments, regional differences in their home countries, healthy food access, class, and political leanings, US diets are also diverse. What is the baseline for US culture and US diets when the country is so culturally, politically, and economically diverse by region? Moreover, people in the USA engage in different food fads and lifestyles, from low-carbohydrate to veganism to paleo diet, to name just a few. Many people in the USA have dietary restrictions based on their religious beliefs and practices. The so-called US diet differs by regional foodways and cuisines. Furthermore, Latin American eateries can be found in most cities in the USA. So, if we are to engage in meaningful dietary acculturation research, it is so important to document both (or more) representations of ethnic cultures or foodways that are being compared because ethnic foodways and healthy eating practices are not universal. In the *comiendo bien (eating well)* study (Martínez, 2010, 2013, 2015), some Latinx immigrant parents were acculturating to the Mediterranean diet, whereas others were adopting to California organic fanaticism, and many just continued to eat their ethnic meals while integrating other ethnic cuisines and junk food along the way.

Moreover, if acculturation is a process that can lead to different health outcomes, we need to study it through developmental stages and throughout the life course, especially when it comes to dietary changes and obesity research. The prevalence of overweight/obesity is higher among Latino children of all ages, but especially children 2 to 11 years old, compared with children in other racial/ethnic groups. At different developmental stages, children adapt food preferences and have more control of what and how they eat as they become older, more independent, and attend school. Thus, simply inquiring about their generation status, nativity, time in the USA, or language and ethnic preferences will not tell us much about what positive or negative dietary practices are changing as a result of eating more US-based foods. In terms of adults' dietary changes and their weight outcomes, we need to collect longitudinal data on dietary changes that consider different stages of their adulthood. For instance, people who are single and working long hours are possibly not paying as much attention to their meals as adults who are rearing children. Also, when children become adolescents and are more independent, they start "acculturating" to other foodways they encounter at school and at their social gatherings (Martínez, 2016). Given all of these factors, we will not know how US foodways that US-born Latinx persons and Latinx immigrants encounter are changing their diets if we do not examine the process longitudinally and with consideration of stages in their development or in their life course, as is the case with adults.

The new context and the modes of incorporation that migrants face in the host society are also important in understanding how their foodways and dietary practices change in the USA. The new foodways that Latinx persons are integrating into their diets are not exclusively "American" foodways, nor are they exclusively about food. For instance, the reduction of work breaks and meal times at low-wage, low-occupational status jobs in the USA may change regular meal patterns from those in the home countries of Latinx immigrants. Latinx immigrants' inadequate housing, with little to no functioning kitchen appliances, may also affect their ability to prepare meals for their families. The lack of meal preparation forces them to eat prepared and take-away foods, which are generally not as healthy as home-cooked meals (Martínez, 2010, 2013, 2015). In relation, unauthorized, temporary, and newly legalized immigrants are not allowed to participate in food assistance programs such as Supplemental Nutrition Assistance Program, and are less likely to enlist their qualifying US-citizen children for fear of public charge in their future immigration applications or the purview of Immigration Customs Enforcement (Kalil & Chen, 2008; Van Hook & Balistreri, 2006). Therefore, when we measure ethnic affiliation from extant acculturation scales, it does not indicate context, modes of incorporation, or the structural conditions in which US-born Latinx persons and Latinx immigrants have to negotiate their ethnic foodways and health practices for those of the USA. Following are suggestions of ways in which this could be done.

Future Needs and Priorities for Acculturation and Latinx Health Research

This chapter commenced by indicating the disjuncture in Latinx health research between researchers in favor of acculturation as a theoretical framework and important covariate and researchers who disdain the use of acculturation in Latinx health research. Despite reservations in the use of acculturation, researchers are often left in a conundrum of whether to abandon the construct or preserve it in our research for the sake of publishing and/or receiving external funding. To address this issue, this chapter provided a brief overview of acculturation theories and measures from anthropology, sociology, and psychology in order to identify areas of expansion for current acculturation and health research. This information was later used to provide an example of how to examine the relationship between acculturation and diet and obesity among US-born Latinx persons and Latinx immigrants. In that section, I tried to demonstrate how complicated it is and what theories and measurements would be needed to understand what dietary and foodways changes are occurring or becoming "more American" at different levels of the social ecology. We have come to learn that processes of acculturation are occurring for Latinx immigrants and their children, which may or may not shape health behaviors and health outcomes. However, the variables we often measure as proxies of acculturation—language acquisition, ethnic affiliation, or adaptation to "U.S. cultural values, beliefs, and customs"—do not represent changes caused by structural conditions of migratory settlement, the developmental stages and life course of the participants, or transnational processes.

Should we eliminate acculturation in the examination of the Latinx population and Latinx health research? Yes and no. Yes, we should reduce the use of dominant measures and their recalcitrant assumptions, conceptualizations, and operationalization(s) of acculturation in the extant Latinx health discourse. Moreover, we need to stop making acculturation the silver bullet for understanding health disparities and protective factors among US-born Latinx persons and Latinx immigrants in the USA. Our differences are not necessarily cultural in nature, as they are more structural in history. However, it may be worthwhile to examine acculturation as a complicated, multilevel process. We have fallen short on theorizing what people are acculturating *from* and *to* and how processes of acculturation are related to a specific health outcome. We learned from the review of acculturation theories that it is a fluid process. This means that people's cultural practices and beliefs vary by the situation, historical moment, and personal characteristics. If we are to know what people are acculturating to and from, we need knowledge about their pre-migration structural positions and their pre-migration attitudes, beliefs, and practices to discern what US traits they are adapting to in US-American culture.

The larger problem lies in the fact that we place too much weight on acculturation as a variable for Latinx health research (Carter-Pokras & Bethune, 2009; Carter-Pokras et al., 2008; Martínez, 2013; Viruell-Fuentes, 2007). In several empirical articles and systematic reviews (Abraído-Lanza et al., 2006; Flórez and Abraído-Lanza 2017; Carter-Pokras & Bethune, 2009; Carter-Pokras et al., 2008; Thomson and Hoffman-Goetz, 2009; Lopez-Class et al., 2011), scholars adamantly point out that not all Latinx individuals are immigrants or share a common history and represent a multiethnic, multiracial, and multilingual diverse group. Even knowing that US-born Latinx persons and Latinx immigrants are culturally heterogeneous, there cannot be a universal measurement of acculturation that is specific to one or more Latinx subgroups; rather, the measure must be modified to control for the diverse contexts that Latinx individuals are coming from and adapting to in the USA.

First, if we continue to apply acculturation measures in Latinx health research, we need to examine modes of incorporation and how the United States' federal, state, and local governments have created policies to exclude Mexican-origin and Latinx persons from fully participating in American society. As researchers, we will continue to place the emphasis on Latinx persons' beliefs and behaviors and not on how those beliefs and behaviors are shaped by institutional forms of racism, such as residential segregation and immigration policies (Abraído-Lanza et al., 2006; Aranda & Vaquera, 2015; Miranda et al., 2011; Viruell-Fuentes, 2007). The geographic location and modes of incorporation of receiving society allow us to both account and control for structural factors related to causing a health outcome or influencing a "cultural" practice. For example, Schwartz et al., (2015) sampled Latinx adolescents from different geographic contexts because they acknowledge that acculturation differs between large cities and small towns and according to the history of immigration (recent or not). Similarly, Waters and Jiménez, (2005) suggest comparing assimilation between cities that are traditional immigrant gateways and so-called new destinations because the latter often lack the institutional arrangements and historic ethnic enclaves that are found in immigrant gateways. The receiving population may not have the macro-level resources to facilitate the Latinx immigrants' integration into their US locality.

Schwartz and Unger (2016) also point out that we must carefully distinguish voluntary immigrants (authorized or unauthorized), refugees, political asylees, and temporary migrants (e.g., migrant farmworkers). This comparative work has rarely been conducted in Latinx health research, and yet, is so important in terms of understanding if and how pre-immigration experiences facilitate or encumber immigrants' ability to adjust to a new country. Having a refugee or asylum status may improve the modes of incorporation and context of reception. For example, in the USA, persons with these political designations have access to federally funded means-tested programs such as housing subsidies, Temporary Assistance for Needy Families, and Supplemental Nutrition Assistance Program benefits. Albeit, the resources are available for only eight months, which has been criticized for not being sufficient for cultural adjustment, but it is more than what most new immigrants receive.

Pre-immigration context and the immigrants' structural position in Latin America help researchers identify if the change in a health outcome, beliefs, values, or behaviors is a result of migration and settlement to the USA, or was already occurring in Latin America. In other words, we can tease out if the changes in health values, beliefs, behaviors, and outcomes are a result of acquiring a new culture or from retaining one's previous culture. Also, inquiring about migrants' pre-immigration contexts would help us discern what it is about the US context that causes changes in health outcomes. For example, Latinx immigrants may not gain more health literacy about nutrition in the USA because they were already participating in nutrition education and health promotion interventions in Latin America. If we are to continue to examine acculturation as an attribute, we must control for these macro-level and meso-level conditions. Examining acculturation as a process requires different models, qualitative techniques, and longitudinal data that control for changes in the host society, and changes that could modify the adaptation to certain cultures throughout a person's life course (Abraído-Lanza et al. 2016; Schwartz & Unger, 2016).

In early anthropologic and sociologic theories of acculturation, there was an emphasis to examine how persons from the dominant culture, in our case, the white population, adopt to heterogeneous immigrant ethic cultures. As the sociologic review demonstrated, intermarriage is underexamined in relation to Latinx acculturation-health research. One of the reasons intermarriage may be of interest to health researchers is that marrying a person from the host society creates social, cultural, and financial capital for immigrants, and can expedite learning a new language and identity roles and expectations. Similarly, Thomson and Hoffman-Goetz (2009) point out the need for acculturation and health research to examine immigrants' and their progeny's interpersonal social networks.

Currently in the USA, 16 million people live with an unauthorized person, whether it be parents, siblings, or extended family (Mathema, 2017). Of these 16 million people, 5 million are minors (Mathema, 2017). Assimilation even differs between family members, particularly siblings, who may have different immigration status from one another and may even display different racial phenotypes. In our study examining chronic stressors in relation to biomarkers for stress and inflammation in

Mexican-origin families, we found that members of the same family often did not identify with the same racial category, in part because family members had different interpretations of race and identified with different racial categories. This finding may be related to the fact that the Latinx population is largely made up of mixed-race persons, and members of a family can be phenotypically distinct from one another, with even siblings having different skin tones, facial features, and hair texture.

First, researchers must stop homogenizing Latin American and Latinx individuals and assuming that they are premodern or culturally inferior or that they are engaging in traditional practices that are perceived by biomedical researchers as positive, such as *familism* and traditional diets. Abandoning premodern assumptions about Latin American and Latinx persons also negates global processes that modernize transnational familial and cultural ties, which could bring them together in peaceful cultural exchanges (e.g., tourism), but that can also create global oppressions in populations across borders (modernizing of food systems, raising the price of healthy foods, and thus increasing the prevalence of obesity in the developing world).

Second, if health researchers insist on giving acculturation prominence in Latinx health research, it should be through complicated processes, in which they examine whether health outcomes differ by segmented forms of acculturation and assimilation. Moreover, given that many Latinx persons are in mixed-status homes and belong to mixed-race families (different racial phenotypes), it is important to evaluate whether immigration status and race shape differences in acculturation trajectories and health outcomes more generally.

The study of acculturation processes also requires the evaluation of how white, European, and US-born Latinx persons acculturate, adapt, and co-opt Latin American subcultures. As I write this chapter, a reggaeton song by Luis Fonsi and Daddy Yankee, "Despacito," was the second-longest leading number-one song of all time (Trust, 2017). This is a present-day example of acculturation of Latin American subcultures and demonstrates how acculturation is not a unilinear process. As Jeffrey Pilcher so beautifully writes in *Planet Taco* (2013), people around the globe have adapted Mexican food to represent their desires and local foodways. Moreover, there is active co-optation of Latinx culture in many arenas, including the use of indigenous medicine as boutique alternative medicine.

Third, the examination of acculturation in relation to Latinx health favors mixed-methods approaches because qualitative methods can illuminate processes of cultural change, and multilevel quantitative designs allow us to examine the effect of acculturation occurring at the individual, group, and society levels. Although acculturation processes emanate and are shaped by the larger society, particularly US racial formation, immigration, and economic policy (Aranda & Vaquera, 2015), individuals are affected by these differently and change and engage behaviors distinctly from one another as a result of their age, gender, socioeconomic position, age at migration, social networks, and other individual-level positions and interactions. As, Rudmin (2009) writes, "… the difficulties of specifying cultures are compounded by within culture variation" (p. 109). Therefore, it remains important to provide nuanced descriptions about the consequences of acculturation on the health outcomes for Latinx individuals. Groups, such as families and friendship networks, are important to study in order to better understand acculturative learning (Rudmin, 2009) in the intergenerational transmission of health practices and the acculturative learning of risky or protective behaviors from peers (Fox et al., 2015). Nevertheless, the genesis of acculturation and reception to assimilate are necessary to study at the collective level. This would also force us to examine multiple aspects of culture and ways of doing.

Does acculturation exist? Yes, absolutely. Adjustment processes occur to both immigrants and members of the receiving society that result from moving to a new country—even a new neighborhood. However, *how* this process is related to a specific health outcome, and their mechanisms, needs to be clearly identified in the construction of the study, not only to ensure internal validity but also to truly move the field of Latinx health forward by not overshadowing the disparities that do exist among Latinx individuals, and the Hispanic paradox. In addition, we must create structural interventions that ensure that all Latinx individuals, citizens, or immigrants, have the ability to engage in healthy behaviors and achieve well-being.

References

Abraído-Lanza, A. F., Dohrenwend, B. P., Ng-Mak, D. S., & Turner, J. B. (1999). The Latino mortality paradox: A test of the "salmon bias" and healthy migrant hypotheses. *American Journal of Public Health, 89*(10), 1543–1548.

Abraído-Lanza, A. F., Armbrister, A. N., Flórez, K. R., & Aguirre, A. N. (2006). Toward a theory-driven model of acculturation in public health research. *American Journal of Public Health, 96*(8), 1342–1346.

Abraído-Lanza, A. F., Echeverría, S. E., & Flórez, K. R. (2016). Latino immigrants, acculturation, and health: Promising new directions in research. *Annual Review of Public Health, 37,* 219–236.

Acevedo-Garcia, D., Soobader, M. J., & Berkman, L. F. (2007). Low birthweight among US Hispanic/Latino subgroups: The effect of maternal foreign-born status and education. *Social Science and Medicine, 65*(12), 2503–2516.

Akresh, I. R. (2007). Dietary assimilation and health among Hispanic immigrants to the United States. *Journal of Health and Social Behavior, 48*(4), 404–417.

Alba, R., & Nee, V. (2003). *Remaking the American mainstream: Assimilation and contemporary immigration.* Cambridge, MA: Harvard University Press.

Anderson, B. (1991). *Imagined communities: Reflections on the origin and spread of nationalism* (Revised ed.). London: Verso.

Anderson, W. (2006). *Colonial pathologies: American tropical medicine, race, and hygiene in the Philippines.* Durham, NC: Duke University Press.

Appadurai, A. (1996). *Modernity al large: Cultural dimensions of globalization* (Vol. 1). Minneapolis, MN: University of Minnesota Press.

Aranda, E., & Vaquera, E. (2015). Racism, the immigration regime, and the implications for racial inequality in the lives of undocumented young adults. *Sociology of Race and Ethnicity, 1,* 88–104.

Ayala, G. X., Baquero, B., & Klinger, S. (2008). A systematic review of the relationship between acculturation and diet among Latinos in the United States: Implications for future research. *Journal of the American Dietetic Association, 108*(8), 1330–1344.

Balcazar, A. J., Grineski, S. E., & Collins, T. W. (2015). The Hispanic health paradox across generations: The relationship of child generational status and citizenship with health outcomes. *Public Health, 129*(6), 691–697.

Bacio, G. A., Mays, V. M., & Lau, A. S. (2013). Drinking initiation and problematic drinking among Latino adolescents: Explanations of the immigrant paradox. *Psychology of Addictive Behaviors, 27*(1), 14.

Barnett, H. G., Broom, L., Siegel, B. J., Vogt, E. Z., & Watson, J. B. (1954). Acculturation: An exploratory formulation. The Social Science Research Council Summer Seminar on Acculturation, 1953. *American Anthropologist, 56,* 973–1000.

Bhatia, S., & Ram, A. (2009). Theorizing identity in transnational and diaspora cultures: A critical approach to acculturation. *International Journal of Intercultural Relations, 33*(2), 140–149.

Bermúdez-Parsai, M., Geiger, J. L. M., Marsiglia, F. F., & Coonrod, D. V. (2012). Acculturation and health care utilization among Mexican heritage women in the United States. *Maternal and Child Health Journal, 16*(6), 1173–1179.

Berrigan, D., Dodd, K., Troiano, R. P., Reeve, B. B., & Ballard-Barbash, R. (2006). Physical activity and acculturation among adult Hispanics in the United States. *Research Quarterly for Exercise and Sport, 77*(2), 147–157.

Berry, J. W. (1980). Acculturation as varieties of adaptation. In A. M. Padilla (Ed.), *Acculturation: Theory, models and some new findings* (pp. 9–25). Boulder, CO: Westview Press.

Berry, J. W., Phinney, J. S., Sam, D. L., & Vedder, P. (2006). *Immigrant youth in cultural transition: Acculturation identity and adaptation across national boundaries.* London: Lawrence Eribaum.

Berry, J. W., Evans, C., & Rawlinson, H. (1972). *Post-secondary educational opportunity for the Ontario Indian population.* Toronto: Ontario Government Bookstore.

Blue, L., & Fenelon, A. (2011). Explaining low mortality among US immigrants relative to native-born Americans: The role of smoking. *International Journal of Epidemiology, 40*(3), 786–793.

Bohon, S. A., & Conley, M. E. (2015). *Immigration and population.* Hoboken, NJ: Wiley.

Bostean, G. (2013). Does selective migration explain the Hispanic paradox? A comparative analysis of Mexicans in the US and Mexico. *Journal of Immigrant and Minority Health, 15*(3), 624–635.

Carter-Pokras, O., Zambrana, R. E., Yankelvich, G., Estrada, M., Castillo-Salgado, C., & Ortega, A. N. (2008). Health status of Mexican-origin persons: Do proxy measures of acculturation advance our understanding of health disparities? *Journal of Immigrant and Minority Health, 10*(6), 475–488.

Carter-Pokras, O., & Bethune, L. (2009). Defining and measuring acculturation: A systematic review of public health studies with Hispanic populations in the United States. A commentary on Thomson and Hoffman-Goetz. *Social Science & Medicine, 69*(7), 992–995.

Clarke, A. E. (2005). *Situational analysis: Grounded theory after the postmodern turn.* Thousand Oaks, CA: Sage Publications.

Chirkov, V. (2009). Critical psychology of acculturation: What do we study and how do we study it, when we investigate acculturation? *International Journal of Intercultural Relations, 33*(2), 94–105.

Coatsworth, J. D., Maldonado-Molina, M., Pantin, H., & Szapocznik, J. (2005). A person-centered and ecological investigation of acculturation strategies in Hispanic immigrant youth. *Journal of Community Psychology, 33*(2), 157–174.

Cuellar, I., Harris, L. C., & Jasso, R. (1980). An acculturation scale for Mexican American normal and clinical populations. *Hispanic Journal of Behavioral Sciences, 2,* 199–217.

Cuellar, I., Arnold, B., & Maldonado, R. (1995). Acculturation rating scale for Mexican Americans-II: A revision of the original ARSMA scale. *Hispanic Journal of Behavioral Sciences, 17*(3), 275–304.

Daviglus, M. L., Pirzada, A., Durazo-Arvizu, R., Chen, J., Allison, M., Avilés-Santa, L., et al. (2016). Prevalence of low cardiovascular risk profile among diverse Hispanic/Latino adults in the United States by age, sex, and level of acculturation: The Hispanic Community Health Study/Study of Latinos. *Journal of the American Heart Association, 5*(8), e003929.

Delavari, M., Sønderlund, A. L., Swinburn, B., Mellor, D., & Renzaho, A. (2013). Acculturation and obesity among migrant populations in high income countries—A systematic review. *BMC Public Health, 13*(1), 458.

DuBois, W. E. B. (1903). *The souls of black folk.* New York: New American Library.

Doucerain, M. M., Segalowitz, N., & Ryder, A. G. (2016). Acculturation measurement: From simple proxies to sophisticated toolkit. In S. J. Schwartz & J. B. Unger (Eds.), *Oxford handbook of acculturation and health* (pp. 97–118). New York: Oxford University Press.

Executive Order No. 13767 (2017). Border security and immigration enforcement improvements. 82 FR, p. 8793.

Fernández-Kelly, P. (2008). Gender and economic change in the United States and Mexico, 1900–2000. *American Behavioral Scientist, 52*(3), 377–404.

Flegal, K. M., Carroll, M. D., Ogden, C. L., & Curtin, L. R. (2010). Prevalence and trends in obesity among US adults, 1999–2008. *Journal of the American Medical Association, 303*, 235–241.

Flórez, K. R., & Abraído-Lanza, A. (2017). Segmented assimilation: an approach to studying acculturation and obesity among Latino adults in the United States. *Family & Community Health, 40*(2), 132–138.

Fox, M., Entringer, S., Buss, C., DeHaene, J., & Wadhwa, P. D. (2015). Intergenerational transmission of the effects of acculturation on health in Hispanic Americans: A fetal programming perspective. *American Journal of Public Health, 105*(S3), S409–S423.

Glazer, N., & Moynihan, D. P. (1963). *Beyond the melting pot: The Negroes, Puerto Ricans, Jews, Italians, and Irish of New York City* (Vol. 13). Cambridge, MA: MIT Press.

Goode, J., Theophano, J., & Curtis, K. (1984). A framework for the analysis of continuity and change in shared sociocultural rules for food use: The Italian-American pattern. In L. K. Brown & K. Mussell (Eds.), *Ethnic and regional foodways in the United States: The performance of group identity* (pp. 66–88). Knoxville, TN: University of Tennessee Press.

Gordon, M. M. (1964). *Assimilation in American life: The role of race, religion, and national origins*. Oxford University Press on Demand.

Haderxhanaj, L. T., Rhodes, S. D., Romaguera, R. A., Bloom, F. R., & Leichliter, J. S. (2015). Hispanic men in the United States: Acculturation and recent sexual behaviors with female partners, 2006–2010. *American Journal of Public Health, 105*(8), e126–e133.

Hawkes, C., Blouin, C., Henson, S., Drager, N., & Dubé, L. (2009). *Trade, food, diet and health: Perspectives and policy options*. Hoboken, NJ: Wiley.

Hazuda, H. P., Stern, M. P., & Haffner, S. M. (1988). Acculturation and assimilation among Mexican Americans: Scales and population-based data. *Social Science Quarterly, 69*(3), 687.

Hill, J. H. (1998). Language, race, and white public space. *American Anthropologist, 100*(3), 680–689.

Hill, J. H. (2015). Tom Horn is studying Spanish: Neo-liberal theories of language and culture and the struggle for symbolic resources (pp. 77–102). In *Visiones de Acá y Allá: Implicaciones de la politica antimigrante en las comunidades de origen mexiano en Estados Unidos y México* by Carlos Vélez-Ibáñez, Roberto Sánchez Benítez, and Mariángela Rodríguez Nicholls (Eds). México: Universidad Nacional Autónoma de México y Universidad Autónoma de Ciudad Juárez.

Hunt, L. M., Schneider, S., & Comer, B. (2004). Should "acculturation" be a variable in health research? A critical review of research on US Hispanics. *Social Science and Medicine, 59*, 973–986.

Isasi, C. R., Ayala, G. X., Sotres-Alvarez, D., Madanat, H., Penedo, F., Loria, C. M., ... & Van Horn, L. (2015). Is acculturation related to obesity in Hispanic/Latino adults? Results from the Hispanic Community Health Study/Study of Latinos. *Journal of Obesity, 2015*, 186276.

Kalil, A., & Chen, J. (2008). Mother's citizenship status and household food insecurity among low-income children of immigrants. In H. Yoshikawa & N. Way (Eds.), *Beyond the family: Contexts of immigrant children's development* (pp. 43–62). San Francisco, CA: Jossey-Bass.

Kaur, J., Lamb, M. M., & Ogden, C. L. (2015). The association between food insecurity and obesity in children—The National Health and Nutrition Examination Survey. *Journal of the Academy of Nutrition and Dietetics, 115*(5), 751–758.

Kim, U. (1989). Acculturation of Korean immigrants to Canada: Psychological, demographic and behavioural profiles of emigrating Koreans, non-emigrating Koreans and Korean-Canadians (Doctoral dissertation, ProQuest Information & Learning).

Koneru, V. K., de Mamani, A. G. W., Flynn, P. M., & Betancourt, H. (2007). Acculturation and mental health: Current findings and recommendations for future research. *Applied and Preventive Psychology, 12*(2), 76–96.

Lara, M., Gamboa, C., Kahramanian, M. I., Morales, L. S., & Bautista, D. E. (2005). Acculturation and Latino health in the United States: A review of the literature and its sociopolitical context. *Annual Review of Public Health, 26,* 367–397.

Lee, H. C. (2008). Flexible acculturation. *Social Thought & Research, 49*–73.

Livingston, G., & Brown, A. (2017). Intermarriage in the U.S. 50 Years After Loving versus Virginia. Pew Research Center, 18 May 2017. Retrieved from http://www.pewsocialtrends.org/2017/05/18/intermarriage-in-the-u-s-50-years-after-loving-v-virginia/.

Lopez-Class, M., Castro, F. G., & Ramirez, A. G. (2011). Conceptions of acculturation: A review and statement of critical issues. *Social Science and Medicine, 72*(9), 1555–1562.

López, E. B., & Yamashita, T. (2017). Acculturation, income and vegetable consumption behaviors among Latino adults in the US: A mediation analysis with the bootstrapping technique. *Journal of Immigrant and Minority Health, 19*(1), 155–161.

Lupton, D. (2012). *Medicine as culture: Illness, disease and the body* (3rd ed.). London: Sage.

Mainous, A. G., Diaz, V. A., & Geesey, M. E. (2008). Acculturation and healthy lifestyle among Latinos with diabetes. *Annals of Family Medicine, 6*(2), 131–137.

Markides, K. S., & Coreil, J. (1986). The health of Hispanics in the southwestern United States: An epidemiologic paradox. *Public Health Reports, 101*(3), 253–256.

Marin, G., Sabogal, F., Marin, B. V., Otero-Sabogal, R., & Perez-Stable, E. J. (1987). Development of a short acculturation scale for Hispanics. *Hispanic Journal of Behavioral Sciences, 9*(2), 183–205.

Marin, G., & Gamba, R. J. (1996). A new measurement of acculturation for Hispanics: The Bidimensional Acculturation Scale for Hispanics (BAS). *Hispanic Journal of Behavioral Sciences, 18*(3), 297–316.

Martínez, A. D. (2010). *Comiendo bien*: A situational analysis of the transnational processes involved in transforming healthy eating among Latino immigrant families in San Francisco. Doctoral dissertation. University of California, San Francisco.

Martínez, A. D. (2013). Reconsidering acculturation for dietary change research among Latino immigrants: Challenging the preconditions of US migration. *Ethnicity and Health*.

Martínez, A. D. (2015). The juxtaposition of *comiendo bien* and nutrition: The state of healthy eating for Latino immigrants in San Francisco. *Food, Culture, and Society, 18*(1), 131–149.

Martínez, A. D. (2016). *Comiendo bien*: The production of *Latinidad* through the performance of healthy eating among Latino immigrant families in San Francisco. *Symbolic Interaction, 39*(1), 66–85.

Mathema, S. (2017). *Keeping families: Together why all Americans should care about what happens to unauthorized immigrants*. Center for American Progress, Washington, DC, 16 March 2017. Retrieved from https://www.americanprogress.org/issues/immigration/reports/2017/03/16/428335/keeping-families-together/.

Mazur, R. E., Marquis, G. S., & Jensen, H. H. (2003). Diet and food insufficiency among Hispanic youths: Acculturation and socioeconomic factors in the third National Health and Nutrition Examination Survey. *American Journal of Clinical Nutrition, 78*(6), 1120–1127.

Miranda, P. Y., Schulz, A. J., Israel, B. A., & González, H. M. (2011). Context of entry and number of depressive symptoms in an older Mexican-origin immigrant population. *Journal of Immigrant and Minority Health, 13*(4), 706–712.

O'Brien, M. J., Alos, V. A., Bueno, A., & Whitaker, R. C. (2014). Acculturation and the prevalence of diabetes in US Latino adults, National Health and Nutrition Examination Survey 2007–2010. *Preventing Chronic Disease, 11,* E176.

Otero-Sabogal, R., Sabogal, F., Perez-Stable, E. J., & Hiatt, R. A. (1995). Dietary practices, alcohol consumption, and smoking behavior: Ethnic, sex, and acculturation differences. *Journal of the National Cancer Institute. Monographs, 18,* 73–82.

Nederveen Pieterse, J. (2007). Global multiculture, flexible acculturation. *Globalizations, 4*(1), 65–79.
Palloni, A., & Arias, E. (2003). *A re-examination of the Hispanic mortality paradox*. Center for Demography and Ecology, University of Wisconsin-Madison, Working Paper, (2003-01).
Palloni, A., & Arias, E. (2004). Paradox lost: Explaining the Hispanic adult mortality advantage. *Demography, 41*(3), 385–415.
Park, R. E., & Burgess, E. W. (1925). *The city: Suggestions for the study of human behavior in the urban environment*. Chicago: University of Chicago Press.
Park, R. E. (1928). Human migration and the marginal man. *American Journal of Sociology, 33,* 881–893.
Park, R. E., & Tristram, E. (1939). *Race relations and the race problem: A definition and an analysis*. Durham, NC: Duke University Press.
Park, R. E., & Tristram, E. (1950). *Race and culture*. Glencoe, IL: The Free Press.
Pérez-Escamilla, R. (2009). Dietary quality among Latinos: Is acculturation making us sick? *Journal of the American Dietetic Association, 109*(6), 988–991.
Pilcher, J. M. (2013). *Planet taco: A global history of Mexican food*. Oxford University Press.
Portes, A., & Rumbaut, R. G. (2001). *Legacies: The story of the immigrant second generation*. Berkeley, CA: University of California Press.
Razum, O., & Twardella, D. (2002). Time travel with Oliver Twist. *Tropical Medicine & International Health, 7*(1), 4–10.
Redfield, R., Linton, R., & Herskovits, M. J. (1936). Memorandum for the study of acculturation. *American Anthropologist, 38*(1), 149–152.
Riosmena, F., Wong, R., & Palloni, A. (2013). Migration selection, protection, and acculturation in health: A binational perspective on older adults. *Demography, 50*(3), 1039–1064.
Rosaldo, R. (1989). *Truth and culture: The remaking of social analysis*. Boston: Beacon Press.
Rudmin, F. W. (2003). Critical history of the acculturation psychology of assimilation, separation, integration, and marginalization. *Review of General Psychology, 7*(1), 3.
Rudmin, F. (2009). Constructs, measurements and models of acculturation and acculturative stress. *International Journal of Intercultural Relations, 33*(2), 106–123.
Savas, L. S., Vernon, S. W., Atkinson, J. S., & Fernández, M. E. (2015). Effect of acculturation and access to care on colorectal cancer screening in low-income Latinos. *Journal of Immigrant and Minority Health, 17*(3), 696–703.
Schwartz, S. J., Montgomery, M. J., & Briones, E. (2006). The role of identity in acculturation among immigrant people: Theoretical propositions, empirical questions, and applied recommendations. *Human Development, 49*(1), 1–30.
Schwartz, S. J., & Zamboanga, B. L. (2008). Testing Berry's model of acculturation: A class latent analysis approach. *Cultural Diversity and Ethnic Minority Psychology, 14*(4), 275–285.
Schwartz, S. J., Unger, J. B., Baezconde-Garbanati, L., Benet-Martínez, V., Meca, A., Zamboanga, B. L., ... & Soto, D. W. (2015). Longitudinal trajectories of bicultural identity integration in recently immigrated Hispanic adolescents: Links with mental health and family functioning. *International Journal of Psychology, 50*(6), 440–450.
Schwartz, S. J., & Unger, J. (2016). Acculturation and health: State of the field and recommended directions. In S. J. Schwartz & J. B. Unger (Eds.), *Oxford handbook of acculturation and health* (pp. 1–14). New York: Oxford University Press.
Scribner, R. (1996). Paradox as paradigm—The health outcomes of Mexican Americans. *American Journal of Public Health, 86*(3), 303–305.
Serafini, K., Wendt, D. C., Ornelas, I. J., Doyle, S. R., & Donovan, D. M. (2017). Substance use and treatment outcomes among Spanish-speaking Latino/as from four acculturation types. *Psychology of Addictive Behaviors, 31*(2), 180–188.
Strauss, A. L. (1993). *Continual permutations of action*. Piscataway, NJ: Aldine Transaction.
Sullivan, S., Schwartz, S. J., Prado, G., Huang, S., Pantin, H., & Szapocznik, J. (2007). A bidimensional model of acculturation for examining differences in family functioning and behavior problems in Hispanic immigrant adolescents. *Journal of Early Adolescence, 27*(4), 405–430.

Szapocznik, J., Scopetta, M., Kurtines, W., & Arnalde, M. A. (1978). Theory and measurement of acculturation. *InterAmerican Journal of Psychology, 12,* 113–130.

Teruya, S. A., & Bazargan-Hejazi, S. (2013). The immigrant and Hispanic paradoxes: A systematic review of their predictions and effects. *Hispanic Journal of Behavioral Sciences, 35,* 486–509.

Thomas, D., & Thomas, D. S. (1928). *The child in America: Behavior problems and programs.* New York: Knopf.

Thomas, W. I., & Znanecki, F. (1923). *A Polish peasant in Europe and America.* Chicago: University of Chicago Press.

Thomson, M. D., & Hoffman-Goetz, L. (2009). Defining and measuring acculturation: A systematic review of public health studies with Hispanic populations in the United States. *Social Science and Medicine, 69*(7), 983–991.

Trust, G. (2017 August). 'Despacito' ties for second-longest-leading hot 100 No. 1 of all time & Cardi B hits top 10. *Billboard.* Retrieved from https://www.billboard.com/articles/columns/chart-beat/7898293/despacito-number-one-14-weeks-hot-100-record.

Van Hook, J., & Balistreri, K. S. (2006). Ineligible parents, eligible children: Food stamps receipt, allotments, and food insecurity among children of immigrants. *Social Science Research, 35,* 228–251.

Vélez-Ibáñez, C. G. (2017). *Hegemonies of language and their discontents: The Southwest North American region since 1540.* University of Arizona Press.

Viruell-Fuentes, E. A. (2007). Beyond acculturation: Immigration, discrimination, and health research among Mexicans in the United States. *Social Science and Medicine, 65*(7), 1524–1535.

Viruell-Fuentes, E. A., Miranda, P. Y., & Abdulrahim, S. (2012). More than culture: Structural racism, intersectionality theory, and immigrant health. *Social Science and Medicine, 75*(12), 2099–2106.

Viruell-Fuentes, E. A., Morenoff, J., Williams, D. R., & House, J. (2011). Self-rated health, language of interview, and the other Latino health puzzle. *American Journal of Public Health, 101*(7), 1307–1314.

Williams, C. L., & Berry, J. W. (1991). Primary prevention of acculturative stress among refugees: Application of psychological theory and practice. *American Psychologist, 46*(6), 632.

Waldram, J. B. (2009). Is there a future for "culture" in acculturation research? An Anthropologist's perspective. *International Journal of Intercultural Relations, 33*(2), 173–176.

Wallace, P. M., Pomery, E. A., Latimer, A. E., Martinez, J. L., & Salovey, P. (2010). A review of acculturation measures and their utility in studies promoting Latino health. *Hispanic Journal of Behavioral Sciences, 32*(1), 37–54.

Waters, M. C., & Jiménez, T. R. (2005). Assessing immigrant assimilation: New empirical and theoretical challenges. *Annual Review of Sociology, 31,* 105–125.

Waters, M. C., Tran, V. C., Kasinitz, P., & Mollenkopf, J. H. (2010). Segmented assimilation revisited: Types of acculturation and socioeconomic mobility in young adulthood. *Ethnic and Racial Studies, 33*(7), 1168–1193.

Zambrana, R. E., & Carter-Pokras, O. (2010). Role of acculturation research in advancing science and practice in reducing health care disparities among Latinos. *American Journal of Public Health, 100*(1), 18–23.

Zentella, A. C. (2003). José can you see: Latin@ responses to racist discourse. In D. Sommer (Ed.), *Bilingual games: Some literary investigations* (pp. 50–66). New York: Macmillan.

Chapter 16
Health Is Political: Advocacy and Mobilization for Latinx Health

Carlos E. Rodríguez-Díaz

Abstract Health is political. In this chapter, the role of politics in Latinx health is outlined, and frameworks are suggested to promote Latinx health. This chapter includes an exploration of the political nature of health followed by an overview of what are referred to as health disparities and health inequities. The social determinants of health framework and proven strategies to improve Latinx health are briefly outlined. Systemic changes for Latino health promotion are suggested, including an example of contemporary actions taken to address health inequities present in Puerto Rico. This chapter is written with the desire to effect change to improve Latinx health and well-being.

Keywords Latinx politics · Puerto Rico · Advocacy · Community-based participatory research · Health disparities

Health is political. While scientific evidence continues to demonstrate the impact of public policies on community and population health, it is profoundly contradictory, and in fact, worrisome that there remains limited discussion about how politics, power, and ideology underpin the health of Latinx communities and promote health disparities (Ortega, Rodríguez, & Vargas Bustamante, 2015; Philbin, Flake, Hatzenbuehler, & Hirsch, 2018). The attention to health disparities and the introduction of the social determinants of health framework by the World Health Organization (WHO) may have contributed to the misconception that these issues have been adequately recognized and understood and are being successfully addressed. However, it can be argued that attention to the role of sociopolitical factors on Latinx health has been confined to academic circles and theory and has focused attention on health disparities as outcomes rather than on existing structural inequities that produce these health disparities within many communities and populations. Furthermore, few structural-level interventions have been designed and implemented to address the political context to reduce health disparities, and increase health equity among Latinx communities and improve the health of Latinx populations.

C. E. Rodríguez-Díaz (✉)
Department of Prevention and Community Health, George Washington University, Washington, DC, USA
e-mail: carlosrd@gwu.edu

In this chapter, the role of politics in Latinx health is outlined and frameworks that can be applied to promote Latinx health and well-being are suggested. This chapter includes an exploration of the political nature of health followed by an overview of what are often referred to as health disparities and health inequities. The social determinants of health framework and proven strategies to improve Latinx health are briefly outlined. Final thoughts on systemic changes to increase health equity and reduce health disparities among Latinx persons are provided, including an example of contemporary actions taken to address health inequities present in Puerto Rico. This chapter is written with the desire to effect change to improve Latinx health and well-being.

Politics and Health

Despite of how obvious the political nature of health may seem to some people, including public health activists and their scientist and practitioner colleagues, the fact is, overall, the political nature of health is not widely acknowledged, understood, or researched. As posited by Bambra, Fox, and Scott-Samuel (2005), health is political because under a neoliberal economic system some social groups—like Latinx persons in the context of the United States—have fewer economic and social resources (e.g., safe housing, quality education, and jobs that pay a living wage) than others. These economic and social resources are often referred to as "social determinants of health" and can be most effectively influenced by political interventions. Thus, the health of an individual, community, and population relies on political actions or inactions.

While health is understood as a human right (WHO, 2017), power is exercised to shape economic, social, and political systems; these systems influence health and changing the conditions under which people can be healthy requires political awareness and struggle. Thus, the health of Latinx persons in the United States is influenced by Latinx persons having less power to shape economic, social, and political systems. There are many factors that may contribute to Latinx communities having less power. Factors that are less explored and acknowledged are the role of Latinx cultural values in understanding US politics; overall negative experiences within state, federal, and international political arenas; and idiomatic and language nuances of the political jargon (Beltrán, 2010; Magaña, 2014; Vargas-Ramos & Stevens-Arroyo, 2012). Central, though, to the health and well-being of Latinx persons in the United States is the Latinx population being marginalized as a minority group; the limited access to political power among Latinx persons; and the fact that this limited access to power is systematically reinforced in a society dominated by configurations of class and status.

This lack of power and the ongoing subjugation of Latinx persons must be recognized and addressed in order to be inclusive of diverse Latinx voices and experiences to improve the overall health status of the Latinx population in the United States. Furthermore, as freedom, mobility, migration, and citizenship are challenged (as they are currently being challenged in the United States), initiating a discussion of politics, ideology, and health can receive a negative reception from those with power and perhaps within some Latinx communities themselves, including those Latinx persons who have some, albeit limited, power. However, there remains an ongoing need to highlight and explore how health, like almost all other aspects of human life, is political.

Health Disparities

Health disparities among Latinx populations have been and continue to be well documented in the literature. This edited volume represents a compilation of some the most pressing and emerging issues facing Latinx communities and populations in the United States. However, the conversation is nascent, not because the Latinx population is new; indeed, it is not. Rather, the conversation is nascent because of multiple "isms", including racism and classism that subtly and not so subtly influence the conversation. Critical questions remain:

- Are we doing enough?
- Can a book dedicated to Latinx health move the needle?
- What needs to change?
- Should the realities of politics play a more prominent role in how we conceptualize and address Latinx health in the United States?

The thesis of this chapter is that health, like most critical issues facing us in the twenty-first century, is political. If we care about the health of Latinx communities and the overall Latinx population, we must think differently; we must accept that politics plays a prominent role in health and well-being. We must "deal with" politics. Politics must become part of the space in which scientists and public health practitioners work.

According to the US Department of Health and Human Services (USDHHS, 2018), a health disparity can be defined as:

> A particular type of health difference that is closely linked with social, economic, and/or environmental disadvantage. Health disparities adversely affect groups of people who have systematically experienced greater obstacles to health based on their racial or ethnic group; religion; socioeconomic status; gender; age; mental health; cognitive, sensory, or physical disability; sexual orientation or gender identity; geographic location; or other characteristics historically linked to discrimination or exclusion.

This definition frames the difference in health status based on comparing or contrasting population groups, for example, comparing gay to non-gay men or residents living in rural to urban areas. This definition is widely used in developing U.S. national and local public health strategies, including programs, interventions, and research supported at the national level by the Health Resources and Services

Administration (HRSA) and the National Institutes of Health (NIH), as examples, and at the local level by the U.S. Centers of Disease Control and Prevention (CDC) and state governments and municipalities. This definition is used in nationwide health promotion and disease prevention plans like Healthy People, in which, for example, race and ethnicity are considered among the demographic factors used to "assess health disparities in the US population" (USDHHS, 2018). However, beyond having comparison-based benchmarks to assess health disparities, there remain incomplete understandings and thus inadequate action plans to address the structural factors, which include (or are influenced by) racism and xenophobia, as examples, that underlie health disparities within Latinx communities and populations.

Furthermore, there remains a need for increased understanding of the health inequities experienced by Latinx populations. Health inequities are the unnecessary, avoidable, unjust, and unfair distribution of health determinants (WHO, 2018). A health equity approach, thus, is rooted in the understanding of health inequalities, the "differences in health status or in the distribution of health determinants between different population groups" (WHO, 2018). Further, the WHO posits, "some health inequalities are attributable to biological variations or free choice and others are attributable to the external environment and conditions mainly outside the control of the individuals concerned" (WHO, 2018). Simply, health inequities result from not changing the critical and modifiable social determinants of health that produce negative outcomes. Health equity refers to the, "Attainment of the highest level of health for all people. Achieving health equity requires valuing everyone equally with focused and ongoing societal efforts to address avoidable inequalities, historical and contemporary injustices, and the elimination of health and healthcare disparities" (USDHHS, 2011).

These definitions, however, are insufficient, and overall, they are not well operationalized. For example, what are those "societal efforts" needed to eliminate health and healthcare disparities? What exactly must be done to ensure health, increase equity, and reduce disparities among Latinx populations? The strategies to reach health equity are largely unknown, have been poorly tested, or have not been disseminated.

Most references used in official documents of the U.S. federal government stress the identification of health disparities by population comparisons, not their solutions. This emphasis on the identification of health disparities guides critical research, but offers very little in terms of interventions and improved health. Moreover, this approach does not prioritize structural-level interventions that are required to reduce inequities. To increase health equity and reduce health disparities, structural-level interventions are needed. Yet, structural-level interventions take intense political will and long-term commitment. Because health is political, health is influenced by ideologies, and those with power have greater likelihood to influence how health is prioritized, defined, measured, and experienced. Furthermore, the outcomes of interventions designed to increase health equity and reduce disparities are distal. They will not be attained in 2–5 years; rather, their outcomes will take decades.

Attention to the Social Determinants of Health

Health is influenced by multiple factors including biology and genetics, individual behaviors, access to needed health services, social factors, and policies. From a socioecological lens (Ansari, Carson, Ackland, Vaughan, & Serraglio, 2003; McLeroy, Bibeau, Steckler, & Glanz, 1988), factors that influence health can be divided into intrapersonal, interpersonal, institutional, community, and policy levels. Some of these factors are not easily modifiable, like gene expression at the intrapersonal level. However, some factors can be influenced and changed in order to improve health outcomes.

In 2008, the WHO published a seminal work on social determinants of health entitled, *Closing the Gap in a Generation: Health Equity through Action on the Social Determinants of Health*. This document was the product of years of work by a diverse group of public health leaders, academics, and advocates who comprised the Commission on Social Determinants of Health. They had three years to "gather and review evidence on what needs to be done to reduce health inequalities within and between countries and to report its recommendations for action to the Director-General of the WHO" (WHO, 2008).

Social determinants of health are the conditions in which people are born, grow, work, play live, and age, and the wider set of forces and systems shaping the conditions of daily life. These forces and systems include economic policies and systems, development agendas, social norms, social policies, and political systems (WHO, 2008).

The Commission made three key recommendations:

1. Improve daily living conditions;
2. Tackle the inequitable distribution of power, money, and resources; and
3. Measure and understand the problem and assess the impact of action.

While members of the Commission recommended certain activities such as the creation of health-promoting policies, strengthening governance that is supportive of all, and a stronger focus on social determinants in public health research, solutions to the health inequities illustrated in the report tended to be underdeveloped. Moreover, the report acknowledged that morbidity and mortality are not random. This problem, the non-randomness of morbidity and mortality throughout the world, is resolvable. However, this is not just a scientific problem; the data are clear. Instead, this is a political problem, requiring not only multi- and transdisciplinary approaches to produce public health innovations (i.e., solutions) but also political commitment. Therefore, to improve the health of Latinx persons, communities, and populations, political will and commitment are needed, and we all must be political agents.

The Power Within Us

Leadership is essential to improve the conditions under which so-called minority groups (e.g., those that comprise a traditionally marginalized population) can enjoy their best health. Political agency—or the capacity to effect social change—is critical to improve Latinx health. The experiences of discrimination, racism, and xenophobia, and where these experiences intersect, should be recognized as a hallmark of oppression of Latinx persons, communities, and populations. Strict identification laws, for example, have differentially negative impacts on the turnout of racial and ethnic minorities in U.S. elections (Hajnal, Lajevardi, & Nielson, 2017); immigration enforcement has led to emotional and behavioral problems among immigrant school-age students (Gándara & Ee, 2018); and delayed and limited response in the aftermath of natural disasters have deepened humanitarian crises (e.g., Hurricanes Irma and Maria) (Brown et al., 2018; Rodríguez-Díaz, 2018).

Several effective strategies designed to influence the politics of health and positively influence the structural factors that affect Latinx health have been identified. Here, three of these strategies are described; health advocacy, community mobilization, and community-based participatory research (CBPR). Examples of how they can be harnessed to improve health are provided.

Health Advocacy

Health advocacy includes taking public positions to support or provide recommendations to promote health. These positions and recommendations may affect factors at any level (or multiple levels) of the socio-ecological model described previously. The advocacy approach in health is not new and is critical to overcome major barriers to public health (Chapman, 2001; Sundwall, 2018; Wise, 2001). Since the *Ottawa Charter for Health Promotion* in 1996 (WHO, 1996), health advocacy has been proposed as a main tool for health promotion because of its usefulness in influencing political, economic, cultural, environmental, behavioral, and biological factors. Despite multiple and conflicting definitions and usage, the two main goals underpinning advocacy are (1) the protection of vulnerable populations and (2) empowerment of disadvantaged populations (Carlisle, 2000).

Latinx populations in the United States have used advocacy to challenge discrimination and invisibility in multiple sectors, including immigration and housing (Mann et al., 2016). Recognizing how Latinx populations are likely to experience housing insecurity, food insecurity, educational inequity, and poverty, several organizations representing Latinx populations in the United States have served as a platform for these efforts. For example, since 1968, UNIDOS US (previously known as National Council for the La Raza [NCLR]; https://www.unidosus.org/) has been a nonpartisan voice for Latinx persons, serving communities through research, policy analysis, and advocacy in the areas of civil rights, immigration, education, economy, health, and housing. Similarly, through community-based programs, the League of United Latin

American Citizens (LULAC; https://lulac.org/) advances the economic conditions, educational attainment, political influence, housing, health and civil rights of Latinx persons, communities, and populations in the United States.

Further, advocacy to influence health outcomes within Latinx populations has been widely applied and studied. Health advocacy as a strategy has been used differently through self- (Dryden, Demarais, & Arsenault, 2017) and collective efficacy (Ramirez et al., 2015), intersectoral partnerships (Pérez-Escamilla et al., 2017), coalitions, and citizen science (a form of community-engaged research) (Winter et al., 2016), among many others.

The TransLatinx Coalition successfully uses health advocacy as a strategy to promote Latinx health. Globally, transgender populations are among the most disproportionately marginalized by institutional and structural conditions that produce profound health disparities and inequities (Logie et al., 2017; Reisner et al., 2016; Su et al., 2016). The indicators of health disparities and inequities experienced by transgender men and women are worse and amplified among those who are also racial and ethnic minorities (Martinez et al., 2016; Muñoz-Laboy, Severson, Levine, & Martínez, 2017; Padilla, Rodríguez-Madera, Vargas-Diaz, & Ramos-Pibernus, 2016; Rhodes et al., 2015). Thus, the TransLatinx Coalition has organized and advocated for the specific needs of transgender Latinx persons, including both immigrants and residents, in the United States. Their work has contributed to increased visibility of Latinx transgender persons, empowerment of Latinx transgender persons and their allies to influence policy-making, and access to primary healthcare, including HIV prevention, care, and treatment for Latinx transgender persons.

Health advocacy requires visibility, and visibility is a cost that not all members of a group or population can afford, particularly in times of particularly oppressive political discourse and profound racism, discrimination, and xenophobia. Competencies to safely and successfully engage in health advocacy in support of marginalized communities and populations should be incorporated in the training of healthcare, public health, and other aid professions. Similarly, health advocacy should be a fundamental tool in strategies intended to support empowerment, particularly those groups made socially vulnerable, including immigrants, women, sexual and gender minorities, and older adults, among others.

Community Mobilization

Community mobilization is a process for reaching different sectors of a community or population and building partnerships in order to address a prioritized public health issue. Community mobilization is especially important for the Latinx population because they are so diverse and do not necessarily share political or health priorities (Beltrán, 2010). Community mobilization often facilitates a group of people to transcend their differences to meet on equal terms for a participatory decision-making process. Usually, community mobilization provides for ownership and sustainability of actions and involves key stakeholders, community leaders, community members, and others who can be affected by the issue been addressed.

Community mobilization for health has been documented among Latinx populations to address issues such as sexuality education (Plastino, Quinlan, Todd, & Tevendale, 2017), chronic diseases (Williams et al., 2017), HIV prevention (Ovalle et al., 2017), and exposure to environmental risks (Vélez-Vega et al., 2016). As an example of this approach in public health, the Latino Commission on AIDS has been implementing community mobilization efforts for several years. HIV continues to disproportionally affect Latinx communities in the United States. Latinx persons represent nearly 18% of the US population, yet they account for about 25% of the total number of new HIV infections (CDC, 2018). In addition, promoting the dissemination of evidence-based community-level interventions, the Latino Commission on AIDS engages communities through existing networks such as the Latino Religious Leadership Conference and Reunion Latina, health briefings and legislative educational activities, and Latinx-specific disease awareness days in order to reach Latinx communities disproportionately affected by HIV and other sexually transmitted infections.

Effective community mobilization requires strong and charismatic leadership and the involvement of critical stakeholders. Challenges can be addressed with initiatives to reinforce leadership and capacity-building strategies within Latinx communities. Emerging initiatives include the use of social media to provide information and to organize and mobilize.

Community-Based Participatory Research (CBPR)

CBPR is considered a partnership approach to research that equitably involves community members, organization representatives, and researchers in all aspects of the research process. It enables all partners to contribute their expertise with shared responsibility and ownership; it enhances the understanding of a given phenomenon; and it integrates the knowledge gained with action to improve the health and well-being of community members, such as through interventions and policy change (Israel, Schulz, Parker, & Becker, 1998; Rhodes et al., 2014). CBPR represent an evidenced approach to conduct research that is not only relevant to the communities, but also appropriate for sustainable change. It is complicated, takes time, and may not be an approach suitable for all kinds of research issues and for all research partnerships. However, it is a research approach that has proven to not only elucidate health issues of importance to diverse, Latinx populations, but also propel structural interventions in the form of policy and changes to the built environment.

In Puerto Rico, several structural issues producing health inequities among lesbian, gay, bisexual, and transgender (LGBT) populations have been addressed in collaboration with CBPR initiatives coordinated through community–academic partnerships. For over five years a community–academic partnership has been documenting the health needs, priorities, and assets; experiences of discrimination; and the preferred modalities for intervention implementation among Puerto Rican LGBT populations (Rodríguez-Díaz, Jovet-Toledo, et al., 2016; Rodríguez-Díaz, Martínez-Vélez, et al., 2016). As a result, several public health programs and research initiatives funded by non-governmental and governmental agencies have been developed. Among these programs and initiatives is Project Trans Tanamá which is aimed at reducing new HIV infections among transgender and gender-non-conforming individuals. The strategies applied in this project are grounded in building community by facilitating social support. As a result, the program is also increasing health-promoting practices such as access to competent transgender primary care and HIV preventative services.

Arte con Salud, another project that has emerged out of an existing community–academic partnership in Puerto Rico, facilitates sexual negotiation skills and safer sexual practices among adult women (Noboa-Ortega, Figueroa-Cosme, Fieldman-Soler, & Miranda-Diaz, 2017). This program builds health-promoting skills among women at risk for HIV infection and has demonstrated the benefits of bridging community members and representatives from universities (i.e., investigators and staff). This project mirrors many other initiatives of improving Latinx health in the United States through community–academic partnerships and CBPR (De Las Nueces, Hacker, DiGirolamo, & Hicks, 2012; Rhodes, 2014; Rhodes et al., 2018).

Toward Sustainable Latinx Health

There are many challenges to overcome in order to achieve Latinx health equity. However, tools exist to improve the health status of Latinx communities and populations in the United States. Certainly, it may seem that there is interest by global agencies like the WHO to promote population health by promoting "health in all policies" (WHO, 2014). This approach is founded on health-related rights and obligations and is designed to ensure accountability of policymakers for population health at all levels of policy-making. As a first step to improve Latinxo equity, health in all policies must be visible and explicit at all levels. Moreover, it is important to decentralize government functions and facilitate the empowerment of local grassroots organizations in community and population health and well-being. The most efficient and sustainable social changes are likely to happen if multiple generations of multiple marginalized groups with different experiences bring attention to the structural challenges and actively participate in or support the actions needed to bring about change, and thus, health equity.

Personal Experience: Being a Latinx Puerto Rican in the Maelstrom of Politics and Health

In September 2017, the history of over 3.5 million residents of Puerto Rico changed dramatically. Hurricanes Irma and Maria made landfall in the islands of Puerto Rico (e.g., Culebra, Vieques, and Puerto Rico) causing thousands of deaths and significant damage to infrastructure and accentuating the negative impact of years of political subjugation by the United States. There is ample evidence of the slow, incomplete, and incompetent response to the emergency caused by the natural disasters (Klein, 2018; Rodríguez-Díaz, 2018). In the aftermath of these hurricanes, migration from the islands to the continental United States increased, and further austerity measures were imposed by the Puerto Rican government in response to the oversight imposed by the US Congress. It is important to know that Puerto Rico has no voting representation in the U.S. Congress. U.S. citizens, and particularly those of the Puerto Rican diaspora, have played a significant role in responding to the emergency in Puerto Rico, and most importantly, in executing the political pressure needed to demand a more comprehensive response.

The experience of Puerto Rico in the aftermath of the hurricanes, if for nothing else, provides evidence of how colonialism—a political tool of oppression—is an ultimate social determinant of health. Certainly, the political relationship of Puerto Rico and the United States has been discussed, analyzed, and criticized for over a century. However, as a response to the aftermath of the hurricanes in Puerto Rico, several groups such as the Puerto Rican Diaspora Summit have *advocated* for changes in the laws and political agreements that situate Puerto Rico as a property that belongs to but is not part of the United States. Likewise, *community mobilization* has been harnessed in Puerto Rico and in many states of the United States. Further, *CBPR* projects have emerged to document the magnitude of the sociopolitical problems in Puerto Rico in the aftermath of these hurricanes and to assess the impact of actions taken as part of the response and recovery. The outcomes of these efforts aligned with advocacy, community mobilization, and CBPR are still in process, and their positive transformations are yet to be realized. Nonetheless, these actions are stirring the public discussion about colonialism, power imbalances, and how to respond even under the precarious circumstances of the island.

Conclusions

As we turn to the future, we must consider how our politics and policies can play a role in changing the health status of the diverse Latinx population in the United States. It is not enough to study disparities; rather, we must develop the consciousness and the tools to change the underlying factors (i.e., social determinants of health) associated with health equity. It is only through more informed policies that community and population health can be improved. Some of the tools exist, including advocacy, community mobilization and CBPR, and others will need development and refinement. However, there is no choice but to effect change in order to make political change and improve the health status and the conditions under which next generations will have a healthier world.

References

Ansari, Z., Carson, N. J., Ackland, M. J., Vaughan, L., & Serraglio, A. (2003). A public health model of the social determinants of health. *International Journal of Public Health, 48*(4), 242–251.

Bambra, C., Fox, D., & Scott-Samuel, A. (2005). Towards a politics of health. *Health Promotion International, 20*(2), 187–193.

Beltrán, C. (2010). *The trouble with unity: Latino politics and the creation of identity*. Oxford University Press.

Brown, P., Vélez-Vega, C. M., Murphy, C. B., Welton, M., Torres, H., Rosario, Z., ... Meeker, J. D. (2018). Hurricanes and the environmental justice island: Irma and Maria in Puerto Rico. *Environmental Justice, 11*(4), 148–153.

Carlisle, S. (2000). Health promotion, advocacy and health inequalities: A conceptual framework. *Health Promotion International, 15*(4), 369–376.

Centers for Disease Control and Prevention. (2018). *HIV among Hispanics/Latinos*. Retrieved from https://www.cdc.gov/hiv/group/racialethnic/hispaniclatinos/index.html.

Chapman, S. (2001). Advocacy in public health: Roles and challenges. *International Journal of Epidemiology, 6*(1), 1226–1232.

De Las Nueces, D., Hacker, K., DiGirolamo, A., & Hicks, L. S. (2012). A systematic review of community-based participatory research to enhance clinical trials in racial and ethnic minority groups. *Health Services Research, 47*(3), 1363–1386.

Dryden, E. M., Demarais, J., & Arsenault, L. (2017). Effectiveness of IMPACT: Ability to improve safety and self-advocacy skills in students with disabilities. *Journal of School Health, 87*(2), 83–89.

Gándara, P, Ee, J. (2018*). U. S. immigration enforcement policy and its impact on teaching and learning in the Nation's schools*. University of California—The Civil Rights Project. Retrieved from https://www.civilrightsproject.ucla.edu/research/k-12-education/integration-and-diversity/u.s.-immigration-enforcement-policy-and-its-impact-on-teaching-and-learning-in-the-nations-schools.

Hajnal, Z., Lajevardi, N., & Nielson, L. (2017). Voter identification laws and the suppression of minority votes. *The Journal of Politics, 79*(2), 363–379.

Israel, B. A., Schulz, A. J., Parker, E. A., & Becker, A. (1998). Review of community-based research: Assessing partnership approached to improve public health. *Annual Review of Public Health, 19*, 173–202.

Klein, N. (2018). *The battle for paradise: Puerto Rico takes on the disaster capitalist*. Haymarket Books.

Logie, C. H., Wang, Y., Lacombe-Duncan, A., Jones, N., Ahmed, U., Levermore, K., ... Newman, P. A. (2017). Factors associated with sex work involvement among transgender women in Jamaica: A cross-sectional study. *Journal of the International AIDS Society, 20*, 21422.

Magaña, L. (2014). *Arizona, immigration, and politics*. Kendall Hunt Publishing.

Mann, L., Simán, F. M., Downs, M., Sun, C. J., Urquieta de Hernandez, B., García, M., ... Rhodes, S. D. (2016). Reducing the impact of immigration enforcement policies to ensure the health of North Carolinians: Statewide community-level recommendations. *North Carolina Medical Journal, 77*(4), 240–246.

Martinez, O., Wu, E., Levine, E. C., Muñoz-Laboy, M., Spadafino, J., Dodge, B., ... Fernandez, M. I. (2016). Syndemic factors associated with drinking patterns among Latino men and Latina transgender women who have sex with men in New York City. *Addiction Research and Theory, 24*(6), 466–476.

McLeroy, K. R., Bibeau, D., Steckler, A., & Glanz, K. (1988). An ecological perspective on health promotion programs. *Health Education Quarterly, 15*(4), 351–377.

Muñoz-Laboy, M., Severson, N., Levine, E., & Martinez, O. (2017). Latino men who have sex with transgender women: The influence of heteronormativity, homonegativity and transphobia on gender and sexual scripts. *Culture, Health, and Sexuality, 19*(9), 964–978.

Noboa-Ortega, P., Figueroa-Cosme, W. I., Fieldman-Soler, A., & Miranda-Diaz, C. (2017). Implementing a randomized controlled trial through a community-academia partnered participatory research: Arte con Salud research-informed intervention. *Puerto Rico Health Sciences Journal, 36*(2), 86–91.

Ortega, A. N., Rodríguez, H. P., & Vargas Bustamante, A. (2015). Policy dilemmas in Latino health care and implementation of the Affordable Care Act. *Annual Reviews of Public Health, 18*(36), 525–544.

Ovalle, I., Loza, O., Peralta-Tores, D., Martinez, J., Hernandez, K., & Mata, H. (2017). Increasing our advocacy capacity through HIV community mobilization: Perspective from emerging and mid-career professionals. *Health Promotion Practice, 18*(1), 11–14.

Padilla, M. B., Rodriguez-Madera, S., Varas-Diaz, N., & Ramos-Pibernus, A. (2016). Transmigrations: Border-crossing and the politics of body modification among Puerto Rican transgender women. *International Journal of Sexual Health, 28*(4), 261–277.

Pérez-Escamilla, Lutter, C. K., Rabadan-Diehl, C., Rubinstein, A., Calvillo, A., Corvalán, C, ... Rivera, J. A. (2017). Prevention of childhood obesity and food policies in Latin America: From research to practice. *Obesity Reviews, 18*(S2).

Philbin, M. M., Flake, M., Hatzenbuehler, M. L., & Hirsch, J. S. (2018). State-level immigration and immigrant-focused policies as drivers of Latino health disparities in the United States. *Social Science and Medicine, 199,* 29–38.

Plastino, K., Quinlan, J., Todd, J., & Tevendale, H. D. (2017). Stakeholder education and community mobilization garner support for se education. *Journal of Adolescent Health, 60*(3S), S24–S29.

Ramirez, A. G., Gallion, K. J., Despres, C., Aguilar, R. P., Adegbe, R. T., Seidel, S. E., & McAlister, A. L. (2015). Advocacy, efficacy, and engagement in an online network for Latino childhood obesity prevention. *Health Promotion Practice, 16*(6), 878–884.

Reisner, S. L., Poteat, T., Keatley, J., Cabral, M., Mothopeng, T., Dunham, E., ... Baral., S. D. (2016). Global health burden and needs of transgender populations: A review. *Lancet, 388,* 412–436.

Rhodes, S. D. (Ed.) (2014). *Innovations in HIV prevention research and practice through community engagement.* Springer.

Rhodes, S. D., Alonzo, J., Mann, L., Sun, C. J., Simán, F. M., Abraham, C., & García, M. (2015). Using photovoice, Latina transgender women identify priorities in a new immigrant-destination state. *International Journal of Transgenderism, 16*(2), 80–96.

Rhodes, S. D., Mann, L., Alonzo, J., Downs, M., Abraham, C., Miller, C., ... Reboussin, B. A. (2014). CBPR to prevent HIV within ethnic, sexual, and gender minority communities: Successes with long-term sustainability. In S. D. Rhodes (Ed.), *Innovations in HIV Prevention Research and Practice through Community Engagement* (pp. 135–160). New York, NY: Springer.

Rhodes, S. D., Tanner, A. E., Mann-Jackson, L., Alonzo, J., Horridge, D., Van Dam, C. N., ... Andrade, M. (2018). Community-engagement research as an approach to expedite advances in HIV prevention, care, and treatment: A call for action. *AIDS Education and Prevention, 30*(3), 243–253.

Rodríguez-Díaz, C. E. (2018). Maria in Puerto Rico: Natural disaster in a colonial archipelago. *American Journal of Public Health 18*(1), 30–32.

Rodríguez-Díaz, C. E., Jovet-Toledo, G. G., Vélez-Vega, C. M., Ortiz-Sánchez, E. J., Santiago-Rodríguez, E. I., Vargas-Molina, R. L., … Mulinelli-Rodríguez, J. J. (2016). Discrimination and health among lesbian, gay, bisexual, and trans in Puerto Rico. *Puerto Rico Health Sciences Journal, 35*(3), 154–159.

Rodríguez-Díaz, C. E., Martínez-Vélez, J. J., Jovet-Toledo, G. G., Vélez-Vega, C. M., Hernández-Otero, N. O., Escotto-Morales, B. M., Mulinelli-Rodríguez, J. J. (2016). Challenges for the well-being of and health equity of gay, lesbian, bisexual and trans people in Puerto Rico. *International Journal of Sexual Health, 28*(4), 286–295.

Su, D., Irwin, J. A., Fisher, C., Ramos, A., Kelly, M., … Coleman, J. D. (2016). Mental health disparities within the LGBT population: A comparison between transgender and nontransgender individuals. *Transgender Health, 1*(1), 12–21.

Sundwall, D. N. (2018). Public health advocacy in the tumultuous times of the Trump administration. *American Journal of Public Health, 108*(4), 449–450.

UNIDOS US. (2018). *We are UNIDOS U.S.* Retrieved from https://www.unidosus.org/about-us/.

US Department of Health and Human Services. (2011). *National stakeholder strategy for achieving health equity.* USDHHS—Office of Minority Health. Available https://minorityhealth.hhs.gov/npa/files/Plans/NSS/CompleteNSS.pdf.

US Department of Health and Human Services. (2018). *Disparities.* Retrieved from https://www.healthypeople.gov/2020/about/foundation-health-measures/Disparities.

Vargas-Ramos, C., & Steven-Arroyo, A. N. (2012). *Belssing la política: The Latino religious experience and political engagement in the United States.* ABC-CLIO, LLC.

Vélez-Vega, C. M., Brown, P., Murphy, C., Figueroa, A., Cordero, J. F., & Alshawabkeh, A. (2016). Community engagement and research translation in Puerto Rico's Northern Karst Region: The PROTECT Superfund Research Program. *NEW SOLUTIONS: A Journal of Environmental and Occupational Health Policy, 26*(3), 475–495.

Williams, A. N., Konopken, Y. P., Keller, C. S., Gonzalez Castro, F., Arcoleo, K. J., Barraza, E., … Shaibi, G. Q. (2017). Culturally-grounded diabetes prevention program for obese Latino youth: Rationale, design, and methods. *Contemporary Clinical Trials, 54,* 68–76.

Winter, S. J., Goldman Rosas, L., Padilla Romero, P., Sheats, J. L., Buman, M. P., Baker, C., & King, A. C. (2016). Using citizen scientist to gather, analyze, and disseminate information about neighborhood features that affect active living. *Journal of Immigrant and Minority Health, 18*(5), 1126–1138.

Wise, M. (2001). The role of advocacy in promoting health. *Global Health Promotion, 8*(2), 69–74.

World Health Organization. (1996). *The Ottawa Charger for Health Promotion.* Retrieved from http://www.who.int/healthpromotion/conferences/previous/ottawa/en/.

World Health Organization. (2008). *Social determinants of health.* Retrieved from http://www.who.int/social_determinants/thecommission/finalreport/about_csdh/en/http://www.who.int/healthpromotion/conferences/previous/ottawa/en/.

World Health Organization. (2014). *Health in all policies: Helsinki statement.* Framework for country action. Retrieved from http://www.who.int/healthpromotion/frameworkforcountryaction/en/.

World Health Organization. (2017). *Human rights and health.* World health organization. Retrieved from http://www.who.int/news-room/fact-sheets/detail/human-rights-and-health.

World Health Organization. (2018). *Health Impact Assessment (HIA)—Glossary of terms.* Retrieved from http://www.who.int/hia/about/glos/en/index1.html.

Index

A

Acculturation, 11, 29, 31–34, 54–56, 58, 68, 72, 73, 79, 99–102, 108, 109, 117, 179, 180, 299, 300, 312, 321–343

Adolescent, 45, 46, 49, 52, 55, 57, 58, 64, 68, 72, 73, 75, 76, 97–99, 101, 102, 104–118, 225, 277, 287, 333, 338, 340

Advocacy, 8, 35, 83, 134–136, 138, 206, 209, 354, 355, 358, 359

Affordable Care Act, 8, 74, 83, 162, 181, 239–248, 254, 258, 262, 263

Assimilation, 11, 73, 101, 322, 325–329, 333, 337, 340–342

B

Bisexual, 3, 4, 54, 77, 83, 177, 178, 185, 217–219, 223, 225, 226, 264, 356

C

Caregivers, 50, 69, 84, 85, 146, 155, 156, 159, 161–163

Care recipients, 146, 156

Children, 6, 9, 25, 29, 45, 46, 48–50, 52, 53, 55, 56, 58, 59, 63–87, 102, 108–110, 127, 129, 130, 132, 134, 136, 137, 149, 153, 156, 169–171, 173, 182–184, 208, 241, 243, 253, 254, 259–262, 264, 272, 276, 277, 281, 282, 284, 285, 287, 289, 326–328, 330, 335, 338, 339

Community-based participatory research, 3, 10, 12, 37, 38, 206–208, 219, 229, 354, 356–359

Cultural congruence, 157

Culture, 2, 8, 21, 22, 31, 33, 45, 46, 53–55, 58, 59, 72, 73, 75, 76, 97, 98, 101, 102, 104, 106, 108–110, 112, 115, 116, 132, 138, 154, 156, 180, 203–205, 208, 218, 262, 273, 299, 321–336, 338, 340–343

D

Demographics, 1, 5, 6, 8, 10, 11, 21, 30, 129, 130, 203, 280, 352

Disability, 6, 127–139, 145, 146, 148, 149, 152–155, 157, 159, 241, 243, 254, 351

Discrimination, 3, 4, 31, 32, 34, 45, 54–56, 58, 67–69, 71, 75, 76, 79, 99, 104, 109, 117, 130, 132, 133, 163, 177, 180, 205, 220–225, 229, 230, 232, 259, 261, 288, 295–297, 299, 300

Disparities, 2, 4, 10, 11, 19–21, 23–26, 29–31, 35, 37, 38, 45, 46, 52, 54, 58, 63, 64, 67, 72, 74, 75, 79, 118, 129–131, 151, 162, 172, 174, 185, 204, 217, 220, 224, 227–231, 246, 254, 259, 263, 264, 271–275, 286, 323, 334–336, 340, 343, 349–352, 355, 358

E

Empowerment, 103, 115, 127, 128, 132, 133, 135–138, 354, 355, 357

Evidence-based intervention, 58, 74, 97, 118

G

Gay, 3, 4, 54, 77, 82, 177, 178, 185, 217–219, 223, 225, 226, 264, 351, 356

Gender minority, 217–219, 227, 355

© Springer Nature Switzerland AG 2020
A. D. Martínez and S. D. Rhodes (eds.), *New and Emerging Issues in Latinx Health*, https://doi.org/10.1007/978-3-030-24043-1

H

Hazard, 172–174, 182, 183, 197, 199–202, 277, 280, 289

Health
- -behavior theories, 19, 20, 33
- child-, 64
- -disparities, 10, 19, 20, 31, 35, 37, 38, 45, 46, 54, 64, 72, 74, 75, 118, 174, 204, 217, 220, 229, 231, 259, 263, 271, 272, 274, 275, 323, 334, 340, 349–352, 355
- environment-health nexus, 275, 276, 287
- -insurance reform, 239, 247, 248
- Latinx-, 3, 4, 11–13, 34, 35, 37, 38, 118, 228, 232, 255, 264, 321–324, 330–332, 339–343, 349–351, 354, 357
- mental health epidemiology, 20, 97
- migrant-, 206
- occupational-, 204–209, 254
- social determinants of-, 7, 12, 46, 63, 66, 67, 87, 185, 271, 349, 350, 352, 353
- -threat, 169, 170, 172, 179, 183–186
- worker-, 197, 203, 205

Healthcare coverage, 80, 83

I

Immigrant, 1, 4, 5, 7–11, 23, 30, 31, 34, 38, 45, 46, 48, 50–52, 55–57, 64, 65, 67–74, 77–79, 83–87, 97, 100–102, 108, 109, 136, 162, 163, 169–186, 199, 200, 202, 204, 220, 221, 224, 228, 241, 243, 244, 253–264, 273, 274, 280, 281, 284, 285, 295, 301–307, 310, 312, 314, 321–332, 334–341, 343, 354, 355

Immigration enforcement, 8–10, 74, 230, 253–255, 257, 258, 260–264, 295, 354

Immigration policies, 74, 108, 163, 170, 181, 182, 204, 221, 253, 254, 257–259, 261, 263, 302, 303, 309, 310, 312, 313, 326, 328, 340

Industry, 81, 171–174, 197–204, 206–209, 226, 247, 275, 330

Intersectionality, 220, 224, 264, 295, 300, 306, 313

Intersectionality theory, 295, 300, 313

Intersex, 217, 219, 223

Intervention, 10, 12, 19, 20, 32–39, 53, 58, 74, 99, 105, 106, 110–113, 115–118, 127, 128, 132, 133, 136–139, 158, 160, 161, 175, 178, 183, 185, 186, 197, 203, 205–208, 219, 229, 231, 253, 262–264, 272, 283, 288, 323, 341, 343, 349–352, 356, 357

L

Latino, 1–4, 20–22, 24, 48, 50, 52, 72, 73, 98, 117, 134, 147, 148, 150, 159, 169–186, 273, 300, 323, 330, 331, 337, 338, 349, 356, 357

Latinx, 1–13, 19–38, 45–59, 63–81, 83–87, 97–118, 127–132, 134, 136–139, 145–147, 149–163, 197–209, 217, 219–232, 239–241, 243, 245, 246, 248, 253–255, 257, 259, 260, 263, 264, 271–275, 277–289, 295, 296, 298, 301, 302

Latinx adults, 24–29, 51, 54, 129, 132, 146, 152, 160–162, 240, 241, 245, 246, 272, 301, 302, 304, 307, 335

Latinx aging, 5, 145–147, 155, 159–161, 163

Latinx children & adolescents, 52

Latinx chronic disease, 7, 19–21, 23, 27, 28, 32–35, 58, 160

Latinx politics, 10, 349–351

Latinx population, 1, 2, 4, 5, 7–13, 19–26, 28–33, 35–38, 45, 46, 51, 52, 54, 57, 58, 64, 70–72, 80, 87, 97–100, 103, 105, 109, 116–118, 127–131, 138, 145–147, 149–152, 154, 155, 157, 159–161, 163, 197, 201, 227, 239, 243, 245, 246, 248, 253, 254, 259, 263, 271–274, 288, 301, 303, 304, 308–310, 326–328, 334, 336, 338, 340, 342, 350, 351, 355, 358

Lesbian, 3, 54, 77, 82, 217–219, 223, 225, 226, 231, 264, 356

M

Migrant, 1, 4, 5, 9, 66, 77, 81, 82, 169–171, 173, 174, 176, 179, 182, 205, 206, 208, 209, 255, 273, 303, 321, 325, 328, 336, 338, 341

Migration, 10, 21, 33, 34, 36, 50–52, 56, 58, 73, 78, 79, 99, 107, 109, 110, 115, 117, 155, 170, 172, 180, 184, 186, 255, 273, 275, 302, 303, 306, 325, 329, 335–337, 340–342, 350, 358

Modifiable risk factors, 19

O

Obesity, 19, 20, 23, 24, 26–32, 36, 67, 72, 73, 80–82, 129, 150, 174, 179, 180, 221,

Index   365

226, 227, 232, 272, 276, 277, 288, 307, 321, 324, 334–339, 342

P
Physical activity, 24, 26–29, 35–37, 66, 82, 137, 161, 271, 272, 277–285, 287–289, 322
Prevention, 19, 20, 26–29, 31, 33–36, 58, 74, 79, 99, 105, 106, 110–118, 160, 163, 175–178, 185, 207, 220, 254, 255, 352, 355, 356
Puerto Rico, 3, 21, 24, 48, 52, 349, 350, 356–358

Q
Queer, 3, 217–219, 223, 264

R
Racism, 3, 31, 34, 58, 75, 184, 220, 224, 225, 259, 263, 295, 296, 298–300, 303, 308–314, 328, 338, 340, 351, 352, 354, 355
Residential segregation, 274–276, 295, 310, 340

S
Sexual minority, 54, 225, 227, 231, 264
Social determinants, 7, 10–12, 34, 45, 63, 66, 67, 71, 73, 78, 87, 185, 262, 264, 271, 323, 349, 350, 352, 353, 358
Social vulnerability, 146, 147, 157, 159, 163
Socio-ecological aka social ecological theory, 33, 36, 106, 107, 271, 353, 354
Structural, 4, 12, 37, 71, 87, 106, 155, 156, 169, 170, 175, 176, 178, 183–186, 203, 205, 207, 228, 231, 232, 264, 275, 295, 296, 299, 301, 303, 309, 310, 312, 314, 323, 327, 328, 333, 334, 336, 339–341, 343, 349, 352, 354–357
Substance use, 46, 48, 51, 52, 55, 58, 66, 75, 97–118, 222, 225, 226, 322

T
Transgender, 3, 54, 77, 82, 177, 217–219, 221–226, 228, 230, 264, 355–357
Transnational, 38, 170, 180, 321, 325, 328, 336, 337, 339, 342

U
United States, 1–10, 12, 21, 23, 25–33, 35, 38, 45, 52, 57, 58, 63, 64, 66, 68–71, 73, 75, 78–81, 85, 86, 97–102, 104, 105, 109, 114–116, 127, 129, 130, 145–147, 153, 154, 160, 162, 163, 169–174, 176–181, 183, 184, 217, 220, 221, 223, 224, 226–228, 239, 240, 253–256, 263, 273, 274, 295, 298–300, 302, 303, 311, 321, 323, 324, 326, 329, 331, 334–339, 341, 350, 354, 357, 358
Urban environments, 271, 273–276, 278–280, 283, 285–289, 337

V
Vulnerability, 56, 68, 77, 82, 104, 105, 118, 146, 147, 157, 159, 163, 169, 170, 172, 173, 176, 177, 179, 182–186, 203, 205, 253–255, 259, 260, 264, 308

W
Well-being, 6, 11, 12, 35, 37, 39, 46, 50, 55, 63, 66, 68–70, 73, 76–78, 83, 84, 87, 97–99, 111, 118, 131–133, 146, 156, 162, 170, 180, 184, 217, 219–221, 224, 228, 230–232, 253, 254, 258, 259, 261–263, 279, 343, 349–351, 356, 357
Women, 7, 21–25, 27, 29–31, 67, 71, 101, 103–105, 115, 116, 128, 132, 138, 146–151, 154, 155, 158, 159, 163, 169, 170, 173, 175, 177, 178, 182, 183, 185, 197, 198, 201, 205, 208, 218, 219, 224, 226, 228, 231, 241, 259, 260, 264, 272, 279–289, 301, 304–308, 330, 355, 357

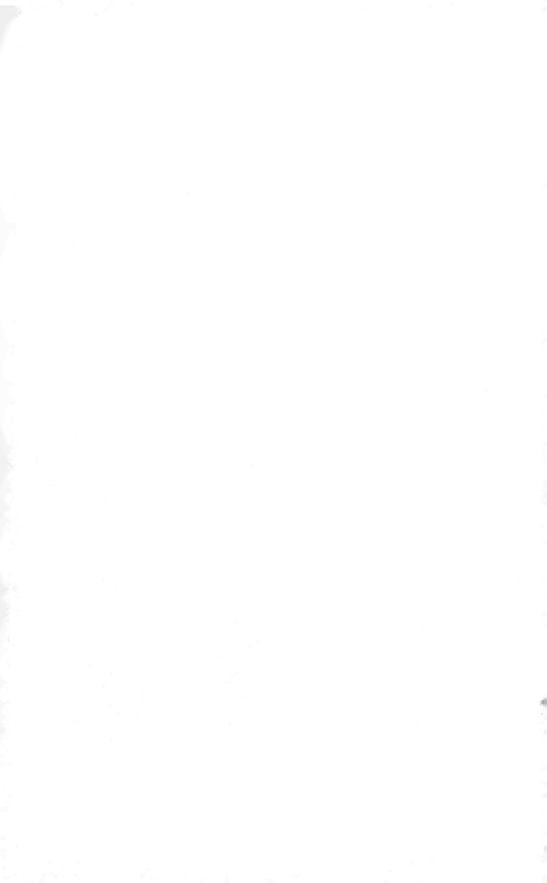

Printed in the USA
CPSIA information can be obtained
at www.ICGtesting.com
CBHW070237150924
14526CB00003B/22